Legal Marijuana

Legal Marijuana

*Perspectives on Public Benefits,
Risks and Policy Approaches*

Edited by JOAQUIN JAY GONZALEZ III
and MICKEY P. McGEE

McFarland & Company, Inc., Publishers
Jefferson, North Carolina

ALSO OF INTEREST AND FROM MCFARLAND: *Cybersecurity: Current Writings on Threats and Protection,* edited by Joaquin Jay Gonzalez III *and* Roger L. Kemp (2019); *Eminent Domain and Economic Growth: Perspectives on Benefits, Harms and New Trends,* edited by Joaquin Jay Gonzalez III, Roger L. Kemp *and* Jonathan Rosenthal (2018); *Small Town Economic Development: Reports on Growth Strategies in Practice,* edited by Joaquin Jay Gonzalez III, Roger L. Kemp *and* Jonathan Rosenthal (2017); *Privatization in Practice: Reports on Trends, Cases and Debates in Public Service by Business and Nonprofits,* edited by Joaquin Jay Gonzalez III *and* Roger L. Kemp (2016); *Immigration and America's Cities: A Handbook on Evolving Services,* edited by Joaquin Jay Gonzalez III *and* Roger L. Kemp (2016); *Corruption and American Cities: Essays and Case Studies in Ethical Accountability,* edited by Joaquin Jay Gonzalez III *and* Roger L. Kemp (2016)

LIBRARY OF CONGRESS CATALOGUING-IN-PUBLICATION DATA

Names: Gonzalez, Joaquin Jay, III, editor. | McGee, Mickey P., 1949– editor.
Title: Legal marijuana : perspectives on public benefits, risks and policy
approaches / edited by Joaquin Jay Gonzalez III and Mickey P. McGee.
Description: Jefferson, North Carolina : McFarland & Company, Inc., 2019 |
Includes bibliographical references and index.
Identifiers: LCCN 2018042639 | ISBN 9781476673097
(softcover : acid free paper) ∞
Subjects: LCSH: Marijuana—Government policy—United States. |
Marijuana—Law and legislation.
Classification: LCC HV5822.M3 L35 2019 | DDC 362.29/55610973—dc23
LC record available at https://lccn.loc.gov/2018042639

BRITISH LIBRARY CATALOGUING DATA ARE AVAILABLE

ISBN (print) 978-1-4766-7309-7
ISBN (ebook) 978-1-4766-3469-2

Front cover image © 2019 iStock

Printed in the United States of America

*McFarland & Company, Inc., Publishers
Box 611, Jefferson, North Carolina 28640
www.mcfarlandpub.com*

Jay and Mick dedicate this book to Golden Gate University's
Executive Master of Public Administration students

Acknowledgments

We are grateful for the support of the Mayor George Christopher Professorship at Golden Gate University, the Bibbero Trust, and GGU's Pi Alpha Alpha Chapter. We appreciate the encouragement from Dean Gordon Swartz and our wonderful colleagues at the GGU Edward S. Ageno School of Business, the Department of Public Administration, and the Executive MPA Program.

Our heartfelt thanks goes to the contributors listed in the back section and the individuals, organizations, and publishers below for granting permission to reprint the material in this volume and the research assistance. Most waived or reduced fees as an expression of their support for practical research and information sharing that benefits our community.

American Society for Public Administration
Berkshire Eagle
Charleston Gazette-Mail
The Columbian
Gary A. Craft
Deseret News
East Bay Times
Elko Daily Free Press
eRepublic
Dereck Glover
Golden Gate University Library
Governing
Government Technology
Guardian
Paul D. Harney
Hawk Eye
Herald-Tribune
Michelle F. Hong
Professor Jim Hynes
International City/County Management Association
Kaiser Health News
Mark Kennedy

Shelley McGee
Mercury News
Michigan Lawyers Weekly
Dr. Patrick Murphy
National Institute on Drug Abuse
National Institutes of Health
Niles Daily Star
Ontario Public Health Association
PA Times
Beth Payne
Samira Perry
Pew Charitable Trusts
PM Magazine
Seth Poe
Public Policy Institute of California
RAND Corporation
Professor Alan Roper
San Francisco State University
Stateline
U.S. Department of Veteran Affairs
U.S. Drug Enforcement Agency
U.S. Food and Drug Administration
University of San Francisco Library
Lichao Zhang

Table of Contents

Preface

The legalization of marijuana has spread rapidly throughout the United States. The nation's capital, Washington, D.C., is on board—from just a handful of states ten years ago to now more than half of them, legalization of medicinal and adult use recreational marijuana is trending upwards. In Canada, it is legal to use and distribute, nationally. Thousands of cities and towns are following suit. Legalization seems to be a win-win situation. Citizens who need pot for health and recreation are relieved. Hence, business is brisk. Many governments welcome cannabis as a much-needed cash cow. But not everyone thinks it's a win-win scenario. The surge has created discussions and debates between and among citizens, cities, states, and the federal government. Using easy-to-read language, this compilation explains the basics of marijuana legalization, the benefits and concerns, the policies and actions, as well as the future of this controversial issue.

Basics

Part I provides the essentials of marijuana's legalization. In the first chapter, KQED reporter John Sepulvado narrates the seed-to-sale process and necessary technology needed for efficient revenue collection in Colorado. Then Professor Donald F. Kettl, in Chapter 2, describes how local pot laws conflict with national policies. Following in Chapter 3 are graduate student Dereck Glover and Professor Mickey P. McGee's examination of the colorful history of U.S. cannabis policy legislation including the national mood shifts on medical and recreational use. Their historical piece is followed by a National Institute on Drug Abuse review of the changes in marijuana policies across states and why marijuana has gained greater social acceptance.

Two chapters from the U.S. Drug Enforcement Agency (DEA) and one chapter from the U.S. Food and Drug Administration (FDA) underscore the federal government's firm stand –marijuana's sale and use are NOT legal. Chapter 5 outlines the DEA's position that smoked marijuana is not medicine and that it is not safe for use. Chapter 6 elaborates on this DEA position and their opposition to wholesale legalization. Chapter 7 presents a list of ten questions and answers provided by the FDA on marijuana product safety, applications and approval, research, and therapy.

Benefits and Concerns

Part II consists of a collection of thirty-two chapters which are meant to move readers from the basics to the benefits and concerns of marijuana legalization.

Opportunities and Benefits. In Chapter 8, *The Hawkeye* contributor William Smith lays down the competing arguments on both sides of the medicinal and recreational marijuana debate in Iowa. Using a New York University study, *Kaiser Health News* (KHN) writer Carmen Heredia Rodriguez, in Chapter 9, discusses the aging baby boomer generation and their use of marijuana as a drug of choice for various medical ailments. In Chapter 10, *Tryon Daily Bulletin* managing editor Ted Yoakum reviews the benefits advocated by government on increased municipal revenues versus business sale's taxes, permits and licensing fees versus citizen's concerns over increased usage among teenagers, overdoses caused by edibles, and increased law enforcement. In Chapter 11, accounting firm partner Kevin Harper examines the responsibilities of California cities and counties in terms of enforcing and managing the new and legal marijuana industry. Closing this section is senior researcher Beau Kilmer's elaboration of a RAND Corporation study on the various benefits and consequences of legalizing marijuana to including increased tax revenues from sales, the suppression of its black market, and an increase in consumption within and outside Vermont.

Business. This section includes reviews of some of the risks and rewards faced by businesses in the marijuana industry. Business editor Gordon Oliver, in Chapter 13, describes the personal dangers faced by marijuana entrepreneurs particularly the absence of a safe place to deposit a primarily cash-only business. In Chapter 14, *Stateline* staff writer Sophie Quinton continues with the banking problems created by federal law prohibiting banks and credit unions from accepting legalized marijuana profits. *Governing* staff writer J.B. Wogan, in Chapter 15, tells the story of Andrew Freedman, Colorado's first and only "marijuana czar" and his consulting services to states seeking their guidance and advice on areas such as taxing and regulations. While Douglas Levy describes the emerging and evolving areas of legal practice around cannabis-based work to include lobbying, legislation, rulemaking, intellectual property, land use and zoning, labor and employment, product safety and taxation in Chapter 16. Teaming up in Chapter 17 are entrepreneur-activist Samira J. Perry and Professor Mickey P. McGee who provide interesting data from government officials, marijuana business owners and public citizens about the financial gains and medical values versus arrest and prosecution as well as enforcement/addiction resource support expenses.

Health. Seven papers illustrating some of the health issues connected to medicinal and recreational marijuana use are included in this section. In Chapter 18, *Kaiser Health News* reporter Shefali Luthra writes about the knowledge gap which exists for medical professionals. Then Anna Gorman, a *Kaiser Health News* colleague, explores the connection between California's decision to legalize marijuana and increase tobacco use in Chapter 19. Sarah Varney, also from *Kaiser Health News*, reports in Chapter 20 about studies showing a sharp increase in marijuana use among pregnant women. In Chapter 21, National Institute on Drug Abuse (NIDA) Director Nora D. Volkow connects the effects of cannabis use with intelligence. In Chapter 22, Juliet Akhigbe et al. share excerpts from their Ontario Public Health Association Cannabis Task Group findings. Paula Gordon, another *Kaiser Health News* reporter, in Chapter 23, asks five health related questions concerning marijuana legalization. Finally, in Chapter 24, senior economist

Rosalie Liccardo Pacula expounds on her RAND study on medical marijuana and opioid deaths.

Youth. What about its effects on the youth? *Kaiser Health News*'s Anna Gorman reviews how legalization of recreational marijuana and the accompanying advertising affect challenges youth drug education and prevention programs in Chapter 25. And National Institute on Drug Abuse Director Nora D. Volkow, comments on youth drug use and attitudes of middle and high school students in Chapter 26.

Workplace. Workplace concerns related to legalization of marijuana are discussed in Chapter 27 by attorney-mediator Joe Jarret. While management consultants William Kirchhoff and Stephen Zimney, in Chapter 28, urge public managers to customize their thinking on marijuana adaptation protocols to face and manage the complexities associated with the use of medical marijuana in the workplace.

Veterans. In Chapter 29, *Kaiser Health News* columnist Michelle Andrews describes the growing problems veterans faced when talking with VA doctors about use of medicinal marijuana. Meanwhile in Chapter 30, Psychiatry Professors Marcel O. Bonn-Miller and Glenna S. Rousseau add to the conversations regarding the juxtaposition of veteran's suffering PTSD and their cannabis use.

Stoned driving. *Berkshire Eagle* contributor Andy Metzger, in Chapter 31, points out salient points on both sides of the debate on legalization of marijuana and echoes opponent's warnings that it would result in greater dangers on roadways and create new problems for law enforcement officers on determining driver impairment. In Chapter 32, *Governing* reporter Daniel C. Vock provides a clear picture cited study findings related to the connection between stoned driving and vehicle accidents. Journalists Stephanie O'Neill and Ben Markus, in Chapter 33, add to the discussion on how to enforce laws against stoned drivers. Driving under the influence of marijuana, just like alcohol, is illegal. In Chapter 34, *Stateline* staff writer Sarah Breitenbach helps to increase reader understanding of methods other than the conventional blood test for detecting drugged driving exist.

Concerns and challenges. In Chapter 35, *Deseret News* beat writer Deborah Sutton suggests that states are lining up to legalize use of medical marijuana and adult use of small amounts of recreational pot to evaluate the whether the costs versus the benefits of legalization is worth the fiscal and social risks. *Elko Press* reporter Dylan Woolf Harris, in Chapter 36, outlines the challenges faced by the City of Elko, Nevada, and the public reluctance spurred by issues such as damage to public lands caused by pot farms, law enforcement policies and drug- and alcohol-free workplace. In Chapter 37, *Herald-Tribune* Editor Diane Raver examines the dangers of increased marijuana-related fatalities, increased use among youth and adults with increase in people in drug treatment programs and increased cost for public health and safety as well as the lower use of law enforcement resources and costs, revenue generation through taxation. *Stateline* writer Rebecca Beitsch in Chapter 38 describes Arizona's Department of Health Services lottery process used to grant licenses to open medical marijuana dispensaries. Public policy analysts Patrick Murphy, Henry McCann and Van Bustic focus on the cultivation aspect, the growing of the marijuana plants and include analyses of new statewide requirements regarding cultivation operations the price of doing business; legal versus illegal paths for growing and risks and rewards of compliance in Chapter 39.

Policies and Actions

Legalized pot does not mean no regulation for its use, sale, etc. Part III provides fifteen chapters on recreational and medicinal marijuana's regulation, enforcement, and bans.

Regulation. In Chapter 40, professor and coeditor Mickey P. McGee examines and analyzes primary data collected from public officials and citizens in Monterey County, California, as well as reviews the various California marijuana-related legislation and selected excerpts from two city ordinances on policies to regulate commercial and personal cultivation. Harvard Professor Stephen Goldsmith, in Chapter 41, relates Colorado's use of an advanced tracking and data-analytics to provide an effective and efficient system to safely and securely control the flow of the drug across the state.

In Chapter 42, *Governing* writer Dylan Scott describes how Colorado dispensaries provide medical marijuana to patients under the watchful eye of state regulators and other states have found Colorado's model useful to emulate to regulate their own marijuana system. Management adviser-author William Kirchhoff, in Chapter 43, explains that most government drugs and alcohol policies are insufficient to effectively manage the many "what if's" of employee use of medical and recreational marijuana.

International City/County Management Association Public Information Director Michelle Frisby, in Chapter 44, talks about the first government-owned marijuana store established by the City of North Bonneville, Washington, which was modeled after a similar store operated at Seattle's Pike Place Market. Meanwhile, grad student Seth Poe and Professor Alan R. Roper, in Chapter 45, provide a comprehensive review and analysis of current and potential risks of marijuana advertising on minors and suggest what government could do to regulate and to restrict targeted advertising. In Chapter 46, policy analysts Patrick Murphy and John Carnevale outline a practical framework to develop recreational marijuana regulations from lessons learned in Colorado, Washington and other states.

Enforcement. Career law enforcer Gary A. Craft and Professor Mickey P. McGee collaborate on two chapters for this section: Chapter 47 examines and analyzes data collected from the experiences of several district attorneys and investigators/inspectors from selected California counties and Chapter 48 delves into police chiefs' perspectives on the California's Health & Safety Code §11362.77 which permitted the cultivation, transportation, possession and furnishing of marijuana for medical purposes.

In Chapter 49, professor and coeditor Joaquin Jay Gonzalez III invites you to examine the August 29, 2013, memo from the Obama Administration (Memo #1) and the January 4, 2018, memo from the Trump Administration (Memo #2). Professor Jim Hynes, in Chapter 50, describes the City of Berkeley's cannabis policy, administrative and land use regulations governing access to cannabis, and enforcement of municipal codes and how it allows reasonable and healthy access to cannabis, promote public safety and prevent negative community impacts. In Chapter 51, *Kaiser Health News* editors Anna Gorman and Phil Galewitz shine a light on the conflict between federal law and state sovereign rights and believes that not much would change because the federal government lacks resources to suppress cannabis production and consumption.

Bans. Politics Professor David Schultz, in Chapter 52, believes it is the right time to reframe the U.S. drug policy that criminalize marijuana's use to one that treats it as a public health problem. In Chapter 53, public finance reporter Liz Farmer reviews state actions like withholding revenue from pot production and sales hoping cities will abandon their bans. In Chapter 54, Silicon Valley journalist Khalida Sarwari reports on how the City of Santa Clara, California, is in no rush to issue the required business licenses to sell recreational marijuana.

Future

We conclude with six chapters on the future of legalized pot beginning with two from Golden Gate University Professor Alan R. Roper. In Chapter 55, he addresses the connection between legalization of marijuana, an increase in consumer demand and electrical power followed by Chapter 56 where he differentiates between traditional farming operations and marijuana production. Photojournalist Zoe Sullivan describes how some Native American nations are considering the possibility of legalizing marijuana to create a new revenue streams in Chapter 57.

Free-lance writer Barbara Feder Ostrov, in Chapter 58, describes how marijuana is distributed and used as sacrament in Rastafari/Native American styled churches and government efforts to close these churches. In Chapter 59, web reporter Ana B. Ibarra introduces the California Department of Public Health website "Let's Talk Cannabis," which contains important information relevant to youth, parents, pregnant women, pet owners, drivers, among others. In Chapter 60, journalist Dave Boucher reminds us that in spite of the massive surge that the future of legalized pot, even the less contentious medical kind, will continue to be uncertain in many states.

Appendices

Useful appended documents include: "Glossary of Legalized Marijuana Terms," "City of Portland Ordinance No. 186857," "U.S. Drug Enforcement Agency Drug Fact Sheet," "Federal Trafficking Penalties for Marijuana, Hashish and Hashish Oil, Schedule I Substances," and "VA and Medical Marijuana—What Veterans Need to Know."

Legalized Marijuana was penned by practitioners, advocates, scholars, journalists, citizens, and entrepreneurs. The editors and contributors provide a starting point and recommendations for states to understand and then prioritize the next steps for regulating legal pot should that be the case in their states. The U.S. Controlled Substance Act of 1970 (CSA) looms large in many of these essays. The CSA is the "elephant in the room" for state-level legalization in the U.S. The "murky federal-state relationship" and the January 2018 Trump Administration memoranda which repealed the previous administration's low priority enforcement leave the question of federal prosecution open. Swimming through the muck of shifting politics and policies is not new for North America's cities and towns. Information about the Basics, the Benefits and Concerns, the Policies and Action, and the Future will inform and educate you on the impact of legalization of marijuana on local, state, regional and federal governments, businesses, society, and citizens.

1. Legalized Pot Pushes Colorado Revenue Department into New Territory[*]

JOHN SEPULVADO

There's the one with the police officer holding a marijuana plant. Or the one with buildings in the dense fog. Or the one about Colorado's and Washington's professional football teams playing in the "Super Bowl."

Since Colorado voters legalized marijuana in 2012, pot memes about the Rocky Mountain (High) State have been good for a laugh and steady streams of clickbait for the sites posting them. The memes play on old stereotypes of silly stoners over-indulging on weed.

Yet Colorado's pot vendors have to run highly organized and savvy businesses if they want to sell legally in the state.

"This isn't 'Cheech and Chong,'" said Daria Serna, communications director for the Colorado Department of Revenue (DOR). The DOR, which traditionally focuses on tax policy and collection for the state, has become the lead agency on legalized marijuana enforcement in Colorado.

"Never in a million years did I think I would know this much about marijuana, but it's become an important part of our service," Serna said. "So we're going to do the best we can, and we hope we can become a model for other states and countries."

To help blaze this new trail down the legalized pot road, Colorado's state bureaucracy is turning to trusted technologies to ensure public and consumer safety.

"Seed-to-Sale" Tracking

When voters approved recreational cannabis in November 2012, state officials wanted to ensure marijuana plants weren't stolen, lost or ending up in the hands of criminals or children.

To help with tracking, Colorado regulators expanded a system that was implemented

---

*Originally published as John Sepulvado, "Legalized Pot Pushes Colorado Revenue Department into New Territory," *Government Technology*, January 28, 2014. Reprinted with permission of the publisher.

when the state legalized medical marijuana in the 1990s. Known as the Marijuana Inventory Tracking Solution (MITS), owners of the retail and medical operations must affix radio frequency identification (RFID) tags to plants once they sprout.

Incarnations of RFID technology have been around for about 50 years, and have been used to track everything from Soviet airplanes to cars passing over toll bridges.

"RFID is basically seed-to-sale monitoring, a way for us to prevent plant diversion," Serna said.

The system allows state regulators to visit a marijuana storehouse, stand a few feet away, and get a complete inventory using a simple Motorola handheld receiver.

The system is manufactured by Franwell, a central Florida company specializing in tracking devices for agricultural uses. Colorado contracted the marijuana tracking to Franwell for about $1.2 million.

As for owners and operators, the price of the RFID tags for shop owners ranges from $0.25 to $0.45.

"Generally, growers find the costs reasonable and are supportive of tracking mechanisms," said Brian Vicente, executive director of Sensible Colorado, a marijuana advocacy group.

"Everything is under camera, so we don't necessarily agree that theft is an issue, and sometimes the system can be a little clunky. It's just a tag on the plant. But it's important at the dawn of this new industry to work with regulators so people know it's safe."

Meanwhile, the demand for Franwell's RFID tags has been huge, according to a Franwell employee. The company's been so busy with requests from Colorado, "nobody got a Christmas break," she said.

Testing for Safety and Potency

If the number of companies making foods featuring a hearty serving of THC is any indication, the edible market in Colorado is huge and growing. But while pot-laced brownies, lollipops and soda may be popular with consumers, at least one group won't touch them with a yardstick: U.S. Food and Drug Administration (FDA) regulators.

Because marijuana is considered to be an illegal narcotic by the federal government, FDA officials are steering clear of the edible business in Colorado. That leaves the DOR in the business of food safety and monitoring.

While marijuana vendors that prepare food items have to follow state and local food safety regulations just like any other café or bakery, Colorado officials believe the FDA is unlikely to spearhead potential foodborne illness investigations involving pot. So the DOR is introducing rules about product testing in July, according to CannLabs CEO Genifer Murray.

Like the RFID technology used to track the plants, Murray said the testing techniques used for edibles have a long history in the food service industry.

"The instrumentation, it's nothing new," Murray said. "It's just that methods that are different. We've been looking at plants for a long time, and marijuana is just another plant."

Murray declined to detail the testing process, other than to say it's very accurate and fast. But beyond microbial testing for foodborne pathogens, labs like Murray's also will look to test the potency of edibles so vendors can properly package their product for consumers.

"Especially tourists," Murray said. "They may not know just how potent edibles are, that if too much is consumed, the highs can last 24 hours or longer. Potency can be horribly detrimental in edibles, so that needs to be clearly labeled."

A Cash Business

After pot has been tagged, tracked, analyzed, and finally sold, shop owners are finding themselves with huge bundles of stone-cold cash. But unlike other cash-based businesses, vendors have nowhere to put it.

That's because banks, which are federally regulated, won't take their money.

"It's not ideal," said Vicente. "Some banks are coming around, and it seems they might take the money in the near future. But as long as the Department of Revenue accepts it, I think cash will be OK."

It's normal for owners to bring the DOR large amounts of cash to pay for fees, licensing and taxes. As a result, the agency has been awash in cash, leaving clerks there to rely on technology first invented almost 100 years ago.

"We use cash counting machines," said DOR Spokeswoman Serna. "They hand over the cash, and we put it into a cash counting machine. We look at the total, they look at it, then the state gives them a receipt. …Having cash is not unusual for us, and that will continue until something is done at the banking level."

For security reasons, Serna declined to comment about what happens to the cash after it's counted.

"I can assure you," she added, "there's not a big room full of cash just sitting around."

2. Local Pot Laws Conflict with National Policies Worldwide*

DONALD F. KETTL

Has The Dude, the pot-smoking character played by Jeff Bridges in the film *The Big Lebowski*, become Seattle's new poster child? In December, using small quantities of marijuana became legal in Washington state, and the Seattle Police Department (SPD) responded by posting Bridges' picture on its website with the caption, "The Dude abides, and says 'take it inside.'"

Under the referendum passed by voters in November, state residents can possess small amounts of pot, but not in public. The SPD's advice: "Under state law, you may responsibly get baked, order some pizzas and enjoy a 'Lord of the Rings' marathon in the privacy of your home, if you want to."

Breckenridge, Colo., might have beaten them to it. For years, newspaper reporters have long referred to the town as "the Amsterdam of the Rockies," where some residents quietly encouraged tourists to come for "our great outdoor beauty—and then relax with a joint at the end of the day." Now, residents in Colorado have also joined with Washington, voting to legalize the possession of small quantities of pot.

But if voters in Colorado and Washington decriminalized the possession of marijuana, federal law remains clear and inflexible. National drug policy still classifies pot as a Schedule I drug, along with heroin, ecstasy and LSD, with "no currently accepted medical use in the United States" and "a high potential for abuse." That has left the Obama administration nothing but tough choices: invoking federal preemption and taking a tough enforcement stand, which would anger many members of the base that just returned the president to the White House; doing absolutely nothing; or artfully threading their way through the dilemma of strong state support for decisions that are in opposition to national policy.

Even Amsterdam has struggled with this tension. The Dutch capital is home to hundreds of "coffee shops," where customers can legally enjoy both java and ganja. In fact, tourist officials estimate that 35 percent of all visitors to Amsterdam stop by a coffee shop. However, the center-right Dutch government in May banned the purchase of pot without a "wietpas" or weed pass, a membership in the coffee shops that is only available

---

*Originally published as Donald F. Kettl, "Local Pot Laws Conflict with National Policies Worldwide," *Governing*, February 2013. Reprinted with permission of the publisher.

to residents. "The objective is to combat the nuisance and crime associated with coffee shops and the trade in drugs," Prime Minister Mark Rutte explained.

The government's crackdown stirred a huge backlash. Amsterdam Mayor Eberhard van der Laan said the ban could push the marijuana trade from the coffee shops into the back alleys, as tourists "swarm all over the city looking for drugs." He said, "This would lead to more robberies, quarrels about fake drugs and no control of the quality of the drugs on the market—everything we have worked toward would be lost to misery."

Ultimately, the Dutch national government found a crack to squeeze through. It insisted on maintaining its policy but left implementation in the hands of local officials. Amsterdam's mayor quickly signaled that he wouldn't be enforcing the ban. The coffee shops were back in smoke-filled business. Lady Gaga celebrated during an Amsterdam concert by smoking a spliff onstage she called "wondrous."

But the national government hadn't finished. In November, it proposed a new ban on "skunk" pot, which contains more than 15 percent of THC (tetrahydrocannabinol, the magic in marijuana). The Dutch justice minister said it was a "hard drug" that created dangerous addiction. The coffee shop industry countered that this could also lead to more danger and crime—"Weak weed in the coffee shops, strong weed on the streets," as a spokesman put it. Tourists would spill back into dangerous back alleys looking for the more potent high that the coffee shops could no longer provide.

For governments everywhere, toking up has raised some exceptionally tough issues. How far can national governments go in enforcing laws out of sync with local officials? How can local officials slide around national policies so they stay in sync with their citizens? In the Netherlands, as in most countries, the battle plays out among governments that are all part of the same (more or less) governmental system. Neighboring governments in France and Germany insisted they would keep their pot bans in place, and the Danish government refused a request from Copenhagen's city council to experiment with Amsterdam-style deregulation. In the Czech Republic, Portugal and Switzerland, the national governments have taken a more Breckenridge-like position. In all these cases, national policy rules the day—to the degree national officials can deal with intransigent local officials and the habits of their citizens.

In the United States, federalism puts an emphasis on local enforcement of laws. The dilemma comes when local laws—and practice—differ with national laws. Seattle's police dealt with this problem by suggesting users not "flagrantly roll up a mega-spliff and light up in the middle of the street," and instead, manage their munchies in the quiet of their own homes. But the Obama administration has to find a road that doesn't abandon federal law when state voters decide they oppose it.

Governing everywhere is much more about finding a common ground between policy goals and different levels—and charting a road to reconcile what officials want and what citizens will actually do. Our system of federalism, as always, adds a special twist.

3. A Brief History of Cannabis Policy Legislation[*]

DERECK GLOVER *and* MICKEY P. MCGEE

The history of cannabis legislation in the United States has a past which begins long before the Controlled Substance Act of 1970 (CSA), which still governs use of cannabis federally today. In 1930, the Department of Treasury created a freestanding branch which would shape the U.S. policy for many years. The newly created Federal Bureau of Narcotics (FBN) was headed up by Harry Anslinger. He would lead the organization from its inception in 1930 until 1962. The appointment of Harry Anslinger was seen as a defining moment in the fight against cannabis. In the beginning of his tenure, Anslinger did not perceive cannabis to be a major threat.

However, by 1935 his perception of cannabis had shifted. He saw cannabis as a major issue facing the United States calling it "killer weed." The 1936 movie *Reefer Madness* was released as a national campaign against cannabis. By 1937, the Federal Bureau of Narcotics had enacted the Marijuana Tax Act (MTA). The MTA was a prohibitive tax which essentially made cannabis illegal. Under the MTA an individual would have to have declare and present their product for inspection prior to sale so it could be recorded for taxation purposes. The MTA would later be challenged and became the basis for measures engineered by Anslinger to limit cannabis over the next several decades. His policy decisions are the basis for the Controlled Substance Act of 1970 (CSA).

Between the enactment of MTA in 1937 and the CSA in 1970, more laws were passed on enforcement, harsher punishment for production, use and distribution of cannabis. This trend of more stringent cannabis regulation would continue throughout Anslinger's tenure. The Boggs Act of 1951 and the Daniel Act of 1956 created mandatory sentences for cannabis related offenses. The government decided to use "deterrence through punishment" as a means for reducing cannabis usage. Although this system was successful in sentencing people to jail time, it did not slow the spread of cannabis use. Mandatory sentencing laws were seen by many as a means of racial profiling and exercising control over the population. Some believe that policies on legalization of marijuana use were used as a way to target and manipulate AfricanAmerican and Hispanic populations. Over the past decades the idea of mandatory sentencing has shifted to more lenient system.

A former Harvard professor, Dr. Timothy Leary, was arrested and charged in 1966

---

*Published with permission of the authors.

for possession of cannabis in Laredo, Texas. Leary was traveling to Mexico from New York while in possession of cannabis. Upon return, his vehicle was inspected and cannabis found. He was charged under the MTA as he could not provide proper documentation to show the purchase of the marijuana. Leary decided to contest the MTA as a violation of his Fifth Amendment rights against self-incrimination. He would argue his case all the way to the U.S. Supreme Court in 1968. The Supreme Court ruled in favor of Leary in 1969, thereby nullifying the MTA of 1937 (https://supreme.justia.com/cases/federal/us/395/6/). The MTA had been the source of policies banning and criminalizing cannabis for nearly three decades. The overturning of the MTA was momentous and left a policy vacuum for cannabis legislation.

The *U.S. v. Timothy Leary* Supreme Court decision rendered the MTA of 1937 unconstitutional was a triggering mechanism for the Nixon administration. The Nixon administration utilized the newly created policy vacuum as an opportunity to create a policy window to reinstate cannabis regulation through legislation. In 1970, the Nixon administration would push through the CSA which was part of the Comprehensive Drug Abuse Prevention and Control Act.

The CSA delivered the largest blow to cannabis by adding cannabis to the Schedule I narcotics list. The Schedule I status placed cannabis on the same level as heroin, creating an obstacle for cannabis legalization and research. President Richard Nixon launched the "War on Drugs" during that same year. The "War on Drugs" became a political tagline, shaping government drug policy moving forward. The CSA came to be more synonymous with the failed "War on Drugs" instead of being an impactful program, helping to stem substance abuse and prevention issues.

Although the Nixon administration was successful in passing the CSA, opposition was strong across the country. Groups like NORML were fighting the legislation at the state level across the country. States across the country began to roll back some of the harsh penalties which had been associated with cannabis and essentially decriminalizing cannabis. In the 1970s, twelve decriminalized cannabis before South Dakota reversed it prior decriminalization in 1978.

Challenging the CSA, California passed the Compassionate Use Act in 1996. After medical use was passed in California, other states would follow suit. Over the next fifteen years, 15 other states and the District of Washington would pass some form of medical cannabis legislation through ballot initiatives. In 2012, Colorado and Washington approved legalized adult-use of recreational cannabis. These first two states were the pioneers challenging the CSA and began a major shift in the national mood. As of this writing, nine states and the District of Washington have passed adult-use legislation though ballot initiative. Twenty-nine and the District of Washington have also approved legalized use of medical cannabis as well.

States and municipal government which currently have legalized adult-use are learning to manage new issues. The added fees and taxes for cannabis purchase and regulatory compliance has developed an environment where big money (Big Cannabis replacing Big Tobacco) is poised to monopolize the market. As more states shift to both medical and adult-use cannabis, governments must ensure they are legislating in a manner which avoids as many of the unintended consequences. Lessons learned must be evaluated and shared among states and policies and legislation adjusted to meet the needs of the citizens. Legalization of adult-use cannabis created unforeseen consequences of driving medical marijuana patients underground and driving the small farmer and distributor out of business.

Although still not federally legal, progress has been made toward acceptance of cannabis as an alternative medicine and recreationally acceptable. It may now be the time for new cannabis legislation allowing access to all and opening more medical testing. Cannabis has slowly changed its long-standing perceptions through activism and education, becoming more widely accepted and achieving legal status across various states. The policy window is now open for other states to use the legislative process to legalize adult-use of recreational marijuana. Legislators are asked today to examine modern and accurate scientific data to make their determination on cannabis regulation.

Conclusion

Though the nation seems to be much more in support of legalization of cannabis, the position of the Trump administration and his Justice Department are in sharp contrast. The U.S. Department of Justice faces lawsuits attempting to overturn the CSA Schedule I narcotic listing for cannabis. As a majority of states begin to tip the balance in favor of cannabis legalization, current and future administrations will be challenged with continued resistance to the will of the people.

4. Marijuana Research Report Series

*Excerpt**

NATIONAL INSTITUTE ON DRUG ABUSE

Changes in marijuana policies across states legalizing marijuana for medical and/or recreational use suggest that marijuana is gaining greater acceptance in our society. Thus, it is particularly important for people to understand what is known about both the adverse health effects and the potential therapeutic benefits linked to marijuana.

Because marijuana impairs short-term memory and judgment and distorts perception, it can impair performance in school or at work and make it dangerous to drive. It also affects brain systems that are still maturing through young adulthood, so regular use by teens may have negative and long-lasting effects on their cognitive development, putting them at a competitive disadvantage and possibly interfering with their well-being in other ways. Also, contrary to popular belief, marijuana can be addictive, and its use during adolescence may make other forms of problem use or addiction more likely.

Whether smoking or otherwise consuming marijuana has therapeutic benefits that outweigh its health risks is still an open question that science has not resolved. Although many states now permit dispensing marijuana for medicinal purposes and there is mounting anecdotal evidence for the efficacy of marijuana-derived compounds, the U.S. Food and Drug Administration has not approved "medical marijuana." However, safe medicines based on cannabinoid chemicals derived from the marijuana plant have been available for decades and more are being developed.

This Research Report Excerpt is intended as a useful summary of what the most up-to-date science has to say about marijuana and its effects on those who use it at any age. The full report is in https://www.drugabuse.gov/publications/research-reports/ marijuana/.

What Is Marijuana?

Marijuana—also called *weed, herb, pot, grass, bud, ganja, Mary Jane,* and a vast number of other slang terms—is a greenish-gray mixture of the dried flowers of *Cannabis*

---

*Originally published as National Institute on Drug Abuse, "Marijuana Research Report Series," https://www.drugabuse.gov/publications/research-reports/marijuana/ (February 2018).

sativa. Some people smoke marijuana in hand-rolled cigarettes called *joints*; in pipes, water pipes (sometimes called *bongs*), or in *blunts* (marijuana rolled in cigar wraps). Marijuana can also be used to brew tea and, particularly when it is sold or consumed for medicinal purposes, is frequently mixed into foods (*edibles*) such as brownies, cookies, or candies. Vaporizers are also increasingly used to consume marijuana. Stronger forms of marijuana include sinsemilla (from specially tended female plants) and concentrated resins containing high doses of marijuana's active ingredients, including honeylike *hash oil*, waxy *budder*, and hard amber-like *shatter*. These resins are increasingly popular among those who use them both recreationally and medically.

The main *psychoactive* (mind-altering) chemical in marijuana, responsible for most of the intoxicating effects that people seek, is *delta-9-tetrahydrocannabinol* (THC). The chemical is found in resin produced by the leaves and buds primarily of the female cannabis plant. The plant also contains more than 500 other chemicals, including more than 100 compounds that are chemically related to THC, called *cannabinoids*.

What Is the Scope of Marijuana Use in the United States?

Marijuana is the most commonly used illicit drug (22.2 million people have used it in the past month) according to the 2015 National Survey on Drug Use and Health. Its use is more prevalent among men than women—a gender gap that widened in the years 2007 to 2014.

Marijuana use is widespread among adolescents and young adults. According to the Monitoring the Future survey—an annual survey of drug use and attitudes among the Nation's middle and high school students—most measures of marijuana use by 8th, 10th, and 12th graders peaked in the mid– to late 1990s and then began a period of gradual decline through the mid–2000s before levelling off. Most measures showed some decline again in the past 5 years. Teens' perceptions of the risks of marijuana use have steadily declined over the past decade, possibly related to increasing public debate about legalizing or loosening restrictions on marijuana for medicinal and recreational use. In 2016, 9.4 percent of 8th graders reported marijuana use in the past year and 5.4 percent in the past month (current use). Among 10th graders, 23.9 percent had used marijuana in the past year and 14.0 percent in the past month. Rates of use among 12th graders were higher still: 35.6 percent had used marijuana during the year prior to the survey and 22.5 percent used in the past month; 6.0 percent said they used marijuana daily or near-daily.

Medical emergencies possibly related to marijuana use have also increased. The Drug Abuse Warning Network (DAWN), a system for monitoring the health impact of drugs, estimated that in 2011, there were nearly 456,000 drug-related emergency department visits in the United States in which marijuana use was mentioned in the medical record (a 21 percent increase over 2009). About two-thirds of patients were male and 13 percent were between the ages of 12 and 17. It is unknown whether this increase is due to increased use, increased *potency* of marijuana (amount of THC it contains), or other factors. It should be noted, however, that mentions of marijuana in medical records do not necessarily indicate that these emergencies were directly related to marijuana intoxication.

What Are Marijuana Effects?

When marijuana is smoked, THC and other chemicals in the plant pass from the lungs into the bloodstream, which rapidly carries them throughout the body to the brain. The person begins to experience effects almost immediately. Many people experience a pleasant euphoria and sense of relaxation. Other common effects, which may vary dramatically among different people, include heightened sensory perception (e.g., brighter colors), laughter, altered perception of time, and increased appetite.

If marijuana is consumed in foods or beverages, these effects are somewhat delayed—usually appearing after 30 minutes to 1 hour—because the drug must first pass through the digestive system. Eating or drinking marijuana delivers significantly less THC into the bloodstream than smoking an equivalent amount of the plant. Because of the delayed effects, people may inadvertently consume more THC than they intend to.

Pleasant experiences with marijuana are by no means universal. Instead of relaxation and euphoria, some people experience anxiety, fear, distrust, or panic. These effects are more common when a person takes too much, the marijuana has an unexpectedly high potency, or the person is inexperienced. People who have taken large doses of marijuana may experience an acute psychosis, which includes hallucinations, delusions, and a loss of the sense of personal identity. These unpleasant but temporary reactions are distinct from longer-lasting psychotic disorders, such as schizophrenia, that may be associated with the use of marijuana in vulnerable individuals.

Although detectable amounts of THC may remain in the body for days or even weeks after use, the noticeable effects of smoked marijuana generally last from 1 to 3 hours, and those of marijuana consumed in food or drink may last for many hours.

How Does Marijuana Produce Its Effects?

THC's chemical structure is similar to the brain chemical *anandamide*. Similarity in structure allows the body to recognize THC and to alter normal brain communication.

Endogenous cannabinoids such as anandamide function as *neurotransmitters* because they send chemical messages between nerve cells (*neurons*) throughout the nervous system. They affect brain areas that influence pleasure, memory, thinking, concentration, movement, coordination, and sensory and time perception. Because of this similarity, THC is able to attach to molecules called *cannabinoid receptors* on neurons in these brain areas and activate them, disrupting various mental and physical functions and causing the effects described earlier. The neural communication network that uses these cannabinoid neurotransmitters, known as the *endocannabinoid system*, plays a critical role in the nervous system's normal functioning, so interfering with it can have profound effects.

For example, THC is able to alter the functioning of the hippocampus and orbito-frontal cortex, brain areas that enable a person to form new memories and shift his or her attentional focus. As a result, using marijuana causes impaired thinking and interferes with a person's ability to learn and perform complicated tasks. THC also disrupts functioning of the cerebellum and basal ganglia, brain areas that regulate balance, posture, coordination, and reaction time. This is the reason people who have used marijuana may not be able to drive safely and may have problems playing sports or engaging in other physical activities.

People who have taken large doses of the drug may experience an acute psychosis, which includes hallucinations, delusions, and a loss of the sense of personal identity.

THC, acting through cannabinoid receptors, also activates the brain's reward system, which includes regions that govern the response to healthy pleasurable behaviors such as sex and eating. Like most other drugs that people misuse, THC stimulates neurons in the reward system to release the signaling chemical *dopamine* at levels higher than typically observed in response to natural stimuli. This flood of dopamine contributes to the pleasurable "high" that those use who recreational marijuana seek.

Is Marijuana Addictive?

Marijuana use can lead to the development of problem use, known as a marijuana use disorder, which takes the form of addiction in severe cases. Recent data suggest that 30 percent of those who use marijuana may have some degree of marijuana use disorder. People who begin using marijuana before the age of 18 are four to seven times more likely to develop a marijuana use disorder than adults.

Marijuana use disorders are often associated with *dependence*—in which a person feels withdrawal symptoms when not taking the drug. People who use marijuana frequently often report irritability, mood and sleep difficulties, decreased appetite, cravings, restlessness, and/or various forms of physical discomfort that peak within the first week after quitting and last up to 2 weeks. Marijuana dependence occurs when the brain adapts to large amounts of the drug by reducing production of and sensitivity to its own endocannabinoid neurotransmitters.

Marijuana use disorder becomes addiction when the person cannot stop using the drug even though it interferes with many aspects of his or her life. Estimates of the number of people addicted to marijuana are controversial, in part because epidemiological studies of substance use often use dependence as a proxy for addiction even though it is possible to be dependent without being addicted. Those studies suggest that 9 percent of people who use marijuana will become dependent on it, rising to about 17 percent in those who start using in their teens.

In 2015, about 4.0 million people in the United States met the diagnostic criteria for a marijuana use disorder; 138,000 voluntarily sought treatment for their marijuana use.

Is Marijuana Safe and Effective as Medicine?

The potential medicinal properties of marijuana and its components have been the subject of research and heated debate for decades. THC itself has proven medical benefits in particular formulations. The U.S. Food and Drug Administration has approved THC-based medications, dronabinol (Marinol) and nabilone (Cesamet), prescribed in pill form for the treatment of nausea in patients undergoing cancer chemotherapy and to stimulate appetite in patients with wasting syndrome due to AIDS.

In addition, several other marijuana-based medications have been approved or are undergoing clinical trials. Nabiximols (Sativex), a mouth spray that is currently available in the United Kingdom, Canada, and several European countries for treating the spasticity and neuropathic pain that may accompany multiple sclerosis, combines THC with another chemical found in marijuana called cannabidiol (CBD). CBD does not have the rewarding properties of THC, and anecdotal reports indicate it may have promise for the treatment of seizure disorders, among other conditions. A CBD-based liquid medication called Epidiolex is currently being tested in the United States for the treatment of two forms of severe childhood epilepsy, Dravet syndrome and Lennox-Gastaut syndrome.

Researchers generally consider medications like these, which use purified chemicals derived from or based on those in the marijuana plant, to be more promising therapeutically than use of the whole marijuana plant or its crude extracts. Development of drugs from botanicals such as the marijuana plant poses numerous challenges. Botanicals may contain hundreds of unknown, active chemicals, and it can be difficult to develop a product with accurate and consistent doses of these chemicals. Use of marijuana as medicine also poses other problems such as the adverse health effects of smoking and THC-induced cognitive impairment. Nevertheless, a growing number of states have legalized dispensing of marijuana or its extracts to people with a range of medical conditions.

An additional concern with "medical marijuana" is that little is known about the long-term impact of its use by people with health- and/or age-related vulnerabilities—such as older adults or people with cancer, AIDS, cardiovascular disease, multiple sclerosis, or other neurodegenerative diseases. Further research will be needed to determine whether people whose health has been compromised by disease or its treatment (e.g., chemotherapy) are at greater risk for adverse health outcomes from marijuana use.

5. Smoked Marijuana Is Not Medicine*

U.S. DRUG ENFORCEMENT AGENCY

Marijuana is properly categorized under Schedule I of the Controlled Substances Act (CSA), 21 U.S.C. § 801, et seq. The clear weight of the currently available evidence supports this classification, including evidence that smoked marijuana has a high potential for abuse, has no accepted medicinal value in treatment in the United States, and evidence that there is a general lack of accepted safety for its use even under medical supervision.

The campaign to legitimize what is called "medical" marijuana is based on two propositions: first, that science views marijuana as medicine; and second, that the DEA targets sick and dying people using the drug. Neither proposition is true. Specifically, smoked marijuana has not withstood the rigors of science–it is not medicine, and it is not safe. Moreover, the DEA targets criminals engaged in the cultivation and trafficking of marijuana, not the sick and dying. This is true even in the District of Columbia and the 19 states that have approved the use of "medical" marijuana.

On October 19, 2009, Attorney General Eric Holder announced formal guidelines for federal prosecutors in states that have enacted laws authorizing the use of marijuana for medical purposes. The guidelines, as set forth in a memorandum from Deputy Attorney General David W. Ogden, makes clear that the focus of federal resources should not be on individuals whose actions are in compliance with existing state laws, and underscores that the Department will continue to prosecute people whose claims of compliance with state and local law conceal operations inconsistent with the terms, conditions, or purposes of the law.

He also reiterated that the Department of Justice is committed to the enforcement of the Controlled Substances Act (CSA) in all states and that this guidance does not "legalize" marijuana or provide for legal defense to a violation of federal law. While some people have interpreted these guidelines to mean that the federal government has relaxed its policy on "medical" marijuana, this in fact is not the case. Investigations and prosecutions of violations of state and federal law will continue. These are the guidelines DEA has and will continue to follow.

---

*Originally published as U.S. Drug Enforcement Agency, "DEA's Position on Marijuana: Smoked Marijuana Is Not Medicine, Part 1," April 2013.

On October 13, 2010, Attorney General Holder again reiterated the Department of Justice's position. In addressing concerns for the possible passing of Proposition 19 in California, a ballot initiative for the legalization of marijuana, he stated that "regardless of the passage of this or similar legislation, the Department of Justice will remain firmly committed to enforcing the CSA in all states. Prosecution of those who manufacture, distribute, or possess any illegal drugs, including marijuana, and the disruption of drug trafficking organizations is a core priority of the Department. Accordingly, we will vigorously enforce the CSA against those individuals and organizations that possess, manufacture, or distribute marijuana for recreational use, even if such activities are permitted under state law."

DEA will continue to conduct its mission to enforce the CSA and other actions as so directed by the U.S. Attorney General.

The Fallacy of Marijuana for Medicinal Use

In 1970, Congress enacted laws against marijuana based in part on its conclusion that marijuana has no scientifically proven medical value. Likewise, the Food and Drug Administration (FDA), which is responsible for approving drugs as safe and effective medicine, has thus far declined to approve smoked marijuana for any condition or disease. Indeed, the FDA has noted that "there is currently sound evidence that smoked marijuana is harmful," and "that no sound scientific studies support medical use of marijuana for treatment in the United States, and no animal or human data support the safety or efficacy of marijuana for general medical use."

The United States Supreme Court has also declined to carve out an exception for marijuana under a theory of medical viability. In 2001, for example, the Supreme Court decided that a "medical necessity" defense against prosecution was unavailable to defendants because Congress had purposely placed marijuana into Schedule I, which enumerates those controlled substances without any medical benefits. *See United States v. Oakland Cannabis Buyers' Cooperative et al.*, 532 U.S. 483, 491–92 (2001).

In *Gonzales v. Raich*, 545 U.S. 1 (2005), the Court had another opportunity to create a type of "medical necessity" defense in a case involving severely ill California residents who had received physician approval to cultivate and use marijuana under California's Compassionate Use Act (CUA). *See Raich*, 545 U.S. at 9. Despite the state's attempt to shield its residents from liability under CUA, the Supreme Court held that Congress' power to regulate interstate drug markets included the authority to regulate wholly intrastate markets as well. Consequently, the Court again declined to carve out a "medical necessity" defense, finding that the CSA was not diminished in the face of any state law to the contrary and could support the specific enforcement actions at issue.

In a show of support for the *Raich* decision, the International Narcotics Control Board (INCB) issued this statement urging other countries to consider the real dangers of cannabis:

Cannabis is classified under international conventions as a drug with a number of personal and public health problems. It is not a "soft" drug as some people would have you believe. There is new evidence confirming well-known mental health problems, and some countries with a more liberal policy towards cannabis are reviewing their position. Countries need to take a strong stance towards cannabis abuse.

The DEA and the federal government are not alone in viewing smoked marijuana as having no documented medical value. Voices in the medical community likewise do not accept smoked marijuana as medicine:

The **American Medical Association (AMA)** has always endorsed "well-controlled studies of marijuana and related cannabinoids in patients with serious conditions for which preclinical, anecdotal, or controlled evidence suggests possible efficacy and the application of such results to the understanding and treatment of disease." In November 2009, the AMA amended its policy, urging that marijuana's status as a Schedule I controlled substance be reviewed "with the goal of facilitating the conduct of clinical research and development of cannabinoid-based medicines, and alternate delivery methods." The AMA also stated that "this should not be viewed as an endorsement of state-based medical cannabis programs, the legalization of marijuana, or that scientific evidence on the therapeutic use of cannabis meets the current standards for prescription drug product."

The **American Society of Addiction Medicine's (ASAM)** public policy statement on "Medical Marijuana," clearly rejects smoking as a means of drug delivery. ASAM further recommends that "all cannabis, cannabis-based products and cannabis delivery devices should be subject to the same standards applicable to all other prescription medication and medical devices, and should not be distributed or otherwise provided to patients…" without FDA approval. ASAM also "discourages state interference in the federal medication approval process." ASAM continues to support these policies, and has also stated that they do not "support proposals to legalize marijuana anywhere in the United States."

The **American Cancer Society (ACS)** "is supportive of more research into the benefits of cannabinoids. Better and more effective treatments are needed to overcome the side effects of cancer and its treatment. However, the ACS does not advocate the use of inhaled marijuana or the legalization of marijuana."

The **American Glaucoma Society (AGS)** has stated that "although marijuana can lower the intraocular pressure, the side effects and short duration of action, coupled with the lack of evidence that its use alters the course of glaucoma, preclude recommending this drug in any form for the treatment of glaucoma at the present time."

The Glaucoma Research Foundation (GRF) states that "the high dose of marijuana necessary to produce a clinically relevant effect on intraocular pressure in people with glaucoma in the short term requires constant inhalation, as much as every three hours. The number of significant side effects generated by long-term use of marijuana or long-term inhalation of marijuana smoke make marijuana a poor choice in the treatment of glaucoma. To date, no studies have shown that marijuana—or any of its approximately 400 chemical components—can safely and effectively lower intraocular pressure better than the variety of drugs currently on the market."

The **American Academy of Pediatrics (AAP)** believes that "[a]ny change in the legal status of marijuana, even if limited to adults, could affect the prevalence of use among adolescents." While it supports scientific research on the possible medical use of cannabinoids as opposed to smoked marijuana, it opposes the legalization of marijuana.

The **American Academy of Child and Adolescent Psychiatry (AACAP)** "is concerned about the negative impact of medical marijuana on youth. Adolescents are especially vulnerable to the many adverse development, cognitive, medical, psychiatric, and addictive effects of marijuana." Of greater concern to the AACAP is that "adolescent marijuana users are more likely than adult users to develop marijuana dependence, and their heavy use is associated with increased incidence and worsened course of psychotic, mood, and anxiety disorders." "The "medicalization" of smoked marijuana has distorted the perception of the known risks and purposed benefits of this drug." Based upon these concerns, the "AACAP opposes medical marijuana dispensing to adolescents."

The **National Multiple Sclerosis Society (NMSS)** has stated that "based on studies to date—and the fact that long-term use of marijuana may be associated with significant, serious side effects—it is the opinion of the National Multiple Sclerosis Society's Medical Advisory Board that there are currently insufficient data to recommend marijuana or its derivatives as a treatment for MS symptoms. Research is continuing to determine if there is a possible role for marijuana or its derivatives in the treatment of MS. In the meantime, other well tested, FDA-approved drugs are available to reduce spasticity."

In 1999, **The Institute of Medicine (IOM)** released a landmark study reviewing the supposed medical properties of marijuana. The study is frequently cited by "medical" marijuana advocates, but in fact severely undermines their arguments.

After release of the IOM study, the principal investigators cautioned that the active compounds in marijuana may have medicinal potential and therefore should be researched further. However, the study concluded that "there is little future in smoked marijuana as a medically approved medication."

For some ailments, the IOM found "…potential therapeutic value of cannabinoid drugs, primarily THC, for pain relief, control of nausea and vomiting, and appetite stimulation."

However, it pointed out that "[t]he effects of cannabinoids on the symptoms studied are generally modest, and in most cases there are more effective medications [than smoked marijuana]."

The study concluded that, at best, there is only anecdotal information on the medical benefits of smoked marijuana for some ailments, such as muscle spasticity. For other ailments, such as epilepsy and glaucoma, the study found no evidence of medical value and did not endorse further research.

The IOM study explained that "smoked marijuana … is a crude THC delivery system that also delivers harmful substances." In addition, "plants contain a variable mixture of biologically active compounds and cannot be expected to provide a precisely defined drug effect." Therefore, the study concluded that "there is little future in smoked marijuana as a medically approved medication."

The principal investigators explicitly stated that using smoked marijuana in clinical trials "should not be designed to develop it as a licensed drug, but should be a stepping stone to the development of new, safe delivery systems of cannabinoids."

Thus, even scientists and researchers who believe that certain active ingredients in marijuana may have potential medicinal value openly *discount the notion that smoked marijuana is or can become "medicine."*

On October 9, 2002, the Coalition for Rescheduling Cannabis petitioned DEA to initiate proceedings for repeal of the rules or regulations that place marijuana in Schedule I of the CSA. The petition requested that it be rescheduled as "cannabis" in either Schedule III, IV or V of the CSA. DEA accepted this petition for filing on April 3, 2003. In accordance with 21 USC 811(b), after gathering the necessary data, the DEA requested a medical and scientific evaluation and scheduling recommendation for cannabis from the Department of Health and Human Services (HHS). HHS concluded that marijuana has a high potential for abuse, has no accepted medical use in the U.S., and lacks acceptable level of safety for use even under medical supervision. On June 21, 2011, the Administrator of DEA denied the petition to reschedule.

The Coalition for Rescheduling Cannabis appealed the DEA denial of the petition and filed a petition for review with the United States Court of Appeals for the District of Columbia Circuit in October 2012, claiming that DEA's final order denying their request was arbitrary and capricious. The Court, in reviewing the petition, noted that adequate and well-controlled studies are wanting not because they have been foreclosed, but because they have not been completed. The Court denied the petition for review.

The Drug Enforcement Administration supports ongoing research into potential medicinal uses of marijuana's active ingredients. As of January 2013:

- There are 125 researchers registered with DEA to perform studies with marijuana, marijuana extracts, and non-tetrahydrocannabinol marijuana derivatives that exist in the plant, such as cannabidiol and cannabinol.
- Studies include evaluation of abuse potential, physical/psychological effects, adverse effects, therapeutic potential, and detection.
- Eighteen of the researchers are approved to conduct research with smoked marijuana on human subjects.

At present, however, ***the clear weight of the evidence is that smoked marijuana is harmful.***

No matter what medical condition has been studied, other drugs already approved by the FDA have been proven to be safer than smoked marijuana.

The only drug currently approved by the FDA that contains the synthetic form of THC is Marinol. Available through prescription, Marinol comes in pill form, and is used to relieve nausea and vomiting associated with chemotherapy for cancer patients and to assist with loss of appetite with AIDS patients.

Sativex, an oromucosal spray for the treatment of spasticity due to Multiple Sclerosis is already approved for use in Canada, New Zealand, Spain, and the United Kingdom. The oral liquid spray contains two of the cannabinoids found in marijuana—THC and cannabidiol (CBD)—but unlike smoked marijuana, removes contaminants, reduces the intoxicating effects, is grown in a structured and scientific environment, administers a set dosage and meets criteria for pharmaceutical products. GW Pharmaceuticals plans to submit Sativex to the FDA in 2014 as a treatment for cancer pain.

Organizers behind the "medical" marijuana movement have not dealt with ensuring that the product meets the standards of modern medicine: quality, safety and efficacy. There is no standardized composition or dosage; no appropriate prescribing information; no quality control; no accountability for the product; no safety regulation; no way to measure its effectiveness (besides anecdotal stories); and no insurance coverage. Science, not popular vote, should determine what medicine is.

6. The Legalization Lobby*

U.S. DRUG ENFORCEMENT AGENCY

The proposition that smoked marijuana is "medicine" is, in sum, false—trickery used by those promoting wholesale legalization.

The Marijuana Policy Project (MPP) has provided funding and assistance to states and localities to promote "marijuana as medicine" initiatives and legislation for many years. In recent years they have also focused on decriminalizing marijuana and encouraging states to change penalties for possession and use from criminal to civil charges. Yet over the past several years their vision statement has clearly indicated they have a much broader goal of legalizing marijuana. At the same time the marijuana legalization proponents are soliciting support for laws allowing marijuana to be used as medicine, they are working toward "a nation where marijuana is regulated similarly to alcohol."

Ed Rosenthal, senior editor of *High Times*, a pro-drug magazine, once revealed the legalization strategy behind the "medical" marijuana movement. While addressing an effort to seek public sympathy for glaucoma patients, he said, "I have to tell you that I also use marijuana medically. I have a latent glaucoma which has never been diagnosed. The reason why it's never been diagnosed is because I've been treating it." He continued, "I have to be honest, there is another reason why I do use marijuana … and that is because I like to get high. Marijuana is fun."

A few wealthy businessmen—not broad grassroots support—started and sustain the "medical" marijuana and drug legalization movements in the United States. Without their money and influence, the drug legalization movement would shrivel. According to National Families in Action, four individuals—George Soros, Peter Lewis, George Zimmer, and John Sperling—contributed $1,510,000 to the effort to pass a "medical" marijuana law in California in 1996, a sum representing nearly 60 percent of the total contributions.

In addition to the continuing support from these businessmen, other contributors have supported the Drug Policy Alliance and the Marijuana Policy Project and their initiatives, including David Bronner, Rick Steves, Sean Parker, Dustin Moskovitz, Richard Lee, Bob Wilson, Jacob Goldfied, and Irwin Mark Jacobs.

In 2000, *The New York Times* interviewed Ethan Nadelmann, Director of the Lindesmith Center (now the Drug Policy Alliance). Responding to criticism that the medical

---

*Originally published as U.S. Drug Enforcement Agency, "DEA's Position on Marijuana: Smoked Marijuana Is Not Medicine, Part 2," April 2013.

marijuana issue is a stalking horse for drug legalization, Mr. Nadelmann stated: "Will it help lead toward marijuana legalization? ... I hope so."

When a statute dramatically reducing penalties for "medical" marijuana took effect in Maryland in October 2003, a defense attorney noted that "[t]here are a whole bunch of people who like marijuana who can now try to use this defense." The attorney observed that lawyers would be "neglecting their clients if they did not try to find out what 'physical, emotional or psychological'" condition could be enlisted to develop a defense to justify a defendant's using the drug. "Sometimes people are self-medicating without even realizing it," he said.

In 2004, Alaska voters faced a ballot initiative that would have made it legal for adults age 21 and older to possess, grow, buy, or give away marijuana. The measure also called for state regulation and taxation of the drug. The campaign was funded almost entirely by the Washington, D.C.–based MPP, which provided "almost all" the $857,000 taken in by the pro-marijuana campaign. Fortunately, Alaskan voters rejected the initiative.

In October 2005, Denver voters passed Initiative 100 decriminalizing marijuana based on incomplete and misleading campaign advertisements put forth by the Safer Alternative for Enjoyable Recreation (SAFER). A Denver City Councilman complained that the group used the slogan "Make Denver SAFER" on billboards and campaign signs to mislead the voters into thinking that the initiative supported increased police staffing. Indeed, the Denver voters were never informed of the initiative's true intent to decriminalize marijuana.

In 2006, the legalization movement funded three state marijuana-related initiatives, which were defeated in the November election. In Colorado, SAFER was behind Amendment 44, which allowed for possession of up to one ounce of marijuana. The amendment was defeated by 60 percent of the vote. In Nevada, Question 7, which was supported by the MPP, sought to permit the manufacture, distribution, and sale of marijuana to adults aged 21 or older. The measure was defeated by 56 percent of the vote. In South Dakota, South Dakotans for Medical Marijuana pushed Measure 4, allowing medical marijuana access. The measure was defeated by 52 percent of the vote.

The legalization movement was more successful at the local level in 2006. MPP-funded local groups were able to pass measures in three California cities: Santa Barbara (Sensible Santa Barbara), Santa Cruz (Santa Cruz Citizens for Sensible Marijuana Policy), and Santa Monica (Santa Monicans for Sensible Marijuana Policy); and in Missoula, Montana (Citizens for Responsible Crime Policy). Residents voted to make marijuana possession the lowest law enforcement priority in their cities.

Three other legalization groups also won local initiatives: the NORML (the National Organization for the Reform of Marijuana Laws) chapter at the University of Arkansas at Fayetteville helped make possession of one ounce or less of marijuana a misdemeanor in Eureka Springs, Arkansas; Americans for Safe Access assisted Albany, CA with passing Measure D, allowing a medical marijuana dispensary in the City of Albany; and the Drug Policy Forum of Massachusetts helped four districts pass non-binding policy statements from voters allowing for possession of up to one ounce of marijuana be a civil violation subject only to a $100 fine (2 districts) and allowing seriously ill patients to possess and grow marijuana with a doctor's recommendation.

In 2007 in Hailey, Idaho, the ballot initiatives to legalize industrial hemp, legalize medical use of marijuana and to allow marijuana laws to receive the lowest enforcement priority passed, but have not been implemented. The initiative to regulate and tax marijuana sales and use failed. Mayor Rick Davis, City Councilman Don Keirn, and Chief of Police Jeff Gunter filed a Declaratory Judgment action alleging that the three initiatives were illegal. "The lawsuit primarily alleges that the three initiatives are illegal because they are contrary to the general laws of the State of Idaho and the United States." Ryan Davidson, director of The Liberty Lobby of Idaho, put the initiatives back on the May ballot, and again they passed. "Davidson's efforts in Hailey are part of a larger grassroots agenda to have marijuana laws reformed statewide and nationally." In March 2009 Blaine County 5th District Court Judge Robert Elgee filed a decision to void the initiatives that would have legalized marijuana use in the city and would have made enforcement of marijuana laws the lowest priority for Hailey police. The judge also voided language in the initiative that would have required individual city officials to advocate for marijuana reform.

In 2008, with support from the Michigan Coalition for Compassionate Care, Michigan became the 13th state to approve marijuana for medicinal purposes.

Massachusetts, backed by the Committee for Sensible Marijuana Policy, replaced criminal penalties for one ounce of marijuana with a civil fine in 2008.

Voters in four districts (15 towns) in Massachusetts, supported by local legalization groups, passed a ballot measure to instruct a representative from each district to vote in favor of legislation that would allow seriously ill patients, with a doctor's written recommendation, to possess and grow small amounts of marijuana for their personal medical use.

In the same year, voters in Fayetteville, Arkansas, supported by Sensible Fayetteville, voted to make adult marijuana possession law the lowest priority for local law enforcement.

In California, Proposition 5, also known as the Non-Violent Offender Rehabilitation Act, and supported by the Drug Policy Alliance, called for more funding for addiction treatment and decriminalization of up to an ounce of marijuana. This initiative did not pass.

The legalizers were also less successful in New Hampshire, where although the state legislature approved a bill to legalize "medical" marijuana, Governor John Lynch vetoed the bill in July 2009, citing concerns over cultivation, distribution and the potential for abuse.

Rhode Island became the third state to allow the sale of marijuana for medicinal purposes. In June 2009, the Rhode Island legislature overrode Governor Circieri's veto of bills that allow for the establishment of three compassionate care centers regulated by the state department of health.

New Mexico opened its first "medical" marijuana dispensary in June 2009, becoming the fourth state to allow "medical" marijuana dispensaries.

In November 2009, Maine became the fifth state to allow dispensaries. The voters also approved the expansion of the "medical" marijuana law, to include defining debilitating medical conditions and incorporating additional diseases that can be included under the law. This effort was funded by the Drug Policy Alliance.

On November 4, 2009, Breckenridge, Colorado citizens voted to decriminalize possession of up to 1 ounce of marijuana for adults over 21 years of age. The measure, however, is symbolic, because pot possession is still against state law. Sean McAllister, a Breckenridge lawyer who pushed for the decriminalization measure said that "the vote shows people want to skip medical marijuana and legalize pot for everyone."

In January 2010, New Jersey became the fourteenth state to allow the use of marijuana for medicinal purposes. With the most restrictive law in the country, only residents with one of twelve chronic illnesses (not including chronic pain) will be able to get a prescription from their doctor to buy up to two ounces a month from one of six dispensaries. Implementation of the program, originally scheduled for October 1, 2010, was extended by the state legislature until January 1, 2011, to give the Governor more time to determine who will grow and dispense marijuana.

In Massachusetts voters in 18 legislative districts approved non-binding measures calling on state lawmakers to pass "medical" marijuana legislation or a bill to regulate marijuana like alcohol. The organizers of these measures included the Drug Policy Forum of Massachusetts, the Massachusetts Cannabis Reform Coalition, Suffolk University NORML and the University of Massachusetts Amherst Cannabis Reform Coalition.

In November 2010, Arizona became the fifteenth state to allow the use of marijuana for medicinal purposes. Proposition 203, the Arizona Medical Marijuana Act, sponsored by the Arizona Medical Marijuana Policy Project with financial support from George Soros, passed with 50.13 percent of the vote. The program, which will be established and implemented by the Department of Health Services, allows residents with certain medical conditions to obtain a doctor's written certification to purchase up to 2.5 ounces of marijuana every two weeks from a state approved dispensary or grow their own if they live 25 miles or more from a dispensary.

In South Dakota residents once again refused to support efforts to legalize marijuana. Measure 13, which sought to authorize the possession, use and cultivation of marijuana by and for persons with specific debilitating medical conditions, was defeated by 63.3 percent of the vote.

In Oregon 58 percent of the voters said no to Measure 74, which would have established a "medical" marijuana supply system and allow for the sale of marijuana and marijuana-laced products in shops throughout the state. The measure was financially backed by billionaire Peter Lewis, a known legalization activist, who resides in Florida.

In California, voters defeated Proposition 19 (The Regulate, Control and Tax Cannabis Act of 2010), which sought to legalize the possession and cultivation of limited amounts of marijuana for use by individuals 21 years of age and older. Had it passed, California would have been the first state to legalize marijuana for recreational purposes. The initiative garnered much debate. Fueled by financial support from legalization activists, including one million dollars each from Oakland cannabis entrepreneur Richard Lee and billionaire George Soros, proponents for the initiative used the media to attempt to sway public opinion. Nine former DEA Administrators called upon U.S. Attorney General Eric H. Holder, Jr., to clarify the federal position and reiterate the law. In response, Attorney General Holder stated the Department of Justice's position: "the Department of Justice will remain firmly committed to enforcing the Controlled Substances Act (CSA) in all states. Prosecution of those who manufacture, distribute or possess any illegal drugs—including marijuana—and the disruption of drug trafficking organizations is a core priority of the Department. Accordingly, we will vigorously enforce the CSA against those individuals and organization who possess, manufacture, or distribute marijuana for recreational use, even if such activities are permitted under state law."

In 2011, Delaware became the 16th state to allow the use of marijuana for medicinal purposes. Senate Bill 17 permits doctor recommended use of marijuana for medical purposes for adults with serious medical conditions. The Delaware Department of Health and Social Services will run the program and marijuana must be purchased from state-licensed and regulated centers that would grow, cultivate and dispense the marijuana. The measure was supported by the MPP.

In Montana, where the 2004 "medical" marijuana program (Initiative 148) was expanding out of control and causing problems throughout the state, legislators began to call for repeal of the law. Governor Schweitzer vetoed the repeal. In response, in 2011 the legislature passed Senate Bill 423, Montana Marijuana Act, which placed additional restrictions on the program, including stricter regulations on businesses and further defining ailments that will qualify under the program. The Governor let the bill pass.

Voters in Kalamazoo, Michigan, passed a ballot initiative making the use or possession of small amounts of marijuana by adults the lowest law enforcement priority; however Police Chief Hadley stated that he still intended to follow state and federal law.

On May 31, 2012, Connecticut became the 17th state to allow the use of marijuana for medical purposes. Public Act No. 12-55, An Act Concerning the Palliative Use of Marijuana, will be run by the Connecticut Department of Consumer Protection. Persons 18 years of age or older with serious qualifying medical conditions and a physician's recommendation can apply for a registration certificate. Access to marijuana will be supplied through licensed dispensaries run by pharmacists. This measure was also supported by the MPP.

In November of 2012, Massachusetts became the 18th state to allow for the use of marijuana for medicinal purposes when it passed Question 3. The program will be run by the Massachusetts Department of Public Health (DPH) and requires persons suffering from debilitating conditions to get a doctor's recommendation before applying for an identification card. Marijuana will be available through DPH-registered "medical marijuana treatment centers." Certain exemptions exist for permission to grow marijuana at home. The ballot initiative was backed by the Committee for Compassionate Medicine and funded in part by Peter Lewis, Chairman of Progressive Insurance, and passed with 63 percent of the vote.

Voters in six legislative districts (45 towns) in Massachusetts approved non-binding measures favoring federal or state marijuana legalization.

Voters in three Michigan cities (Detroit, Flint and Grand Rapids) approved initiatives to decriminalize penalties for marijuana use. However, use and possession are still crimes under state law. In Ypsilanti voters approved a measure to make marijuana enforcement the lowest police priority.

In Chicago, Illinois, the City Council passed an ordinance that allows police to ticket people with small amounts of marijuana instead of arresting them. The intent behind the change is to reduce the amount of paperwork police officers have to do so they can devote their time to more serious law enforcement matters as well as increasing city revenue from ticket fees.

In Arkansas, Arkansans for Compassionate Care, with funding from the Marijuana Policy Project, pushed for passage of Issue 5, Authorize the Use of Marijuana for Medical Purposes. This initiative lost with 48 percent of the vote.

Measure 80, Initiative 9, The Oregon Tax Act Initiative, sought to repeal Oregon's marijuana prohibition and replace it with a system of taxation and regulation. Sponsored by the Yes on Measure 80 Campaign, the initiative lost with 46 percent of the vote. The Measure was led by Paul Stanford, owner of the Hemp and Cannabis Foundation Medical Clinics.

In Montana voters passed Initiative 124 by 66 percent, reaffirming the passage of Senate Bill 423 in 2011. The Marijuana Cannabis Industry Association had submitted the initiative in hopes of repealing Senate Bill 423 and restoring the "medical" marijuana program to the way it was prior to implementation of the Senate Bill.

Rhode Island passed a bill to decriminalize the simple possession of marijuana. Adults apprehended with up to one ounce of marijuana will receive a $150.00 fine, with no arrest, jail time or criminal record.

The year 2012 saw the first state legalize marijuana for recreational purposes. Colorado passed Amendment 64 by 55 percent of the vote, allowing the personal possession and cultivation of marijuana by adults who are 21 and older and for regulated sale of marijuana. It creates a system of state-licensed cultivation, manufacturing and testing facilities, and state-licensed retail stores. This initiative was sponsored by the Campaign to Regulate Marijuana like alcohol, which if funded and staffed by the Marijuana Policy Project, with assistance from SAFER and NORML.

Washington is the second state to legalize marijuana with the passage of Initiative 502 by 55 percent of the vote, allowing for the possession of an ounce of marijuana by adults who are 21 and older and for regulated sales. Washington, unlike Colorado, will not allow home cultivation. This initiative was sponsored by the New Approach Washington, which included support from the Drug Policy Alliance, Peter Lewis, Rick Steves, Harriett Bullitt, former U.S. Attorney John McKay, and former Spokane Regional Health Director Dr. Kim Thorburn.

On July 25, 2007, the U.S. House of Representatives defeated, by a vote of 165–262, an amendment (HR-3093) that would have prevented the DEA and the Department of Justice from arresting or prosecuting medical marijuana patients and providers in the 12 states where medical marijuana was then legal.

Two Congressional initiatives on marijuana also failed in 2008. HR5842, Medical Marijuana Patient Protection Act and HR5843, Act to Remove Federal Penalties for the Personal Use of Marijuana by Responsible Adults, both died in committee.

Three Congressional initiatives were introduced in Congress in 2009: HR2835 Medical Marijuana Patient Protection Act; HR2943 Personal Use of Marijuana by Responsible Adults Act of 2009; and HR3939 Truth in Trials Act. None were passed.

The Consolidated Appropriations Act of 2010 (HR 3288) became law in December 2009 without the "Barr Amendment," a provision that has been included in the Appropriations bill for the District of Columbia since 1999. The Barr Amendment had prohibited "any funds to be used to conduct a ballot initiative which seeks to legalize or reduce the penalties associated with the possession, use, or distribution of any Schedule I substance under the Controlled Substances Act (or any tetrahydrocannabinois derivative)."

The elimination of the Barr Amendment enabled the District of Columbia to implement Initiative 59, a ballot initiative that was approved in 1998 to allow for the use of marijuana for medical treatment. In May 2010, the District of Columbia City Council approved a bill that would allow chronically ill patients to receive a doctor's prescription to use marijuana and buy up to two ounces a month from a city-sanctioned distribution center. The Legalization of Marijuana for Medical Treatment Amendment Act of 2010 became law in July. The District of Columbia government is still working on the details of the program to ensure strict regulatory controls are in place prior to implementation.

In 2011 two Congressional initiatives were introduced. HR 1983, States' Medical Marijuana Patient Protection Act, and HR 2306, Ending Federal Marijuana Prohibition Act of 2011, both died in committee.

In 2012 four members of the U.S. House of Representatives attached an amendment to HR5326, the Commerce, Justice, Science and Related Agencies Appropriations Act, 2013, stating that the Department of Justice could not use funding to attack medical marijuana operations in states that had approved "medical" marijuana. The bill failed.

7. FDA and Marijuana

*Questions and Answers**

U.S. FOOD AND DRUG ADMINISTRATION

1. How is marijuana therapy being used by some members of the medical community?

A. The FDA is aware that marijuana or marijuana-derived products are being used for a number of medical conditions including, for example, AIDS wasting, epilepsy, neuropathic pain, treatment of spasticity associated with multiple sclerosis, and cancer and chemotherapy-induced nausea. To date, the FDA has not approved a marketing application for a drug product containing or derived from botanical marijuana and has not found any such product to be safe and effective for any indication.

2. Why hasn't the FDA approved marijuana for medical uses?

A. To date, the FDA has not approved a marketing application for marijuana for any indication. The FDA generally evaluates research conducted by manufacturers and other scientific investigators. Our role, as laid out in the Federal Food, Drug, and Cosmetic (FD&C) Act, is to review data submitted to the FDA in an application for approval to assure that the drug product meets the statutory standards for approval.

The FDA has approved Marinol and Syndros for therapeutic uses in the United States, including for the treatment of anorexia associated with weight loss in AIDS patients. Marinol and Syndros include the active ingredient dronabinol, a synthetic delta-9-tetrahydrocannabinol (THC) which is considered the psychoactive component of marijuana. Another FDA-approved drug, Cesamet, contains the active ingredient nabilone, which has a chemical structure similar to THC and is synthetically derived.

3. Is marijuana safe for medical use?

A. The FDA has not approved any product containing or derived from botanical marijuana for any indication. This means that the FDA has not found any such product to be safe or effective for the treatment of any disease or condition. Study of marijuana in clinical trial settings is needed to assess the safety and effectiveness of marijuana for medical use.

The FDA will continue to facilitate the work of companies interested in appropriately

---

*Originally published as U.S. Food and Drug Administration, "FDA and Marijuana: Questions and Answers," https://www.fda.gov/NewsEvents/PublicHealthFocus/ucm421168.htm#notapproved (August 2017).

32

bringing safe, effective, and quality products to market, including scientifically-based research concerning the medicinal uses of marijuana.

4. How does FDA's role differ from the role of other federal agencies when it comes to the investigation of marijuana for medical use?

A. Conducting clinical research using marijuana involves interactions with several federal agencies. This includes: a registration administered by the Drug Enforcement Administration (DEA); obtaining the marijuana for research from the National Institute on Drug Abuse (NIDA), within the National Institutes of Health, or another DEA-registered source; and review by the FDA of an investigational new drug (IND) application and research protocol.

Additionally:

- As a Schedule I controlled substance under the Controlled Substances Act, DEA provides researchers with investigator and protocol registrations and has Schedule I-level security requirements at the site marijuana will be studied.
- NIDA provides research-grade marijuana for scientific study. The agency is responsible for overseeing the cultivation of marijuana for medical research and has contracted with the University of Mississippi to grow marijuana for research at a secure facility. Marijuana of varying potencies and compositions is available. DEA also may allow additional growers to register with the DEA to produce and distribute marijuana for research purposes.
- Researchers work with the FDA and submit an IND application to the appropriate division in the Office of New Drugs, in the Center for Drug Evaluation and Research (CDER), depending on the therapeutic indication.

The roles of the three agencies are the same for investigations of marijuana for use as an animal drug product, except that researchers would establish an investigational new animal drug (INAD) file with the Center for Veterinary Medicine to conduct their research, rather than an IND with CDER.

5. Does the FDA object to the clinical investigation of marijuana for medical use?

A. No. The FDA believes that scientifically valid research conducted under an IND application is the best way to determine what patients could benefit from the use of drugs derived from marijuana. The FDA supports the conduct of that research by:

1. Providing information on the process needed to conduct clinical research using marijuana.
2. Providing information on the specific requirements needed to develop a drug that is derived from a plant such as marijuana. In June 2004, the FDA finalized its Guidance for Industry: Botanical Drug Products, which provides sponsors with guidance on submitting IND applications for botanical drug products.
3. Providing specific support for investigators interested in conducting clinical research using marijuana and its constituents as a part of the IND process through meetings and regular interactions throughout the drug development process.
4. Providing general support to investigators to help them understand and follow the procedures to conduct clinical research through the FDA Center for

Drug Evaluation and Research's Small Business and Industry Assistance group.

6. What kind of research is the FDA reviewing when it comes to the efficacy of marijuana?

A. The FDA reviews applications to market drug products to determine whether those drug products are safe and effective for their intended indications. The FDA reviews scientific investigations, including adequate and well-controlled clinical trials, as part of the FDA's drug approval process.

The FDA relies on applicants and scientific investigators to conduct research. Our role, as outlined in the Federal Food, Drug, and Cosmetic Act, is to review data submitted to the FDA in a marketing application to determine whether a proposed drug product meets the statutory standards for approval. Additional information concerning research on the medical use of marijuana is available from the National Institutes of Health, particularly the National Cancer Institute (NCI) and NIDA.

7. How can patients get into expanded access program for marijuana for medical use?

A. Manufacturers may be able to make investigational drugs available to individual patients in certain circumstances through expanded access, as described in the FD&C Act and implementing regulations. For example, GW Pharmaceuticals is currently making a drug product that contains cannabidiol and that is being developed for seizure disorders available through expanded access. Information about this program can be obtained from the company.

8. Does the FDA have concerns about administering a cannabis product to children?

A. We understand that parents are trying to find treatments for their children's medical conditions. However, the use of untested drugs can have unpredictable and unintended consequences. Caregivers and patients can be confident that FDA-approved drugs have been carefully evaluated for safety, efficacy, and quality, and are monitored by the FDA once they are on the market. The FDA continues to support sound, scientifically-based research into the medicinal uses of drug products containing marijuana or marijuana constituents, and will continue to work with companies interested in bringing safe, effective, and quality products to market.

9. Does the FDA have concerns about administering a cannabis product to pregnant and lactating women?

A. As stated above, to date, the FDA has not approved a marketing application for marijuana for any indication. The FDA is also aware that there are potential adverse health effects with use of marijuana in pregnant or lactating women. Published scientific literature reports potential adverse effects of marijuana use in pregnant women, including fetal growth restriction, low birth weight, preterm birth, small-for-gestational age, neonatal intensive care unit (NICU) admission, and stillbirth. Based on published animal research, there are also concerns that use of marijuana during pregnancy may negatively impact fetal brain development.

The American College of Obstetricians and Gynecologists (ACOG) recommends that women who are pregnant or contemplating pregnancy should be encouraged to discontinue marijuana use. In addition, ACOG notes that there are insufficient data to evaluate the effects of marijuana use on breastfed infants; therefore, marijuana use is discouraged when breastfeeding. Pregnant and lactating women should talk with a health care provider about the potential adverse health effects of marijuana use.

10. What is FDA's reaction to states that are allowing marijuana to be sold for medical uses without the FDA's approval?

A. The FDA is aware that several states have either passed laws that remove state restrictions on the medical use of marijuana and its derivatives or are considering doing so. In particular, we know that a number of states are interested in allowing access to cannabinoid oil, or cannabidiol, in an attempt to treat childhood epilepsy. It is important to conduct medical research into the safety and effectiveness of marijuana products through adequate and well-controlled clinical trials. We welcome the opportunity to talk with states who are considering support for medical research of marijuana and its derivatives to provide information on Federal and scientific standards.

8. The Possibilities of Pot*

WILLIAM SMITH

When the Iowa Board of Pharmacy reclassified marijuana in 2010 as a drug with medicinal purposes, supporters of the drug's medical use saw a bit of light at the end of the tunnel.

Two states—Colorado and Washington—already have legalized marijuana for recreational use, even though it flies in the face of federal law. Eighteen states and the District of Columbia have legalized marijuana for medicinal use (counting Colorado and Washington), which also is against federal law. Illinois Gov. Pat Quinn could sign a bill that would legalize the drug for medical use in less than two weeks, if supporters have their way. The Illinois Senate passed The Compassionate Use of Medical Cannabis Pilot Program Act in May.

Just don't expect marijuana to be legalized in Iowa any time soon.

State Sen. Tom Courtney, D–Burlington, has been fighting for the legalization of medical marijuana, and he doesn't have high hopes.

"We will try in the future. The House [of Representatives] changes every two years," he said. "It could be another couple of years."

The Failed Road

There was a bill in the Iowa House and Iowa Senate this year that would have legalized medical marijuana—House File 22 and Senate File 79—and neither made it past the first funnel. Both aimed to legalize medical marijuana for people with a "chronic or debilitating medical condition" such as cancer, glaucoma or HIV.

Courtney was one of the co-sponsors on the bill, and it's still a cause he believes in, on a personal and legislative level.

"Doctor after doctor has told me that if they could have used marijuana, it could have reduced the pain. It doesn't have any side effects to speak of," he said.

It's also a personal cause for Courtney, whose wife, Donna, died of cancer in 2008.

"Marinol pills gave her some relief, but it would have been so much better if she had had legal access to marijuana," Courtney said.

---

*Originally published as William Smith, "The Possibilities of Pot," *The Hawk Eye*, July 2013. Reprinted with permission of the publisher.

Opponents of legalized marijuana say the term "medical marijuana" is no different than marijuana purchased from a drug dealer. State Sen. Tom Sands, R–Wapello, stands resolutely against its legalization.

"I've never supported legalizing anything that is a drug and is wrong to use," Sands said.

Though Sands doesn't want marijuana to be legalized in any form, he doesn't discount testimonials and studies that point to the use of marijuana as an effective way to treat chronic pain. He pointed out the marijuana pill dronabinol—a legal pill that contains the active ingredient of marijuana—as a possible alternative that could make the marijuana legalization discussion moot. A recent study of the drug showed the pain-reducing effects lasted longer than that of smoking marijuana. While smoking the drug decreased pain sensitivity for about 2½ hours, the pill continued to have pain-reducing effects for about 4½ hours. However, the pain-killing effects of the pill took about an hour to kick in, compared with about 15 minutes for smoking marijuana. The study was published in the medical journal *Neuropsychopharmacology*.

"If there is a true medical benefit, there would be more possibility of it coming to the public," Sands said. "I think the public is against it."

Public opinion on medical marijuana has been changing, though. A 2010 poll by the *Des Moines Register* revealed 64 percent of Iowans supported allowing medical uses of marijuana. Nearly half the adults in the country have tried marijuana, and 12 percent of them in the past year, according to a survey by the Pew Research Center. Fifty-two percent of adults favor legalizing marijuana, up 11 percentage points just since 2010. Sixty percent think Washington shouldn't enforce federal laws against marijuana in states that have approved its use.

Sands said legalization of marijuana is a partisan issue. Younger people, who tend to vote more Democratic, are more supportive of legalizing marijuana. Courtney said any future bills to legalize medical marijuana would need bipartisan support, and it just isn't there right now.

"As far as where it goes next year, I would be very surprised if there was any movement," Courtney said. "It's definitely a bipartisan issue. A couple of years ago, I had as much support from Republicans as Democrats."

Sands agreed, though he's not ruling anything out.

"I don't see the possibility, but I never would have thought I would see gay marriage legalized in this state," Sands said.

Cracking Down

Whatever medical advantages marijuana may have, many believe legalizing the drug in any form would have a disastrous effect on the community. Burlington Police Chief Doug Beaird is one of them.

"Iowa law classifies it as a Schedule 1 controlled substance, and there's a big potential for abuse," Beaird said. "That's the law I've known, and that's the law we'll hold up for now."

Like many other cities, possession of marijuana arrests are common, and the Burlington Police Department is in the middle of an investigation into marijuana distribution. Though Beaird wouldn't reveal any details about the investigation, the BPD has been active busting marijuana dealers. Two years ago, narcotics agents seized 120 pounds of marijuana from Buddies Trailer Sales. That led to several other busts, with one being a Burlington man who already tried to bring 24 pounds of marijuana into Burlington while riding an Amtrak train. He was arrested two months ago in Galesburg, Ill.

Despite the busts, there really hasn't been a big change in local marijuana prices, Beaird said. There always will be those who want to smoke, and those who want to sell it to them. Beaird said most of the marijuana is coming from southern Texas, principally the Brownsville and El Paso areas, often hidden in unusual places, including gas tanks and hay bales.

"There hasn't been a big increase in use," he said.

Iowa has the largest racial disparity in the country of arrests in marijuana possession, with blacks being more than eight times as likely to be arrested than whites, even though whites use marijuana at about the same rate, a national American Civil Liberties Union study has found.

When asked about the study, Gov. Terry Branstad said that was no reason to legalize marijuana.

"The problem with marijuana is that it's a gateway drug," Bearid said.

Beaird's biggest problem with legalizing marijuana would be the increase of impaired driving, which is commonly cited by those against legalization.

"How much more prevalent would that become?" Beaird mused.

Treating Marijuana

Impaired driving also is a concern for Melissa Foster, a prevention supervisor for Alcohol and Drug Dependency Services on Mount Pleasant Street. She teaches required classes for locals who have been busted for operating a vehicle while under the influence and has noticed more and more offenders under the influence of marijuana.

"A person under marijuana, their peripheral vision is very impaired. We are seeing an increase in that locally," she said. "Alcohol is still the primary one. Our max class size is 12 participants, and one or two of them are there for marijuana."

Foster agreed marijuana shouldn't be legalized in any form.

"My opinion falls fairly close to the ADDS opinion," she said. "We feel the legalization of marijuana for medical purposes needs to be left up to the medical community. They have access to all the longitudinal research [long-term studies]. There are short-term studies out there that anyone could use for the legalization of marijuana."

Some of those long-term studies already are bearing fruit. According to a new study in the United Kingdom, people who smoke marijuana regularly over long periods of time tend to produce less of a chemical in the brain linked to motivation. Nineteen people in the study used cannabis heavily, each began using the drug between the ages of 12 and 18, and all experienced symptoms of psychosis while under the influence.

Another study, this one conducted on mice, suggested chronic marijuana use may cause inflammation in the brain that leads to problems with coordination, learning and schizophrenia.

"Marijuana is as addictive as any other substance," Foster said. "It has very significant health problems."

While the verdict still is out on how addictive marijuana is, many long-term users have gone to ADDS to wean themselves from the drug. Foster said 20.5 percent of all admitted ADDS clients cited marijuana as their primary drug of choice. About 13 percent said marijuana was their secondary drug of choice, and 4 percent said it was their tertiary drug of choice. Those numbers fall in line with the national average, as the National Survey on Drug Use and Health reported marijuana accounted for 4.5 million of the estimated 7.1 million Americans dependent on or abusing illicit drugs.

Foster said clients report a number of negative withdrawal symptoms after quitting the drug, including anxiety, crankiness, decreased appetite and disturbed sleep patterns.

"Because THC [the main psychoactive substance found in the cannabis plant] has such a slow release from the body, sometimes the side effects are very subtle, and we don't notice them as withdrawal symptoms. Anxiety is a big one I hear from individuals who have stopped smoking," she said.

Foster's main concern about legalizing medical marijuana is the easier access it might provide for youth, whom she interacts with in the schools while teaching drug prevention courses. According to the 2012 youth survey for Des Moines County, 31 percent of all 11th-graders admitted to trying marijuana, and 12 percent have used within 30 days. Two percent of sixth-graders admitted to trying it.

"Des Moines County is slightly higher than the state average (22 percent of 11th graders) in regards to marijuana use. And you see that with alcohol," Foster said.

Benefits

Mike AbouAssaly, a physician at Burlington Area Family Practice in West Burlington, doesn't know if he approves of medical marijuana. He hasn't done enough research to decide.

But he likes what he's seen so far.

"I think we have seen the benefits," he said.

AbouAssaly, who has been running his family practice for 15 years, isn't allowed to prescribe medical marijuana. But he's had three or four patients during his time in Burlington who took it upon themselves to ingest marijuana to ease their pain. In each case, the patients reported the ease of pain without the nasty side effects caused by their prescribed medications.

"[Prescription drugs] are highly addictive and habit-forming medications, and they didn't really control their pain that well, and they caused constipation. But they're legal, because a doctor prescribed them," AbouAssaly said.

In all the cases, the patients ingested marijuana through food rather than smoking it, and AbouAssaly was appreciative they were up-front with him about it. Their insistence on using the drug changed what AbouAssaly prescribed to them.

"There are certainly narcotics you don't want to mix," he said.

Compounds in marijuana can relieve pain, combat nausea and stimulate appetite. Unlike many abused drugs, an overdose of marijuana is not lethal, according to the National Cancer Institute. Although marijuana can be addictive for some, studies have shown the potential for forming an addiction to marijuana is lower than some prescription drugs and other abused drugs.

"I see a growing trend, and a lot of physicians are using it. No one around here, but several of my friends on the West Coast have dabbled in it," AbouAssaly said.

Recreational Use

The first year of the 2014 Iowa Legislature has adjourned, but the legalization of marijuana isn't entirely out of the picture. Legislation introduced this year will carry over to next year, meaning House File 22 and Senate File 79 can be picked up in 2014. This also means SSB 1045, introduced by Gov. Terry Branstad through the Iowa Office of Drug Control Policy, will remain active as well. It strips the power of the pharmacy board to allow medical use of marijuana if the board deems it appropriate.

If medical marijuana becomes a reality for Iowans in the future, that leaves the question—how far away is the legalization of recreational use of marijuana?

Courtney wouldn't hazard a guess on that one, and he isn't sure if he would be in favor of such a bill if it ever came along. But he does want to help those in pain.

"I just think [medical marijuana] ought to be an option," he said. "I'm not saying everyone should jump on it. But it can make people feel better."

9. Seniors Increasingly Getting High, Study Shows[*]

CARMEN HEREDIA RODRIGUEZ

Baby boomers are getting high in increasing numbers, reflecting growing acceptance of the drug as treatment for various medical conditions, according to a study published Monday in the journal Addiction.

The findings reveal overall use among the 50-and-older study group increased "significantly" from 2006 to 2013. Marijuana users peaked between ages 50 to 64, then declined among the 65-and-over crowd.

Men used marijuana more frequently than women, the study showed, but marital status and educational levels were not major factors in determining users.

The study by researchers at New York University School of Medicine suggests more data is needed about the long-term health impact of marijuana use among seniors. Study participants said they did not perceive the drug as dangerous, a sign of changing attitudes.

The study was based on 47,140 responses collected from the National Survey on Drug Use and Health.

Joseph Palamar, a professor at the NYU medical school and a co-author of the study, said the findings reinforce the need for research and a call for providers to screen the elderly for drug use.

"They shouldn't just assume that someone is not a drug user because they're older," Palamar said.

Growing use of the drug among the 50-and-older crowd reflects the national trend toward pushing cannabis into mainstream culture. Over 22 million people used the drug in 2015, according to the Substance Abuse and Mental Health Services Administration.

Eight states have legalized the drug for recreational use as well as medicinal use, according to Marijuana Policy Project, a non-profit advocacy group dedicated to enacting non-punitive marijuana policies across the United States. The drug has also proved to be a financial boon for state economies, generating over $19 million in September in Colorado.

Researchers also uncovered an increasing diversity in marijuana users. Past-year use doubled among married couples and those earning less than $20,000 per year.

---

*Originally published as Carmen Heredia Rodriguez, "Seniors Increasingly Getting High, Study Shows," *Kaiser Health News*, December 6, 2016. Reprinted with permission of the publisher.

More people living with medical conditions also sought out marijuana. The study showed the number of individuals living with two or more chronic conditions who used the drug over the past year more than doubled. Among those living with depression, the rate also doubled to 11.4 percent.

Palamar says the increase among the sick could be attributed to more individuals seeking to self-medicate. Historically, the plant was difficult to research due to the government crackdown on the substance. The Drug Enforcement Administration classifies the plant as a Schedule I substance, "defined as drugs with no currently accepted medical use and a high potential for abuse."

Benjamin Han, assistant professor at the New York University School of Medicine and the study's lead author, fears that marijuana used with prescription drugs could make the elderly more vulnerable to adverse health outcomes, particularly to falls and cognitive impairment.

"While there may be benefits to using marijuana such as chronic pain," he said, "there may be risks that we don't know about."

The push and pull between state and federal governments has resulted in varying degrees of legality across the United States. Palamar says this variation places populations at risk of unknowingly breaking the law and getting arrested for drug possession. The issue poses one of the biggest public health concerns associated with marijuana, Palamar says.

But unlike the marijuana of their youth, seniors living in states that legalized marijuana for medicinal use now can access a drug that has been tested for quality and purity, said Paul Armentano deputy director of NORML, a non-profit group advocating for marijuana legalization. Additionally, the plant is prescribed to manage diseases that usually strike in older age, pointing to an increasing desire to take a medication that has less side effects than traditional prescription drugs.

The study found over half of the users picked up the habit before turning 18, and over 90 percent of them before age 36.

"We are coming to a point where state lawmakers are responding to the rapidly emerging consensus-both public consensus and a scientific consensus—that marijuana is not an agent that possesses risks that qualifies it as a legally prohibited substance," he said.

Kaiser Health News's coverage of end-of-life and serious illness issues is supported by The Gordon and Betty Moore Foundation.

10. Studies Show Benefits, Downsides of Recreational Marijuana[*]

TED YOAKUM

As Michigan prepares for the changes to its medical marijuana industry—and possible decision to legalize the substance recreationally—parts of the country that have already made the decision to "go green" are raking in green (backs) themselves.

In some cases, they are also paying for it.

In 2012, Washington and Colorado became the first states in the country to legalize recreational use of marijuana, following the passage of ballot initiatives during the general election that year. Two years later, voters in Alaska and Oregon followed suit, and in 2016 another four states—California, Nevada, Maine and Massachusetts—also legalized recreational use of the drug, all through ballot initiatives.

While the marijuana industry is still in the infancy in states that legalized marijuana since 2014, Colorado and Washington have served as a test tube for the effects that a regulated marijuana industry has on its citizens, in terms of financial impact and public safety.

Grass Means Cash

Among the groups eyeing these studies is the National Organization for the Reform of Marijuana Laws, a nonprofit dedicated to marijuana advocacy. The organization, which is headquartered in Washington, D.C., with regional affiliates located across the country, was one of the main groups that spearheaded the push for Amendment 64, the ballot proposal that paved the way for legalization in Colorado.

Although the push for recreational use came to a head with the 2012 initiative, which passed by 11 points, the battle for legalization had raged for years, with sporadic successes and failures at the municipal level in the state, including legalization in Denver in 2005.

For advocates with NORML, the case for allowing open use of the drug hinged on a simple premise, of bringing a trade that has existed for decades from the underground into the light. The goal was to end prohibition-style enforcement of marijuana and instead

---

*Originally published as Ted Yoakum, "Studies Show Benefits, Downsides of Recreational Marijuana," *Niles Daily Star*, July 7, 2017. Reprinted with permission of the publisher.

have governments see it the same way they see alcohol: as a substance only adults may consume and that only licensed businesses may sell to customers.

"This wasn't about allowing a marijuana free-for-all," said Paul Armentano, deputy director with NORML. "It was about regulating a market that already exists. It was about providing oversight to transactions that take place every day and allowing governments to take a chunk of that to put to use for the public good."

So far, bringing marijuana into the daylight appears to be paying off for the citizens of Colorado and Washington—at least in terms of dollars.

Figures from the Colorado Department of Revenue show nearly 500 licensed marijuana retail stores, and hundreds more cultivators, product manufacturers and testing facilities, open in the state as of June 1, 2017. Official figures for Washington are harder to come by, though a list of medically endorsed businesses compiled by the state liquor and cannabis board show a similar number of retail establishments operating in the state.

The public sector has also benefited from the boom in sales, as well.

According to a 2016 study by the Drug Policy Alliance, a nonprofit dedicated to ending the "war on drugs," Colorado has earned $207 million in taxes from marijuana, well in excess of the $140 million the industry was expected to generate. Tax revenue in Washington also shattered initial expectations, bringing in $298 million compared to the projections of $162 million.

The sales taxes are not simply expanding the coffers of the state governments, either. Colorado lawmakers are using the funds to pay for school construction, marijuana enforcement and general state needs, while in Washington leaders are using the money to fund substance abuse prevention and treatment programs, youth and adult drug education, community health care services, and academic research and evaluation the drug is having on Washington residents.

Stickier Issues

When it comes to societal effects of legalization, things become a bit murkier.

Opponents of marijuana legalization who argued that permitting adult use of the substance would lead to increased usage among teenagers will find little data to vindicate these claims, at least when it comes to Colorado and Washington. Recent studies by both governments found that usage rates among adolescents have either remained static or even dipped slightly since marijuana was legalized.

There are some areas where marijuana legalization has caused problems, however.

Overdoses caused by edibles, or marijuana infused food products, became a problem in Colorado during the first few years of recreational use, contributing to the death of several individuals.

However, the state has enacted several changes in recent years to combat the problem, requiring packaging on such products to list its potency and contaminant testing information, as well as warnings to keep them away from children.

Employers in Washington and Colorado have also found it harder to find employees who are able to pass drug screenings, according to a recent study by Quest Diagnostics. Prospective employees in the two states demonstrated the largest growth in failure rates for cannabis from 2015 to 2016, increasing 9 percent and 11 percent, respectively.

Even in terms of financials, the impact of marijuana legalization has not been a complete success.

In spite of promises that legalization would bring an end to the era of back alley dealings, the black market for marijuana continues to thrive. In Colorado, marijuana from the state not only drives illegal sales within its borders but in other states as well. In an interview with a Denver news station this past March, officials with the Denver Police Department said they had arrested 242 people for illegally growing, selling or extracting marijuana in the city, and seized nearly $9,000 worth of the substance last year.

This problem may not be impossible to stamp out, though, Armentano said. Colorado lawmakers have passed legislation to bring the effective tax rate of marijuana sales down from 29 to 27 percent, which will hopefully drive product costs down.

"As prices go down, it will be harder and harder for the black market to compete, and that is a good thing," Armentano said. "No one who supported marijuana regulation expected the black market problem to disappear overnight."

In spite of these thorns, public support for legalization remains strong among the populations of the states, Armentano said. A 2015 poll commissioned by Quinnipiac University found that 58 percent of Colorado voters support continued legalization of marijuana, versus 38 percent against, while a study conducted later that year in Washington found that 58 percent of voters supported legalization compared to 37 percent against.

"Those are the big success stories coming from these states," Armentano said. "We proved we could regulate the marijuana industry and that the sky wouldn't fall, and in fact would be a net gain for the public."

Concerns About the Future

Public support for recreational marijuana is also growing across the U.S. A poll conducted last fall by the Pew Research Center found that 57 percent of citizens support legalization, with 37 percent showing opposition.

In spite of growing popular support, Armentano and others in NORML are not entirely optimistic about the future of legalized pot.

Even in several states where voters have recently passed ballot initiatives approving marijuana, such as Maine and Florida, the actual creation of laws and regulations surrounding marijuana use and sale have stalled in the legislature.

There is also the elephant in the room—the fact that federal laws still forbid the use and sale of marijuana. In spite of the flurry of action at the state level, lawmakers in the nation's capitol have remained static on the issue of legalization, and, with both President Donald Trump and Attorney General Jeff Sessions expressing interest in possibly cracking down on the burgeoning marijuana industry, the problem is likely to get worse before it gets better, Armentano said.

"It's an untenable situation, and it has to rectified," he said.

Voters in Michigan may get the chance to decide themselves whether or not to allow recreational use of marijuana next year, as pro-marijuana advocates are pushing for a ballot proposal to legalize the drug on 2018 general election. The Michigan Board of Canvassers approved a petition from the coalition to place the initiative on the ballot, with volunteers now collecting the mandatory 250,000 signatures needed to solidify its place there next year.

Even if the measure makes the ballot, it will face opposition from many powerful groups in the state—including many in the Michigan law enforcement community.

Among those opposing legalization in the state is Cass County Prosecutor Victor Fitz. A past president of the Michigan Prosecutors Association, the prosecutor remains unconvinced that legalizing marijuana will not adversely affect teenagers and children.

Michigan is already burdened with heavy drug use, especially among youth: the state ranks sixth in the national in terms of overall drug use/addiction, 13th in terms of use on school grounds and 15th in terms of teenage drug abuse. The prosecutor also said that many of the drug cases his office handles involve adults who began using marijuana when they were teenagers.

"It's a quality of life issue," said Cass County Prosecutor Victor Fitz. "Do we want what is best for our kids, or do we chase an illusive dollar that may have a tremendous burden on the taxpayer?"

Fitz also expressed concern about other issues involved with expanding the marijuana industry in Michigan, including the possibility of increased robberies of grow operations or dispensaries.

With law enforcement frequently dealing with problems related to drunk driving and underage sales of alcohol, the last thing police, prosecutors and judges need to worry about is another intoxicant becoming more widely available, Fitz said.

"We already have one vice," Fitz said. "Why do we need a second one as well?"

11. Medical Marijuana Emerges from the Shadows[*]

Kevin Harper

The legal marijuana market is one of the fastest growing industries in the United States.[1] Some 54 California cities and counties have accepted the change in society's view of marijuana and have adopted ordinances allowing medical marijuana dispensaries in their jurisdictions.[2]

If marijuana is fully legalized for recreational sale to adults in 2016 as predicted by some analysts, then more local governments will be considering similar actions. Those localities that allow dispensaries stand to gain substantial tax revenues.

California's 2013 marijuana harvest (legal and illegal), for example, was worth $31 billion.[3] Legal medical marijuana sales in California totaled a little over a billion dollars in 2014.[4] If recreational use of marijuana is legalized, a large portion of the annual marijuana harvest will begin generating tax revenues for the state and for the local jurisdictions that allow dispensaries.

Since marijuana remains illegal under federal law, banks fear being implicated as money launderers, so they frequently decline medical marijuana organizations as customers. This puts retailers' safety at risk and creates problems for the collectives when paying taxes and managing employee payroll.

"The crime potential for an all-cash business, whether that's robbery, burglary or assault—violent crimes—or tax evasion, fraud, and skimming—white-collar crimes—is pretty substantial," observed Colorado Representative Ed Perlmutter.[5]

He added that "It is not fair to small businesses and employees in Colorado, and in 33 other states and the District of Columbia, where some form of marijuana is legal or decriminalized, to be forced out of the banking system and discriminated against by the federal government."[6]

In February 2014, the Obama administration allowed the banking industry to do business with legal marijuana sellers.[7] For the first time, legal distributors can set up checking and savings accounts with major banks.

This lays out a path for bringing marijuana commerce out of the shadows and into the mainstream financial system. Banks, however, remain reluctant because nothing in

*Originally published as Kevin Harper, "Medical Marijuana Emerges from the Shadows," *PM Magazine*, June 15, 2015. Reprinted with permission of the publisher.

the guidance protects a bank from future prosecution if a new administration decides to prosecute state-licensed companies for violating federal drug laws, analysts say.[7]

Case History: Richmond

In 2010, the city council of Richmond, California, amended its municipal code to permit up to three medical marijuana collectives in the city. An ordinance approved by citizens in the November 2, 2010, general election requires that a business license tax be collected. The code requires each dispensary to:

- File an application for a permit and pay a nonrefundable permit processing and notification fee.
- Obtain a seller's permit from the California Board of Equalization.
- Demonstrate evidence of a computerized telephonic system for communicating with other dispensaries in the city to ensure a patient does not receive more than one ounce of marijuana per day.
- Provide for monitoring of the property at all times by closed-circuit television.
- Maintain written accounting of all cash, in-kind contributions, reimbursements, compensation, and expenditures received or paid by the dispensary.
- Maintain inventory records of dates and quantities of marijuana cultivated and stored.
- File quarterly business license tax returns and pay 5 percent of gross revenues to the city.

Three dispensaries began operations in the city during 2012. Gross sales for the three dispensaries in calendar 2013, the first full year of operations, totaled approximately $5 million, with approximately 75 percent being generated by the largest. The three dispensaries paid approximately $250,000 of business license tax to the city for calendar year 2013.

Finance Director James Goins decided an audit of the dispensaries was needed to determine whether they were paying the correct amount of business license taxes. My company was engaged to audit the collectives for the period from their inception to December 31, 2013, and to provide Richmond's finance staff with procedures they could use to conduct a reasonableness test of tax amounts remitted by collectives in future quarters.

Insights from the Audits

Audits of the city's three medical marijuana collectives included:

- Reading the city's ordinances.
- Discussing concerns and issues with city finance and police management.
- Requesting and reviewing documents from the collectives that included:
- Revenue reports showing each revenue transaction, including cash collected, credit received, and in-kind contributions received.

- Inventory record showing dates and quantities of marijuana added to inventory and sold each day.
- California sales tax returns.
- Federal income tax returns.
- Bank statements and related bank reconciliations.
- General ledger reports and profit-and-loss statements.
- Narrative description of procedures followed by the collectives related to collection, billing, depositing, and recording revenue.

Testing the reasonableness of reported gross revenues by:

- Verifying the mathematical accuracy of the business tax returns.
- Tracing reported gross revenue to the collective's general ledger report and profit-and-loss statement.
- Reconciling reported gross revenue to revenue per state sales tax returns and federal income tax returns.
- Selecting a sample of individual revenue transactions, tracing to bank statement, and examining supporting documents.
- Reviewing allowable deductions (cash discounts, volume discounts, promotional discounts, inventory clearance discounts, refunds, federal excise tax, and sales and use tax) for reasonableness.
- Reviewing the cash reconciliations for unusual items, verifying mathematical accuracy, and tracing to bank statements and general ledger reports.

Preparing a report, including procedures performed, schedules of gross revenues and tax collected for each collective, and recommendations for improvement in collective procedures or city procedures.

We noted that most sales of marijuana are cash sales. Because medical marijuana collectives often have difficulty establishing banking relationships, most of the collectives' revenues were not deposited in the bank. This created the unusual auditing issues of being unable to confirm cash balances by reviewing bank records and being unable to compare amounts of revenues and expenditures to bank debits and credits.

The three dispensaries began operations in 2012. Two of them are small businesses and like many of the city's other community-based organizations, did not maintain good accounting and inventory records nor document important procedures.

Examples of missing or inadequate accounting information included:

- Lack of inventory records.
- No list of sales transactions.
- Tardy filing of federal tax returns (by two years).
- No federal income tax returns.

Another audit issue is tied to the confidentiality laws regarding patient names. Depending on how the dispensary maintained its records of sales transactions, patient names needed to be removed from documents before being provided to us.

If there is no other field used to identify an individual patient—a unique patient number—then it's not possible to test whether patients are being sold more than one ounce per day or to ensure receipts relate to the transaction being tested.

We noted that the city did not have adequate procedures in place to test the reasonableness of the quarterly business license taxes that were being collected from the collectives. The city also was not complying with the municipal code related to timing of tax collections and assessing late penalties and interest.

As a result of these issues, we were not able to conclude whether the dispensaries were paying the correct amount of business license taxes. Instead, our audit recommendations focused on the issues the city needed to address in order to adequately oversee the dispensaries going forward, including complying with the code, improving communications with the collectives, and testing the reasonableness of the quarterly taxes remitted.

Substantial Tax Revenues

A growing number of California cities and counties are adopting ordinances allowing medical marijuana dispensaries to operate in their jurisdictions and again, because the market for marijuana is large, the tax revenues that will be generated are expected to be substantial. Those localities that allow marijuana dispensaries need to have procedures in place to assure that they comply with local laws and remit the full amount of business taxes owed.

As local governments begin regulating marijuana dispensaries, and as the federal government allows them to participate in the U.S. banking system, it appears that marijuana operations are emerging from the shadows.

California State Law versus Federal Law

Approved by California voters, Proposition 215—the Compassionate Use Act of 1996—allows seriously ill Californians the right to obtain and use marijuana for medical purposes when it has been recommended by a physician.

The California state legislature passed the Medical Marijuana Program Act in 2004, establishing a voluntary identification card program and a legal framework for collectives and cooperatives to distribute medical marijuana. Each county's health department issues optional identification cards for patients.

These identification cards are issued after the county verifies the cardholder's status as a patient or primary caregiver. The cards offer legal protection from arrest for possession of up to eight ounces of usable marijuana and cultivation of up to six mature or 12 immature plants. Only 2 percent of the approximately 500,000 California patients obtained identification cards in fiscal year 2012–13.[8]

The Medical Marijuana Program Act allows patients to form not-for-profit collectives or cooperatives to cultivate and distribute medical marijuana. These cooperatives and collectives may operate dispensaries that sell to qualified patients.

A cooperative or collective must be a not-for-profit organization and properly organized under state law. It cannot purchase marijuana from or sell to nonmembers, but instead can only provide a means for facilitating transactions between members.

Medical marijuana patients must have a recommendation from a licensed physician. Physicians may not prescribe marijuana because the Food and Drug Administration, which regulates prescription drugs, and federal law—the 1970 Controlled Substances Act

(CSA)—make it unlawful to manufacture, distribute, dispense, or possess any controlled substance.

The CSA identified marijuana as a drug with "no currently accepted medical use." Physicians, however, may issue a verbal or written recommendation under state law indicating that marijuana would be a beneficial treatment for a serious or persistent medical condition.

In 2007, the California Board of Equalization confirmed its policy of taxing medical marijuana transactions, as well as its requirement that businesses engaged in such transactions hold a seller's permit. Sales are taxable even if the seller does not make a profit.[9]

Cities and counties have the authority to adopt local ordinances that ban or regulate the location, operation, or establishment of a medical marijuana cooperative or collective in their jurisdictions.[10]

The incongruity between California state law and federal law has given rise to understandable confusion. Congress has provided that states are free to regulate in the area of controlled substances, provided that state law does not positively conflict with the CSA.

Neither Proposition 215 nor the Medical Marijuana Program Act conflict with the CSA because, in adopting these laws, California did not legalize medical marijuana, but instead exercised the state's right to not punish certain marijuana offenses under state law when a physician has recommended its use to treat a serious medical condition.

NOTES

1. Ferner, Matt. "Legal Marijuana Is the Fastest-Growing Industry in the U.S.: Report." Huffington Post, January 26, 2015, http://www.huffingtonpost.com/2015/01/26/marijuana-industry-fastest-growing_n_6540166.html.

2. "California Local Regulations." Americans for Safe Access, March 1, 2013, http://www.safeaccessnow.org/california_local_regulations.

3. Green, Johnny. "California's 2013 Marijuana Harvest Was Worth 31 Billion Dollars." The Weed Blog, June 11, 2014, http://www.theweedblog.com/californias-2013-marijuana-harvest-was-worth-31-billion-dollars.

4. Platt, John. "Another Cause of California's Drought: Pot Farms." Mother Nature Network, April 7, 2014, http://www.mnn.com/earth-matters/climate-weather/stories/another-cause-of-californias-drought-pot-farms.

5. Ferner, Matt. "House Votes to Allow Banking Access for Marijuana Businesses." Huffington Post, July 16, 2014, http://www.huffingtonpost.com/2014/07/16/house-marijuana-banking_n_5592620.html.

6. Migoya, David. "U.S. House OKs Bill That May Open Door to Bank Accounts for Pot Shops." Denver Post, July 17, 2014, http://www.denverpost.com/business/ci_26160270/house-oks-bill-stop-feds-from-using-cash.

7. Douglas, Danielle. "Obama Administration Clears Banks to Accept Funds from Legal Marijuana Dealers." Washington Post, February 14, 2014, http://www.washingtonpost.com/business/economy/obama-administration-clears-banks-to-accept-funds-from-legal-marijuana-dealers/2014/02/14/55127b04–9599–11e3–9616-d367fa6ea99b_story.html.

8. "State Medical Marijuana Programs' Financial Information." Marijuana Policy Project, October 18, 2013, http://www.mpp.org/assets/pdfs/library/State-Medical-Marijuana-Programs-Financial-Information.pdf.

9. Guidelines for the Security and Non-Diversion of Marijuana Grown for Medical Use, published August 2008 by the California Department of Justice.

10. California Assembly Bill 1300, Date of Hearing April 26, 2011.

12. Options and Issues Regarding Marijuana Legalization in Vermont[*]

Beau Kilmer

Legalizing recreational marijuana production, distribution and possession in Vermont could generate significant tax revenues, but also involves costs and important decisions about how best to regulate the substance, according to a new RAND Corporation study.

The report makes clear that if Vermont chooses to remove its prohibition on producing and selling marijuana, lawmakers will have many choices to make about who will supply it, who can buy it, if and how it will be taxed, and how it will be regulated.

The report does not make a recommendation about whether Vermont should change its marijuana laws. Researchers say the goal of the report is to inform, not sway, discussions about the future of marijuana policy in Vermont and other jurisdictions considering alternatives to traditional marijuana prohibition.

The RAND report provides the most-detailed accounting available about the wide number of issues that face state officials—in Vermont and elsewhere—when considering alternatives to traditional marijuana prohibition.

"Our conversation about whether to legalize marijuana must be rooted in facts and be transparent about the uncertainties. This RAND report will serve as a critical foundation for our ongoing discussion about the best course for Vermont," said Vermont Gov. Peter Shumlin. "I continue to support moves to legalize marijuana in Vermont but have always said that we have to proceed with rigorous research and preparation before deciding whether to act. This report will help us do that."

In May 2014, Shumlin signed Act 155 that required the state's secretary of administration to produce a report about the various benefits and consequences of legalizing marijuana. The RAND report was produced for the administration in response to that legislation.

The study examines several supply models that Vermont lawmakers may wish to explore—from permitting those aged 21 and older to grow marijuana for their own use

---

[*]Originally published as Beau Kilmer, "Options and Issues Regarding Marijuana Legalization in Vermont," RAND Corporation, https://www.rand.org/news/press/2015/01/16.html. Reprinted with permission of the publisher.

53

to regulating supply through nonprofit or for-profit corporations, or through a governmental entity. The report also profiles numerous marijuana regulations that could be imposed, such as a THC ceiling on products, a ban on fruit flavors and marijuana-infused candies, mandatory child-resistant packaging, age restrictions on sellers and purchasers, price floors, and a ban on self-service displays, among others.

"It is a false dichotomy to think about marijuana policy in terms of choosing either prohibition or the for-profit commercial model we see in Colorado and Washington," said Beau Kilmer, project leader and co-director of RAND's Drug Policy Research Center. "Jurisdictions considering alternatives to prohibition could limit supply to home production, cooperatives, nonprofit organizations, socially responsible businesses, a public authority or even a state monopoly."

The report estimates that during 2014, Vermont residents likely consumed between 15 metric tons and 25 metric tons of marijuana, and spent between $125 million and $225 million on marijuana. RAND researchers estimate that state and local governments in Vermont now spend less than $1 million each year enforcing current marijuana laws on those aged 21 and older, while regulatory costs associated with legalizing production and retail sales of marijuana would likely exceed that level.

If Vermont legalized marijuana, taxed the product aggressively, suppressed its black market, and consumption increased, tax revenues from sales to Vermont residents could be in the tens of millions of dollars annually, according to the report.

In addition to impacts in the state, legalizing marijuana in Vermont also could have implications for neighboring states. There are nearly 40 times as many regular marijuana users living within 200 miles outside of Vermont's borders as there are living inside Vermont, according to the report.

Vermont could therefore end up supplying large numbers of out-of-state users, directly via tourism or indirectly. This would vastly increase the potential revenue to the state, unless other states in the Northeast also legalized marijuana, researchers say. At that point, the flow of revenue to Vermont from marijuana legalization would depend on whether surrounding states imposed lower taxes, which would not only cut the revenue from out-of-state visitors but also undermine revenues from taxing Vermont's own residents.

The report also warns that cross-border commerce could prompt a federal government response, making all revenue projections highly uncertain.

The report reviews evidence on the public health consequences of marijuana consumption and prohibition, including both the harms and the benefits. The scientific literature identifies some clear acute and chronic health effects, especially of persistent heavy marijuana use. Acute risks include accidents, impaired cognitive functioning while intoxicated, as well as anxiety, dysphoria and panic.

"There are pros and cons to all marijuana policy options, and there is tremendous uncertainty about how different forms of legalization will affect public health and safety," said Jonathan Caulkins, a report coauthor and the Stever Professor of Operations Research and Public Policy at Carnegie Mellon University. "Much will depend on how any marijuana policy change influences the use of other substances such as tobacco, alcohol and prescription opiates."

Longer-term risks of persistent heavy marijuana use include dependence and bronchitis. Some evidence suggests other serious risks for heavy marijuana users, particularly with psychotic symptoms, cardiovascular disease and male testicular cancers.

"While marijuana use is strongly correlated with many adverse outcomes, it is much harder to ascertain whether marijuana use causes those outcomes," said Robert MacCoun, a report coauthor and a professor at Stanford School of Law.

For example, with respect to the ongoing debate about whether marijuana use has long-term effects on intelligence quotient, MacCoun said it is premature to argue that long-term cognitive impairment has been clearly established, but just as premature to argue that the risks are nonexistent.

RAND's study was supported by the State of Vermont and by Good Ventures, a philanthropic foundation that makes grants in consultation with GiveWell, an organization that researches charities and advises donors.

Other authors of the report include Mark Kleiman of UCLA and BOTEC Analysis Corporation, Gregory Midgette and Rosalie Liccardo Pacula of RAND, Pat Oglesby of the Center for New Revenue, and Peter Reuter of the University of Maryland.

The report, "Considering Marijuana Legalization: Insights for Vermont and Other Jurisdictions," is available at www.rand.org.

Since 1989, the RAND Drug Policy Research Center has conducted research to help policymakers in the United States and throughout the world address issues involving alcohol and other drugs. In doing so, the center brings an objective and data-driven perspective to an often emotional and fractious policy arena.

13. Where Will Legal Marijuana Industry STASH Its CASH?*

GORDON OLIVER

Washington's legalized marijuana industry may quickly become a cash cow for many of its first-generation entrepreneurs. But those fledgling business owners face a unique challenge: when the cash starts flowing, they'll have no place to put it.

In one of the most tangled conflicts between state and federal laws over marijuana, the federal government's rules intended to ban banking by the illegal drug industry are trumping voter-approved legalization of marijuana in Washington and Colorado. So far, no Washington bank is willing to navigate through a gray area of federal policies and laws to offer banking services to marijuana growers, distributors, and retailers. Just two credit unions, Numerica in Spokane and Salal in Seattle, say they'll take marijuana business operators as members. But both of those credit unions say they'll serve only growers and distributors, avoiding retailers whose sales to minors or to out-of-state residents could put the credit unions at risk.

"Retailers are in a difficult situation," said Russ Rosendal, Salal's president and chief executive officer. "Hopefully someone will take those retailers on."

The risk of a large cache of cash stashed away in homes and businesses, with financial transactions carried out using money orders or cash, raises major safety concerns in both states. One winner of the state lottery to open a marijuana retail store in Vancouver says he feels like he'll have "a target on my back" in the absence of a place to secure his money. Among his ideas is to move into a gated apartment complex for added personal safety, said the man, who requested anonymity out of concern for his security.

Brian Stroh, whose CannaMan Farms in Orchards is a state-licensed marijuana-growing operation, says safe money management will be his top priority as retail stores open and he begins selling his product to them. Stroh, a former mortgage lending officer, won't reveal his money management plan. But the absence of a safe depository for money is "the piece that's going to get somebody killed," he worries. "You don't have that in your job description."

Bankers say numerous interconnected federal laws prohibiting banking in the illegal drug trade are quite clear, and that the Obama administration's efforts to find a middle

---

*Originally published as Gordon Oliver, "Where Will Legal Marijuana Industry STASH Its CASH?," *The Columbian*, June 8, 2014. Reprinted with permission of the publisher.

ground don't protect banks from federal prosecution. The Department of Justice issued a memo last summer as "a guide to the exercise of investigative and prosecutorial discretion" in the two states that have legalized marijuana. But the memo, written by Deputy Attorney General James M. Cole, reaffirms the federal government's authority to enforce federal drug laws related to banking regardless of state law, and notes that neither the memo nor state laws can be used in a legal defense against federal prosecution.

"The risk of prosecution is still there," said Jenifer Waller, senior vice president of the Colorado Bankers Association.

In the absence of a change in federal law, then, no commercial banks in Washington or Colorado are willing to take their chances.

"It's kind of a risk-reward analysis, and the risk outweighs the reward," said James Pishue, president and CEO of the Washington Bankers Association.

It's not as if bankers and regulators couldn't see this coming. Medical marijuana is now legal in 22 states and the District of Columbia, and banks have no legal protection in providing financial services to medical marijuana providers. "It's no secret that people in the medical marijuana field have been robbed quite often," said Scott Jarvis, director of Washington's Department of Financial Institutions.

Last month, Gov. Jay Inslee and Colorado Gov. John W. Hickenlooper wrote to top federal regulators including Federal Reserve Chair Janet Yellen to request further clarification of federal instructions to bank and credit union examiners regarding banking issues for the recreational marijuana industry. Jarvis hopes that the top regulators, who guide the Federal Crimes Enforcement Network, will address the issue soon.

"We're trying to make it work," Jarvis said of the banking conundrum. "Security is very much on our mind and on the governor's mind."

"Violates Banks' DNA"

A web of rules aim to curtail drug trafficking through the banking system by, among other measures, requiring banks to report large cash transactions and by prohibiting the use of electronic fund transfers for money derived from drug sales.

David Bristol, an attorney at the Vancouver office of Schwabe, Williamson & Wyatt who was chief legal officer for the former First Independent Bank, says bankers' wariness is based in part on the industry's culture. Taking money from people involved in drug dealing that's illegal under federal law "just violates banks' DNA," he said. "Banks have always helped government monitor illegal activity."

Unpleasant memories of the banking industry's recent history with federal regulators also contribute to banks' risk-averse approach to dealing with the marijuana trade, Bristol believes. In the boom years of 2004–2006 leading up to the devastating crash of the nation's financial system, regulators regularly praised bankers for their role in fueling the economy. But when the crash came, that praise turned to criticism.

"Regulators became unpredictable," said Bristol, who helped First Independent recover from a weak financial position before its owners sold to Sterling Bank in 2012. Bankers are now wondering, he says, "should we trust our regulators' words now that they are not going to give us a black eye five years from now?"

Even setting aside the legal issues, the marijuana industry is not a sure-fire sugar daddy for Washington banks, Bristol said. Given today's low interest rates, banks don't make much money on deposits. While marijuana production, distribution, and sales will require short-term funding to even out cash flow, the industry does not require the major capital investments that translate into profitable bank loans, he added.

"It's unclear how banks are going to make money," he said.

Still, Bristol found in his own informal survey that local banking officials are not driven by their own personal or ethical concerns about marijuana legalization, and most would be ready to do business with the industry if legal issues can be resolved.

"Most don't have a moral issue with it, but nobody wants to be first because of the reputational risk," he said.

Credit unions, also federally regulated, face the same legal obstacles as banks. But they are beholden to their members and therefore not beholden to investors. That makes some more willing to take risks, as long as they have support of their members and the board that represents them and can cover costs with appropriate fees.

So far, two Washington credit unions say they're willing to fill part of the void. Salal, with branches in King, Pierce and Snohomish counties, has its origins as a credit union for employees of Seattle health care giant Group Health. "We believe there are clear health benefits around (treating) certain diseases with marijuana," said Rosendal, the credit union's president and CEO.

He noted the credit union's concern for public safety, adding "it's our philosophy to help those individuals banks won't help." Rosendal said the credit union is open to the idea of extending its services to the industry in Western Washington counties outside its core service area.

Spokane-based Numerica credit union says it will also limit its services to growers and distributors, avoiding retailers because of the difficulty of tracking their sales practices. It will offer banking only within its service area, which includes Wenatchee and the Tri-Cities.

"It all comes down to community safety," said credit union spokeswoman Kelli Hawkins. "We feel there's a hazard to the community with all that cash."

In Vancouver, Columbia Credit Union CEO Steve Kenny says his board has discussed the issue and so far is not ready to serve the marijuana industry.

"I have to ask the question: Does it bring value to our members at Columbia Credit Union?" said Kenny. But on the other side, he said the credit union is open to finding a way to serve the industry. "It is a legal business and we do not turn away legal businesses," he said.

An Act of Congress

An industry that deals in cash and money orders, but is obligated to meet state rules and make state tax payments, does not seem sustainable. But with retail sales set to begin as early as next month, no one has a solution to avoid an ugly and dangerous financial mess in the great experiment of marijuana legalization.

"It's going around in a circle and everybody's pointing to the person on the right," said Kenny.

Colorado's Legislature has approved an interim approach of creating what is an uninsured marijuana co-op that would provide money management until federal regulatory issues could be resolved. But the money management system requires Federal

Reserve approval. Such approval seems unlikely, given the Fed's rules, said Waller of the Colorado Bankers Association, since "dealing with an illegal substance is not permissible activity."

That moves the conversation into what is a common cliché: it will take an act of Congress to fix this problem. "We need to get this thing moving at the federal level, because that's where the action is," said Pishue, of the Washington Bankers Association.

U.S. Rep. Denny Heck, a Democrat whose district covers most of Pierce and Thurston counties, is backing a bill sponsored by Rep. Ed Perlmutter, a Colorado Democrat, that would prevent bank regulators from prohibiting or taking action against state-licensed marijuana businesses.

That bill would also provide immunity from federal prosecution or investigation against an institution or its employees based only on their provision of services to those businesses.

Banking associations in both Colorado and Washington favor the bill as a starting point for political action. But with only two states facing the problem, the bill so far has drawn little attention in the House.

Some see hope in an unexpected political movement last month on the equally troubling issue of banking in the medical marijuana industry. The House last month approved a little-noticed amendment to a low-profile bill to restrict the Drug Enforcement Administration from targeting medical marijuana operations in states where it is legal. That measure won support from 49 Republicans, including Washington's Doc Hastings of Pasco, but still faces several procedural hurdles before it can be ratified.

Bristol, the Vancouver attorney, says that in the present void marijuana entrepreneurs will need to prepare for a potentially dangerous situation.

"My recommendation to a retailer in particular is that they have lots of cameras, a panic button to close things down, and that they use an armored car system," Bristol said.

But when asked where the armored car would take the money, Bristol said he simply doesn't know.

14. Why Legal Marijuana Businesses Are Still Cash-Only*

Sophie Quinton

Tim Cullen's marijuana business brought in millions of dollars last year, but he's had a hard time finding a bank to take the money. He's cycled through 14 checking accounts in six years. Recently, he said, a bank shut down all his personal accounts, including college savings for his 3-year-old daughter.

Federal law prohibits banks and credit unions from taking marijuana money. So here in Colorado, everyone involved with the state's legal cannabis industry has a banking problem. Businesses can't get loans, customers have to pay in cash, and state tax collectors are processing bags of bills.

Some community financial institutions have become more open to serving the cannabis industry since the U.S. Treasury and Justice Departments said they won't go after institutions that keep a close eye on their clients and report suspected wrongdoing, such as funding gang activity.

But the big banks refuse to touch the industry, and banking challenges are only going to grow as legal marijuana expands. Nationwide, sales hit $5.4 billion in 2015, according to The ArcView Group, an analysis and investment firm that specializes in the legal cannabis industry.

Twenty-three states allow medical use of marijuana and four also allow recreational use. Voters in Arizona, California, Massachusetts and Nevada may legalize adult use this fall, and Vermont's Senate recently approved a bill that would do so.

States are looking to Colorado—which legalized medical marijuana in 2000, and adult use in 2012—for answers to the banking problem, but the state has few to offer. "We don't truly think we'll see a solution unless there's a federal solution," said Andrew Freedman, Colorado's director of marijuana coordination, who's also known as the state's pot czar.

An Unbanked Industry

Cullen has been an unofficial spokesman for Colorado's cannabis industry ever since he bumped into a CNN camera crew while picking up one of the state's first retail mar-

---

*Originally published as Sophie Quinton, "Why Legal Marijuana Businesses Are Still Cash-Only," *Stateline*, March 22, 2016. Reprinted with permission of the publisher. © The Pew Charitable Trusts.

ijuana licenses, he said. It helps that he's a clean-cut former high school biology teacher who designed his stores with his mom in mind.

"We wanted to look like Restoration Hardware," he said while walking through the main Denver location of Colorado Harvest Company, the marijuana growing and retail business he founded in 2009 and co-owns. That means wood paneling, edibles laid out in glass cases like chocolates, and a scent in the air that's more reminiscent of a day spa than a college dorm.

But even Cullen's squeaky-clean operation makes banks uneasy. The company's current account, with a credit union, only covers basic services such as direct deposit for the company's 70-odd employees and sending tax payments to the state, Cullen said.

An ATM sits in the corner of each of his three stores, because his business can't process credit or debit card payments (credit card companies, like banks, may refuse to touch marijuana money). Every day an armored car swings by to pick up the day's revenue—all cash—and takes it away to be deposited.

About 40 percent of Colorado cannabis businesses lack bank accounts altogether, according to the office of U.S. Rep. Ed Perlmutter, a Democrat who has pushed to improve banking for the cannabis industry. State officials would not comment on that number.

Freedman said a growing number of marijuana businesses seem to be obtaining bank accounts, judging by the declining share of tax revenue that businesses are paying in cash. But the services they're able to access are limited and costly—"which means a lot of people prefer to keep as much as they can in cash," he said.

All the cash floating around makes cannabis businesses targets for crime, Freedman says. Since Colorado fully legalized marijuana in January 2014, the Denver Police Department has logged over 200 burglaries at marijuana businesses, as well as shoplifting and other crimes.

The loose cash also makes it harder for the state to track businesses' finances to make sure they are obeying the law and paying their taxes. And in order to get a bank account, some businesses will funnel their cash through a shell company, Cullen said. "It starts to look a lot like money laundering."

As Cullen's experience shows, accounts can also be tenuous. Sometimes, a financial institution will change its mind about taking marijuana money. Or it might learn of a client's ties to the marijuana industry. Mark Goldfogel, a consultant, said his bank closed accounts he'd held for 14 years after he revealed who his marijuana clients were.

Not Much States Can Do

Colorado's attempts to solve the problem have shown other states how few options they have.

In May 2014, lawmakers authorized a new class of financial institution called a cannabis credit co-operative, which wouldn't have to acquire and maintain deposit insurance. But no such institutions have been formed so far, partly because the Federal Reserve isn't likely to approve them.

Later that year, lawmakers authorized a credit union for the cannabis industry. But the Fed denied the credit union access to a master account, which is necessary for transferring money, and the National Credit Union Administration refused to insure its deposits.

"Even transporting or transmitting funds known to have been derived from the distribution of marijuana is illegal," the Federal Reserve Bank of Kansas City said during a court case the credit union brought and recently lost.

Without a master account, the credit union can't fully function, said Mike Elliott, head of the Marijuana Industry Group, a trade association in Colorado. "It can be a vault. But we don't need a vault," he said.

Officials in other states that allow marijuana have run up against the same barriers. Tax officials in California have floated the idea of a state-run bank, for instance, as have officials in Alaska. But such an institution would still have to use federal wiring services, said George Runner of the California State Board of Equalization.

California already has trouble collecting taxes on medical marijuana, Runner said. "We've had folks come in with hundreds of thousands of dollars" in cash to make a payment. Other than increasing security at tax collection offices, there's not much his office can do about it.

The cannabis industry's banking problems would vanish if Congress were to take marijuana off the federal government's list of most dangerous drugs. Last November, U.S. Sen. Bernie Sanders of Vermont, who is running for the Democratic presidential nomination, became the latest lawmaker to propose the change.

But that's a remote possibility. Perlmutter has introduced a bill—twice—that would take a smaller step, and stop federal regulators from penalizing financial institutions for serving the cannabis industry. He hasn't been able to get a hearing, let alone move the bill out of committee.

Perlmutter and his allies in Congress are now trying to cut off funding for federal enforcement actions against banks and credit unions that serve cannabis businesses.

Finding a Way

The Fed and other regulatory agencies have made it clear that states can't create new financial institutions for the cannabis industry. But because the Obama administration has indicated that it will look the other way when existing institutions serve cannabis clients, businesses like Cullen's do have some options.

Vermont's Department of Financial Regulation has researched the services available to the state's four medical marijuana dispensaries and found some good news. The state's largest credit union serves one dispensary and says it would serve more. Although the credit union doesn't offer marijuana businesses much more than depository accounts, federal regulators confirmed the accounts are insured.

Vermont state Sen. Joe Benning, a Republican who co-sponsored the Senate proposal to legalize marijuana for adult use, said the state's financial institutions should be able to handle the cannabis industry's expansion—at least initially. "You're not going to have to be bringing in wheelbarrows full of cash to make deposits," he said.

In other states, new services have emerged to eliminate cash transactions. In Washington and Oregon, an intermediary company called PayQwick electronically transfers money between marijuana growers, sellers, customers and their financial institutions. PayQwick also files all the paperwork the Treasury Department requires, taking a burden off banks.

Tax collection offices are doing what they can to manage cash collections. Offices in Oregon and Colorado have invested in extra security, such as safety glass and security cameras; businesses are also hiring security guards to help them make their deposits safely.

Auditing cash-only cannabis businesses is tough, but not impossible. In Colorado, the Department of Revenue relies on the state's system for tracking legally grown and sold marijuana plants, Freedman said.

Still, the situation is far from ideal for businesses or for states. It's temporary, too; nobody knows how the next president will enforce federal marijuana policies.

While Colorado waits for Congress to act, state officials will keep meeting with bank and credit union boards and explaining the nuances of federal law, Freedman said. That slow, institution-by-institution campaign may be states' best hope for getting marijuana money off the streets.

"I think it's going to get better. It certainly couldn't be worse," Cullen said of the cannabis industry's banking problem. He takes the sunny view that as more states legalize the drug, it will become something federal lawmakers will no longer be able to ignore.

15. For This Pot Guy, States Are His Biggest Customers[*]

J.B. WOGAN

It's a Wednesday morning in June and Andrew Freedman is taking another meeting. For once, it's at his home office in Denver. Since February, work has taken him to Boston; Chicago; Oakland, Calif.; Sacramento, Calif.; Tallahassee, Fla.; New York City; and Washington, D.C. Like every meeting for Freedman these days, this one's about marijuana.

For nearly three years, Freedman worked for Colorado as the world's first and only state marijuana czar, a temporary position created to help Colorado implement regulations around medical and recreational marijuana. Now he's taking what he learned from that experience and using it for a new consulting business.

The office of Freedman & Koski is a condo in a converted church near Denver's Five Points neighborhood. The conference room doubles as Freedman's living room, which is also his dining room. It has a giant stained-glass window. Freedman has been pining for a whiteboard where he and his business partner, Lewis Koski, can conduct their weekly strategy meetings, but there isn't a practical place to put one.

The first meeting of the day is with a potential client, David Sutton, who is developing a new line of medical marijuana products for temporary pain relief. Sutton hopes Freedman will join his company's board of directors. They both grew up in Denver and know each other from elementary school, but only reconnected recently. Sutton is pulling demo products from his bag and explaining to Koski how customers would apply a THC-infused lotion on the skin. "It doesn't get you high. It's relaxing when you put it on a pulse point," Sutton says. "I don't know if you have any pain where you can…"

"No, thank you," Koski interrupts, shifting uncomfortably in his chair. He smiles. It's a friendly but stern rejection. He doesn't try marijuana products.

Koski is the former director of the marijuana enforcement division within the Colorado Department of Revenue. Before he was a regulator, he was a police officer in suburban Arvada, northwest of Denver. Although he and Freedman helped make legal marijuana a reality in Colorado, they are not advocates for legalization and, as a rule, do not take clients who make money from growing or selling marijuana. Ask about their personal experience with the drug, and they decline to comment. They won't even disclose

---

*Originally published as J.B. Wogan, "For This Pot Guy, States Are His Biggest Customers," *Governing*, August 2017. Reprinted with permission of the publisher.

how they voted on Amendment 64, the ballot measure that brought legalized recreational marijuana to Colorado in 2012. "Not even my wife knows," Koski says.

Since legalization in 2012, Colorado has licensed nearly 700 marijuana cultivation facilities.

After the meeting, Freedman and Koski agree that they can't take Sutton on as a client. "With opportunities like that, we've probably turned down a lot of work," Koski says. Though they market themselves as experts in marijuana policy, they want to maintain a regulator's distance from the industry itself. "We're a good-government company," Koski explains. "We want to do everything we can to protect public health and public safety with the cards we're dealt."

Freedman is quick to point out that they aren't lobbyists, and none of the three founding partners (the third is John Hudak, an academic researcher at the Brookings Institution) has taken a public position for or against legalization. But once voters have decided to legalize marijuana, Freedman says, "we're the technocrats who make it happen."

There's increasing demand for that kind of technocratic expertise. Support for legalizing both medical and recreational marijuana has increased over the past two decades. National polling from Gallup shows that 60 percent of Americans now think the use of marijuana should be made legal, up from 25 percent in the mid–1990s. In the past five years, voters in Alaska, California, Colorado, Maine, Massachusetts, Nevada, Oregon and Washington state have approved the legalization of marijuana for recreational purposes, with a retail market that is—or soon will be—taxed and regulated. Twenty-seven states and the District of Columbia also allow for state-regulated dispensaries of medical marijuana. An estimated 65 million Americans, about one-fifth of the country's population, now live in states with some form of legalization. With the likely expansion of it in more states, annual marijuana sales in North America are projected to grow from $6.7 billion last year to more than $20 billion by 2021.

But this is also a period of uncertainty for the marijuana industry. Under the Obama administration, the U.S. Department of Justice signaled that it wouldn't use its limited resources to prosecute people and businesses that complied with state marijuana laws, so long as they met certain federal criteria such as keeping marijuana out of the hands of minors. But President Trump's administration has cast doubt on whether the federal government will maintain its hands-off approach. As a candidate, Trump sent mixed messages about his position on legal marijuana, calling it "bad" but also suggesting it was an issue best left up to states. Trump's attorney general, Jeff Sessions, is a longtime critic of states that legalized marijuana. In February, White House spokesman Sean Spicer told reporters to expect ramped up enforcement of federal marijuana laws.

Meanwhile, in states where marijuana ballot measures have already passed, many governors and their counterparts at the local level are becoming the reluctant stewards of a policy they once opposed. But after voters approve a marijuana measure, officials look for advice from the few places with some experience in taxing and regulating legal marijuana. Colorado Gov. John Hickenlooper says his office has fielded calls from more than 25 states asking for guidance. When he read Freedman's pitch for a consulting firm aimed at meeting that demand, Hickenlooper encouraged him to pursue the idea. "This is going to be one of the great social experiments of the 21st century, and it's going to require taking all of the experience and the knowledge that we create, and building upon that," he says. Citing Freedman's prior role as a convener across agencies and businesses, and among legislators and other outside interest groups, Hickenlooper says Freedman is uniquely suited to provide insights about the implementation details. "His understanding of the process and how it works would be invaluable to other states."

Freedman and Koski launched their consulting firm in January.

Freedman, 34, hadn't planned on becoming the world's first marijuana czar. About seven years ago, he graduated from Harvard Law School and had a job lined up with a private law firm in Washington, D.C. But the job didn't start right away, so Freedman was toying with the idea of spending those few months learning to surf in Australia. The year after undergrad, he had managed to pack in a lot: teaching English in India, working at a peace camp in Israel and volunteering at a women's rights center in Thailand. But his older brother talked him out of embarking on yet another international adventure and persuaded him to instead work on Hickenlooper's first campaign for governor.

Following the gubernatorial race, he became chief of staff for then–Lt. Gov. Joseph Garcia before spearheading an ill-fated ballot measure that sought to raise billions in new tax dollars for public education. Despite several years in state government, Freedman was a novice on marijuana policy when Hickenlooper's chief of staff recruited him to be the director of marijuana coordination. He was so unfamiliar with the industry that he hadn't been to a grow facility until he visited one on the job. In a way, that lack of experience was an asset. The governor's chief of staff told Freedman the state needed someone who was seen as neutral on the question of legalization.

Though Freedman's official title was never "marijuana czar," the term quickly became shorthand for what he did. In one TV interview, a local anchor pushed Freedman on the term. "We are working very hard not to be called that," Freedman said, in a futile effort to distance himself from the title. As he sees it, policy czars, as a rule, lack authority. And drug czars in particular are meant to be adversaries of illicit substance use. By contrast, Freedman did have authority—he spoke for the governor—and he didn't see himself as an antagonist to the marijuana industry. His role was to help in setting up rules for legitimate businesses and customers to safely use a legal product. The anchor called him the pot czar anyway, and it stuck.

The title may help Freedman and Koski market their new business. While other states have tapped someone to oversee marijuana regulation and enforcement, Colorado is the only one to have created a special position in the governor's office for coordinating policy across executive agencies and the legislature. Freedman will also go down as the last marijuana czar in Colorado. Because most of the initial implementation details have been settled, Hickenlooper, with Freedman's support, asked the legislature to sunset the czar position in June.

Although states have plenty of pro- and anti-legalization advocates, not many people can claim firsthand experience in developing and implementing policy. In addition to their insights from Colorado's rollout, Freedman and Koski also draw from the expertise of Hudak, their third founding partner, who recently published a book on the history of marijuana policy. As a result, in their first five months of business they have already won contracts with Florida, Los Angeles County and Ohio.

Public officials will be hungry for advice, says Beau Kilmer, a drug policy researcher with the RAND Corp., because there isn't a playbook for overseeing a legal marijuana retail market. Early adopters are still learning from their own experiences. "We still don't know the best way to regulate and tax marijuana," he says. In 2015, Kilmer co-authored a report for the state of Vermont on the potential benefits and costs of legalizing marijuana, illustrating the many paths that the state could take and the tradeoffs officials will need to consider. For example, some states may decide to prioritize the elimination of a black market, with looser regulations and fewer protections for public health; others may choose heavier taxes and regulations in an effort to protect public health. "So much comes down to your personal values," Kilmer says, "and your preferences for risk."

Whatever choices state and local governments make, they'll want expert counsel in thinking through competing interests, and he predicts an increasing number of private firms will try to provide those services. "It's a growing industry," Kilmer says. "No pun intended."

Colorado pot regulations require licensed businesses to track every plant from seed to sale with tags and bar codes.

Although officials undoubtedly will try to emulate what worked in Colorado, the consulting business also gives Freedman an opportunity to address misgivings he has about how his own state handled the marijuana rollout. He can fix what he saw as loopholes, and apply some lessons learned.

For example, in the first year of legalization in Colorado, customers—especially out-of-state tourists and first-time users—didn't have enough guidance on recreational products. Children and adults alike were ending up in the emergency room after consuming unsafe concentrations of THC. One visiting college student from Wyoming jumped out of his hotel room after consuming some especially potent pot cookies. *New York Times* columnist Maureen Dowd highlighted the plight of uninformed consumers when she wrote about her own experience underestimating the potency of edibles.

Over time, the legislature made tweaks in the law to address some early oversights. Packaging for marijuana products now must have a universal "THC" diamond symbol, along with a warning that the edibles are for adults over 21 years old and should be kept out of children's reach. In an effort to make edible gummies look less like candy for children, the state has banned gummies in the shape of a fruit, animal or human. Chocolate bars now have to be divided in to squares with equal doses of 10 milligrams of THC, an amount that's considered safe to consume in one sitting.

Freedman also would have liked to see the state put in place public information and youth prevention campaigns before retail stores opened. Today, the state Department of Transportation runs television ads urging residents not to drive while high. Giant billboards warn against using marijuana while pregnant or during breastfeeding. But the state didn't launch those public health and safety campaigns until they could be funded with revenues from retail marijuana sales. That meant residents were buying legal marijuana for eight months before the earmarked money was available for public awareness campaigns.

Another insight from the Colorado experience is that states need to collect better baseline data. For the most part, Colorado officials don't have precise information about how expanded access to legal marijuana has affected the health and safety of residents. For example, before legalization the state didn't require schools to document when they suspended students for marijuana use; instead, the older data only show that suspensions were related to some kind of drug use. When the state examined last year's newer, more precise data, they discovered that roughly two-thirds of student drug suspensions involved marijuana. While they can monitor marijuana suspensions going forward, they'll never know if an increase occurred because of legalization.

The state faces similar problems in measuring the impact of the policy on driving under the influence of marijuana. Before legalization, Colorado didn't have statewide standards for what constituted driving while high. Now the standard is set at five nanograms of active THC per milliliter of blood. Law enforcement has also received training on identifying and charging impaired drivers, so it's likely that the marijuana DUI arrests have gone up. But it's difficult to know how much.

States seem likely to accept most of these good-government recommendations, but Freedman does have at least one controversial idea he's floating with his government clients: He doesn't think surplus revenue from marijuana sales ought to fund schools. In Colorado, the constitutional amendment legalizing recreational marijuana set aside roughly $40 million a year for public school construction projects around the state. That may sound like a lot of money, but it's dwarfed by the current demand for school infrastructure funding in the state, which is roughly $2.8 billion. Freedman worries that the average voter in Colorado is now reluctant to approve funding increases for education because the linking of marijuana revenue to education was so well publicized. "I think that it sets education back," he says. "They're more likely to believe marijuana can save education, and it can't."

States would be better off, he says, using marijuana tax revenues in areas that might see a bigger return on investment. Before he left his job with the state, Freedman helped pitch the Colorado Legislature on the idea that surplus marijuana revenue—in addition to the money already going to school construction—ought to support affordable housing for the homeless. The result was roughly $15 million next year for housing and support services.

There was one last loophole in Colorado's marijuana laws that Freedman wanted to address before he stepped down from his post. The state already had strict regulations for licensed businesses selling marijuana, but it also allowed people to grow up to 99 plants for personal use, so long as they had a note from their doctor. The law allowed people to ask others to assist in growing marijuana plants for medical purposes. No other state allows caregivers or patients to grow more than 16 plants at home. The fact that Colorado had much looser regulations around homegrown medical marijuana had an unintended consequence: Organized crime syndicates were growing large amounts of marijuana in their backyards and then shipping it out of Colorado to sell in other states. Freedman saw it as the Achilles' heel of the state's regulatory system, and he spent the better part of three years working with law enforcement, legislators, marijuana lobbyists, patients and caregivers to address it.

Four separate attempts to close the loophole through legislation had failed. Patients and caregivers had fought any regulations that impeded their legitimate use of homegrown medical marijuana. "It had become my white whale," Freedman says.

Though Freedman officially launched his firm this January, he stayed on with the governor's office for four months on a part-time basis to usher through one last set of bills that might finally address the gray market. Legislators took up the bills in March, and passed them unanimously. The new laws limit the number of homegrown plants to 12, down from 99, but patients and caregivers can appeal to their local governments to receive individual exemptions. The legislature also allocated $6 million a year in grant funds for local law enforcement to find and shut down illegal grow operations.

At the bill signing in June, marijuana business owners, public health advocates, police, patients and caregivers all came to celebrate. It was a diverse set of groups who often lobbied on opposite sides of an issue. As people gathered, Freedman circled the room, shaking hands and smiling. It was his victory lap.

Hickenlooper called the bills an "unlikely compromise" that was emblematic of the way Freedman coordinated across government and private stakeholders for his three years as marijuana czar. "He was able to build relationships with conflicting interests," Hickenlooper says, and persuade the larger community to support changes that protected public health and safety. "One of the [areas] where Andrew exceeded expectations was to help advise this incipient marijuana industry that they needed to be good citizens, that they needed to care about public welfare."

16. Firm Brings Cannabis to the Forefront[*]

Douglas Levy

When putting together Dykema Gossett PLLC's newly launched Cannabis Law practice group, R. Lance Boldrey said he did some surveying.

The results surprised him.

Last November he asked attorneys in the firm's Michigan and out-of-state offices about their legal experience in the marijuana industry.

"We expected to find maybe a few people across the firm who represented clients in this space," Boldrey said. "We did not expect to find we had 28 lawyers or lobbyists who had been or were engaging in substantive cannabis industry projects. And since then, it's been growing."

Boldrey, who chairs the Cannabis Law group from within Dykema's public policy department, said most business for the group centers on lobbying, legislation and rule-making. But other sectors such as intellectual property, land use and zoning, labor and employment, product safety and taxation also make up the group.

"Nearly every area of legal practice has the potential to be involved in cannabis-based work as new laws" evolve, he said.

"It's an industry we've seen as an emerging one, but we've also seen enough work in different pockets of the firm to justify creating a practice group. It took some time for everybody to come to the conclusion that this was an industry that was going to stay and would grow and have a significant demand for legal services."

While attorneys at other large Michigan law firms have cannabis law clients sprinkled within their practice, Boldrey said Dykema is first large law firm in Michigan to classify such a business as a group.

"We're the first to formalize this effort and pull together folks from across the firm to make it a real practice," he said.

---

*Originally published as Douglas Levy, "Firm Brings Cannabis to the Forefront," *Michigan Lawyers Weekly*, June 7, 2016. Reprinted with permission of the publisher.

A Strong Trend Line

Boldrey said the idea for the group began germinating during Michigan's 2008 ballot campaign. Dykema served as election law counsel for the entity that drafted and ran the campaign for the medical marijuana initiative, which got voters' approval.

"But there wasn't a lot of legal work in the area, at least in terms of business law work, until the big change we saw, which was the authorization of adult (recreational] use in Colorado and Washington state," he said. "It started to get people's attention and we started to get more sophisticated clients examining this space."

Other states in which Dykema serves clients also had medical marijuana initiatives approved. Boldrey said 24 states and Washington, D.C., have legalized marijuana for medicinal purposes, while four states and D.C. have legalized marijuana for adult recreational purposes.

"The trend line is accelerating," he said. "There are six states with potential ballot measures in November to legalize for recreational use, and four that will likely have medical marijuana ballot measures, and there are other states moving through their state legislative process. Everyone sees this trend line continuing."

Boldrey said California could end up being the biggest catalyst for nationwide marijuana reform, as it recently enacted medical marijuana regulation and has recreational use on the November ballot.

The only wild card, he said, is the fact that it's still illegal to possess cannabis, which remains a schedule 1 controlled substance.

"All of this activity in all of these state industries are really dependent on the federal government exercising prosecutorial discretion," Boldrey said. "And with a change in administration, there's a possibility things could go the other way."

Pushing for Regulation

Boldrey said a change in administration is just what made things bit of a mess after the 2008 Michigan election.

When the medical marijuana initiative was crafted in 2007 for the 2008 ballot, "there was a real concern that if the initiative was going to provide for (medical marijuana] dispensaries, that would make the initiative a lot more politically challenging to get passed," Boldrey said.

"So the Michigan initiative does not specifically provide for retail sale of marijuana. That was a very intentional choice, and at the time it was crafted, people didn't foresee the political dynamics that we had in the 2008 election," he said.

He explained that in 2007 Hillary Clinton and Rudy Guiliani were considered the presidential front runners—but the political landscape shifted sharply once Barack Obama gained speed and won.

In the aftermath of November 2008, no regulatory framework was put in place for Michigan dispensaries, though Boldrey said a number of efforts could change that.

The House in 2015 passed legislation, House Bill 4877, to create a regulated system, while three recent bills—HBs 4209, 4210 and 4827—concern cannabis extraction, a "seed-to-sale" tracking system and business protections.

"There's some hope that regulated system will be enacted yet this year. That will provide a lot more legal work as well as a much better framework for the industry itself, as well," Boldrey said. "Because instead of having all these dispensaries or caregiver centers that have arisen by virtue of local law enforcement or cities looking the other way, we will actually have a state-license system and we won't have this unregulated activity taking place."

He added, "It'll also give the municipalities a clear and defined role in enacting their own zoning and regulation of dispensaries. It will be a much cleaner system for everyone and it would mirror what we've seen in a lot of other states."

Clients Big and Small

But just because the system isn't "cleaner" doesn't mean cannabis business within it is nonexistent.

And that's where Dykema's practice group comes in, Boldrey said.

For example, on the product safety side, Boldrey said the group as an FDA specialist who's already advised some companies that manufacture cannabis-infused foods—more commonly known as "edibles"—on product labeling issues.

"Those products aren't covered under the food law today, but nevertheless people need to pay attention," he said. "A couple of weeks ago in Colorado, the first products liability suit was filed against an edibles manufacturer and the dispensary that sold the products."

For labor and employment, the group's lawyers advice non-cannabis businesses on the applicability of their drug policies when an employee is a medical marijuana patient.

Boldrey said biggest types of clients are the large-scale growing operations and dispensary associations, in addition to the National Patients Rights Association and some of the dispensary owners guilds, who need lobbying efforts.

"We have folks involved in preparing offering memoranda for California businesses that are raising capital to construct large-scale commercial growing operations," he said.

Meanwhile some of the smaller clients are individuals who need work with employment contracts or joint-venture agreements. Boldrey said one client is in the analytics business and is consulting with Washington state marijuana organizations on their customer bases and other opportunities.

In addition, he said ancillary businesses—particularly those in agriculture—are starting to see cannabis as a business opportunity.

"We met with a Wisconsin-based company that manufactures distilling equipment used for processing oils in the agricultural industry," Boldrey said. "They never in a million years thought of cannabis as an opportunity until some of the cannabis extraction companies discovered their products a few years ago.

"That (cannabis] extraction business base has gone from exactly none of its customer base to 25 percent of their sales today."

Boldrey said that Dykema's own business base must be handled with great care.

He said one of the biggest issues for lawyers to deal with is the ethical issues created by the sale and possession of cannabis remaining illegal under federal law.

"Under MRP 1.2, lawyers cannot counsel or assist a client with violating the law,"

Boldrey said. "So we have to very carefully delineate the services we can provide, such as advising a client on how to be compliant with state law, and the services we cannot provide, such as assisting a client in escaping federal liability.

"This also means doing due diligence on the clients themselves to determine if we want to take them on in the first place."

17. Business and Citizen Thoughts on Legalized Marijuana[*]

SAMIRA J. PERRY *and* MICKEY P. MCGEE

The issue of marijuana legalization within the United States has been a constant stream of uncertainty for the American public as well as its politicians. One of the first publicly documented issues regarding legalization of marijuana is often attributed to The Federal Marihuana Tax Act of 1937 (renamed today as the 1937 Marijuana Tax Act). The popularity of marijuana during the 1930s began to increase within the United States borders pre-prohibition of alcohol. During this time over 16 states made efforts in attempting to ban the substance, but it was not until Congress and the fledgling Federal Bureau of Narcotics began creating a frenzied state for locals by stating that marijuana was primarily used by Black and Mexican men, and caused rape, murder, and mayhem to occur (Rock, 2009).

In 1970, Congress enacted the Controlled Substances Act (CSA) as part of the Comprehensive Drug Abuse Prevention and Control Act of 1970 (21 U.S.C. § 801 et seq.) Gibson states that, the implementation of the CSA was indeed the, "initial foundation of the governments fight against the abuse of drugs and other substances" (Gibson, 1997). This federal law was created with the explicit intent of prohibiting the manufacture, possession, sale, or distribution of marijuana. The law also stipulates the placement of marijuana as a Schedule I controlled substance, which is also deemed to have no reputable, medically confirmed properties thereby deeming it unusable for recreational, medicinal or any other purpose.

The cost of marijuana enforcement in California currently can be estimated at over $200 million per year, as follows:

- State prison (1500 prisoners at $49 K per year—2009 estimation.) $73.5 million
- Jail costs (estimated 40% of prison population) $29.4 million
- Felony prosecution, court and probation (estimated 8500 felony prosecutions (2008)
- SF DA's office estimated $9250 (per case) $78.6 million
- Felony arrests 17,000 arrests (2008) at $732/arrest, $12.4 million
- Misdemeanor court costs: $100 court time/case, 61,000 cases) $6.1 million

---

*Published with permission of the authors.

- Misdemeanor arrests ($300/arrest, offset by fines)—$0
- California Marijuana Suppression Program (OCJP) $3.8 million
Total: $203.8 million

Qualitative Approach

In this essay, we highlight the results of a 2014 qualitative study completed in Northern California which revealed interesting data from nine government business and public citizen key informants. Four of the key informants worked in city/county government with three of them working within the legal system. Two of the key informants owned companies that were strictly related to the cannabis industry. Two key informants were fulltime students. And one key informant was a medical doctor.

The key informants were asked if they've ever been involved in marijuana related policies and/or issues. Four key informants have and/were still actively involved with policy related issues concerning marijuana. Key Informant 5 stated that he owns seventeen (17) growing rooms in Marina, California and is the Co-Owner of Coasterdam Cannabis Collective of Marina (a 501 (c)(3) non-profit organization). Key Informant 7 is the President of Coasterdam Cannabis Collective of Marina (a 501 (c)(3) non-profit organization). At the time of the study, they were both in a legal battle with the City of Marina to rescind the medical marijuana moratorium. They had received a cease and desist order from the police chief demanding that they stop delivering medical marijuana. They have both stated that they were defying his order under the protection of Senate Bill 439. Key Informant 4 stated that he has been a marijuana activist for many years. He follows cannabis related laws and policies. He also writes opinion pieces on cannabis related measures and bills.

Findings

When asked if they thought marijuana and its related industries could be an economic resource, one-hundred percent of the Key Informants acknowledged that legalizing marijuana for recreational use would generate an additional economic resource for the State of California. Four of the Key Informants stated that the criminal risks were far greater than the economic impact. While five of the Key Informants believed the opposite. They stated the risks are minimal compared to the financial rewards.

When asked if they believe that marijuana should be legalized for recreational use, five of the Key Informants believed that marijuana should be legalized for recreational use and the other four Key Informants did not believe marijuana should be legalized for recreational use. All five Key Informants who believed marijuana should be legalized for recreational use also believed it would generate more revenue for the State of California. Key Informant 2 is the County Managing Deputy District Attorney. He supervises sixteen attorneys, oversees criminal cases involving real world marijuana cases and enforces key legislation involving policy related cannabis issues. He stated that, "I do not believe marijuana should be legalized for recreational use. The medical marijuana laws should be re-evaluated to prevent fraud." He was strongly believed that marijuana should not be legalized for recreational use. Based on his field of work as Deputy District Attorney, he concluded that marijuana is a gateway drug which too often leads to the use of more dangerous narcotics. Key Informant 7, a 3rd year law student at the time and President of Coasterdam Cannabis Collective of Marina. She stated that marijuana should be legal, that it "would empty our overcrowded jails from all of the people with marijuana related charges. It would restore the records and lives of those criminally prosecuted and incarcerated."

In terms of suggested policy recommendations legalization of recreational marijuana, Key Informant 6 suggested an immediate implementation of a marijuana sanctuary in Marina. He also stated that the DARE program should be dismantled in schools and adults should stop lying to the youth about marijuana and have honest conversations with them. He also believed that all barriers such as moratoriums should be removed, and tax incentives should be offered to encourage marijuana companies and research startups to come to Marina/Monterey Bay.

Key Informant 9 recommended that reducing the criminal charge for marijuana from a felony to an infraction should be in place on for persons ages 18–21. He also suggests that lobbyists for the big industries should keep markers in place for smaller farmers to sustain through the transitional period, if legislation is passed for marijuana to be used recreationally.

When asked why marijuana issues matter to the public at large, eleven percent believed it does not matter to the public while ninety-nine percent of the Key Informants believe this issue does matter to the public at large. Key Informant 6 stated that marijuana issues matter to the public at large because it will reduce criminal activity in the public sector. Key Informant 7 believed that legalizing marijuana for recreational use does matter to the public because it will reduce incarcerations and lower drug related crime rates. On the other hand; Key Informant 2 stated that he does not believe the marijuana issue is a significant one for the public at large. He believed it was only important to those who want to use it legally and conversely to those who are collateral victims of marijuana abuse.

Key Informant 1, a graduate student with a master's degree in the public administration stated: "I personally have never used marijuana. However, I believe marijuana should be legalized; it would create money for the State of California, which is desperately needed." Key Informant 3, a former City Manager, stated that, "I will not support legalization of marijuana in California." The key informant felt that the actual risks involved in the legalization of marijuana far outweighed the potential benefits. In reference to the legality of alcohol, tobacco, and firearms, he suggested that the public should not concentrate on legalizing avenues for people to kill themselves and/or become burdens on society.

Key Informant 4, a freelance journalist, cannabis activist, and father of the youngest medicinal cannabis patient stated, "Yes, I do believe that cannabis should be legalized for recreational use. The benefits of legalization outweigh the risks on all levels. Prohibition has led to the development of a black market with territorial control and politics just as alcohol prohibition did in the twenties."

Key Informant 6, at the time a 3rd year law student and co-owner of Coasterdam Cannabis Collective of Marina, agreed stating "Yes, cannabis, not just medicinal cannabis, should be treated like alcohol; taxed and regulated for use by anyone over 21—not 18. […] the teenage brain is not fully developed yet and to add high grade cannabis to that could be a costly mistake."

Conclusions and Recommendations

Infrastructures must be in place to carry California into a legalized-marijuana environment to support the industries that would benefit from legalization. Interviews and surveys indicated that there was stronger support for legalization of recreational marijuana and there was significant disagreement on establishing a fair selling price and tax rate.

Removing prohibitions on producing and distributing cannabis will dramatically reduce wholesale prices. The effect on consumption and tax revenues will depend on many design choices, which would include: the tax level, whether there is an incentive for a continued black market, whether to tax and/or regulate cannabinoid levels, whether there are allowances for home cultivation, whether advertising is restricted, and how the regulatory system is designed and adjusted.

The legal production costs of cannabis will be dramatically below current wholesale prices. In fact, production costs will be such that taxes and regulation will be insufficient to raise retail prices to prohibition levels. The expectation, then, is that legalization will increase consumption substantially, but the size of the increase is uncertain since it depends on design choices and the unknown shape of the cannabis demand curve. The primary argument for the legalization of recreational marijuana in California is its financial impact especially the potential revenue gains through taxation combined with offsets from prohibition enforcement.

Note: In November 2016, California voters passed Proposition 64, making California the most recent state in the nation to legalize the recreational use of marijuana. Effective January 1, 2018, Californians age 21 and older may now possess, transport, buy and use up to one ounce of cannabis for recreational purposes. The new law would also allow retail sales of marijuana and impose a 15 percent tax. Non-medical marijuana can only be sold by state licensed businesses. On January 1, 2018, California began issuing sales licenses for recreational retailers.

Proponents for legalized recreational use of marijuana believe that the approval by voters of the nation's most populous state sends an important message in the fight for marijuana legalization across the U.S. Proposition 64 was opposed by most major law enforcement groups, including the California Association of Highway Patrolmen, the Peace Officers Research Association of California and the California Police Chiefs Association. Opponents cited problems including teen drug abuse and impaired driving experienced where recreational use was previously legalized: Colorado, Alaska, Oregon and Washington.

18. As States OK Medical Marijuana Laws, Doctors Struggle with Knowledge Gap[*]

Shefali Luthra

Medical marijuana has been legal in Maine for almost 20 years. But Farmington physician Jean Antonucci says she continues to feel unprepared when counseling sick patients about whether the drug could benefit them.

Will it help my glaucoma? Or my chronic pain? My chemotherapy's making me nauseous, and nothing's helped. Is cannabis the solution? Patients hope Antonucci, 62, can answer those questions. But she said she is still "completely in the dark."

Antonucci doesn't know whether marijuana is the right way to treat an ailment, what amount is an appropriate dose, or whether a patient should smoke it, eat it, rub it through an oil or vaporize it. Like most doctors, she was never trained to have these discussions. And, because the topic still is not usually covered in medical school, seasoned doctors, as well as younger ones, often consider themselves ill-equipped.

Even though she tries to keep up with the scientific literature, Antonucci said, "it's very difficult to support patients but not know what you're saying."

As the number of states allowing medical marijuana grows—the total has reached 25 plus the District of Columbia—some are working to address this knowledge gap with physician training programs. States are beginning to require doctors to take continuing medical education courses that detail how marijuana interacts with the nervous system and other medications, as well as its side effects.

Though laws vary, they have common themes. They usually set up a process by which states establish marijuana dispensaries, where patients with qualifying medical conditions can obtain the drug. The conditions are specified on a state-approved list. And the role of doctors is often to certify that patients have one of those ailments. But many say that, without knowing cannabis' health effects, even writing a certification makes them uncomfortable.

"We just don't know what we don't know. And that's a concern," said Wanda Filer, president of the American Academy of Family Physicians and a practicing doctor in Pennsylvania.

*Originally published as Shefali Luthra, "As States OK Medical Marijuana Laws, Doctors Struggle with Knowledge Gap," *Kaiser Health News*, August 15, 2016. Reprinted with permission of the publisher.

This medical uncertainty is complicated by confusion over how to navigate often contradictory laws. While states generally involve physicians in the process by which patients obtain marijuana, national drug policies have traditionally had a chilling effect on these conversations.

The Federation of State Medical Boards has tried to add clarity. In an Aug. 9 *JAMA* editorial, leaders noted that federal law technically prohibits prescribing marijuana, and tasks states that allow it for medical use to "implement strong and effective … enforcement systems to address any threat those laws could pose to public safety, public health, and other interests." If state regulation is deemed insufficient, the federal government can step in.

That's why many doctors say they feel caught in the middle, not completely sure of where the line is now drawn between legal medical practice and what could get them in trouble.

In New York, which legalized marijuana for medicinal purposes in 2014, the state health department rolled out a certification program last October. (The state's medical marijuana program itself launched in January 2016.) The course, which lasts about four hours and costs $249, is part of a larger physician registration process. So far, the state estimates 656 physicians have completed the required steps. Other states have contacted New York's Department of Health to learn how the training works.

Pennsylvania and Ohio are also developing similar programs. Meanwhile in Massachusetts, doctors who wish to participate in the state medical marijuana program are required to take courses approved by the American Medical Association. Maryland doesn't require training but encourages it through its Medical Cannabis Commission website, a policy also followed in some other states.

Physicians appear to welcome such direction. A 2013 study in Colorado, for instance, found more than 80 percent of family doctors thought physicians needed medical training before recommending marijuana.

But some advocates worry that doctors may find these requirements onerous and opt out, which would in turn thwart patients' access to the now-legal therapy, said Ellen Smith, a board member of the U.S. Pain Foundation, which favors expanded access to medical cannabis.

Education is essential, given the complexity of how marijuana interacts with the body and how little physicians know, said Stephen Corn, an associate professor of anesthesiology, perioperative and pain medicine at Harvard Medical School. Corn also cofounded The Answer Page, a medical information website that provides educational content to the New York program, as well as a similar Florida initiative. The company, one of a few groups to offer teachings on medical marijuana, is also bidding to supply information for the Pennsylvania program, Corn said.

"You need a multi-hour course to learn where the medical cannabis works within the body," Corn said. "As a patient, would you want a doctor blindly recommending something without knowing how it's going to interact with your other medications? What to expect from it? What not to expect?"

But many say the science is too weak to answer these questions.

One reason: the federal Drug Enforcement Agency classifies marijuana as a schedule I drug, the same level as heroin. This classification makes it more difficult for researchers to gain access to the drug and to gain approval for human subjects to participate in studies. The White House rejected a petition this past week to reclassify the drug in a less strict category, though federal authorities say they will start letting more facilities grow marijuana for the purpose of research. (Currently, only the University of Mississippi can produce it, which advocates say limits study.)

From a medical standpoint, the lack of information is troubling, Filer said.

"Typically, when we're going to prescribe something, you've got data that shows safety and efficacy," she said. With marijuana, the body of research doesn't match what many doctors are used to for prescription drugs.

Still, Corn said, doctors appear pleased with the state training sessions. More than 80 percent of New York doctors who have taken his course said they changed their practice in response to what they learned.

But even now, whenever Corn speaks with doctors about medical marijuana, people ask him how they can learn more about the drug's medical properties and about legal risks. Those two concerns, he said, likely reduce the number of doctors comfortable with and willing to discuss marijuana's place in medicine, even if it's allowed in their states.

Though others say this circumstance is starting to ease, doctors like Jean Antonucci in Maine continue to struggle to figure out how marijuana can fit into safe and compassionate medicine. "You just try and be careful—and learn as much as you can about a patient, and try to do no harm," she said.

Kaiser Health News *is a nonprofit news service covering health issues.*
It is an editorially independent program of Kaiser Family Foundation
that is not affiliated with Kaiser Permanente.

19. Could Legalizing Pot Diminish California's Gains Against Smoking?*

Anna Gorman

California's decision to legalize marijuana was touted as a victory for those who had argued that the state needed a system to decriminalize, regulate and tax it.

But the new law, approved by voters on Nov. 8, also could be a boon to the tobacco industry at a time when cigarette smoking is down and cigarette companies are looking for ways to expand their market, according to researchers in Los Angeles County and around the state.

They warn that unless the state proceeds carefully, the legalization of marijuana for recreational use could roll back some of the gains California has made in reducing the use of tobacco.

"There is a concern that there could be a potential renormalization of smoking," said Michael Ong, associate professor at UCLA's David Geffen School of Medicine.

Ong said it will depend on how the initiative is implemented, whether officials follow through on the regulation, and how involved public health officials are with it. "It will be important to make sure that we don't have a setback in terms of what we have done for clean air in California ... and what we have done to reduce tobacco's harms," he said.

Ethan Nadelmann, executive director of the Drug Policy Alliance, which supports marijuana legalization, said there is no evidence that it leads to increased cannabis consumption—or tobacco smoking.

California's adult smoking rate is the second-lowest in the country, at 11.6 percent, according to the California Department of Public Health. The smoking rate dropped by more than 50 percent between 1988 and 2014, cutting health care costs and reducing tobacco-related diseases, according to the department.

The headway against smoking over the past few decades is due to a combination of factors, including tobacco taxes, laws restricting where people can smoke, and broad-based media campaigns and programs to help people quit. Despite the decline in smoking,

---

*Originally published as Anna Gorman, "Could Legalizing Pot Diminish California's Gains Against Smoking?," *Kaiser Health News*, November 18, 2016. Reprinted with permission of the publisher.

the use of e-cigarettes has increased dramatically over the past few years, with nearly 10 percent of adults ages 18 through 24 now using them, according to the department.

Another ballot initiative passed by voters last week could push the smoking rate even lower, experts said. Prop. 56 adds $2 per pack to the tax on cigarettes and increases taxes on electronic cigarettes that contain nicotine and other tobacco products. The money will help pay for health care and increase funding for tobacco control and prevention.

The marijuana initiative, Prop. 64, allows adults ages 21 and over to grow, buy and possess small amounts of marijuana for personal use. It also regulates recreational marijuana businesses and imposes taxes that will help pay for drug education and prevention programs.

Bonnie Halpern-Felsher, pediatrics professor at the Stanford University School of Medicine, said she is concerned that there may not be enough education and prevention written into the proposition, especially targeted at youth.

Marijuana is already the most widely used illegal drug among adolescents. Many young people consider marijuana, and blunts (marijuana rolled with a tobacco leaf wrapper), to be more socially acceptable and less risky than cigarettes, according to a recent study co-authored by Halpern-Felsher. The study also found that youths who saw messages about the benefits of marijuana were more likely to use it.

Blunts, Halpern-Felsher said, are particularly worrisome because they contain nicotine as well as marijuana. She said many young people may not understand the risk of blunts or marijuana, and once they start thinking that smoking one product is acceptable, they may believe it's OK to smoke other things as well. "That's my concern," she said. "I do think people are going to generalize."

From the tobacco industry's point of view, marijuana could serve as a "smoke inhalation trainer," and thus become a gateway to tobacco use, said Robert K. Jackler, a professor at the Stanford School of Medicine.

Jackler, who researches tobacco advertising, said tobacco and marijuana are similarly marketed—as products to help people relax and ease their stress. "There is tremendous overlap potential," he said.

Tobacco companies could easily try to exploit that to enter the marijuana market, Jackler said. They already have enormous influence on state laws and regulations and could try to set up small dispensaries and make marijuana another one of their products.

"The tobacco industry is always looking for replacement products because, at least in America, smoking is down," he said. "This will give them a new entry into the market. They are best equipped to exploit this market opportunity."

In fact, the tobacco industry considered getting into the marijuana market in the 1960s and 70s and could easily do so, said Stanton Glantz, a professor at University of California, San Francisco School of Medicine. Glantz believes that even as the newly approved tobacco tax reduces California's smoking rate further, legalized marijuana will help sustain the tobacco market. He said he expected to see mass marketing and branding of marijuana over time.

Along with some therapeutic benefits of marijuana, there are also health risks, Glantz said. "The likely costs that are going to be incurred by all the marijuana-induced diseases don't come close to being covered by the taxes that are written into Prop. 64," he warned.

The initiative should have included higher taxes, graphic warning labels, provisions to keep demand low and a broad-based education campaign like there is on tobacco, Glantz argued. "The ideal situation is where it's legal so nobody is thrown in jail, but nobody wants to buy it."

Legalization supporters said they don't believe the tobacco industry will get involved in the marijuana market until and unless federal prohibition ends. Marijuana is still illegal under federal law.

Nadelmann, of the Drug Policy Alliance, said it is misguided to conflate the two products. Young people can distinguish between the effects of cigarettes and marijuana, he said.

"Teenagers are actually smarter than most of the adult propaganda," Nadelmann said. "They know smoking cigarettes is really stupid and that smoking marijuana is not such a major issue."

Kaiser Health News is a nonprofit news service covering health issues. It is an editorially independent program of Kaiser Family Foundation that is not affiliated with Kaiser Permanente.

20. As Marijuana Laws Relax, Doctors Say Pregnant Women Shouldn't Partake*

SARAH VARNEY

Two-year-old Maverick Hawkins sits on a red, plastic car in his grandmother's living room in the picturesque town of Nevada City, Calif., in the foothills of the Sierra Nevada. His playpal Delilah Smith, a fellow 2-year-old, snacks on hummus and cashews and delights over the sounds of her Princess Peppa Pig stuffie.

It's playtime for the kids of the provocatively named Facebook group "Pot smoking moms who cuss sometimes."

Maverick's mother, Jenna Sauter, started the group after he was born. "I was a new mom, a young mom—I was 22—and I was just feeling really lonely in the house, taking care of him," she said. She wanted to reach out to other mothers but didn't want to hide her marijuana use.

"I wanted friends who I could be open with," Sauter said. "Like, I enjoy going to the river and I like to maybe smoke a joint at the river."

There are nearly 2,600 members now in the Facebook group. Marijuana, which became legal for recreational use in California this month, is seen by many group members as an all-natural and seemingly harmless remedy for everything from morning sickness to postpartum depression.

Delilah Smith's mom, Andria, is 21 and a week away from her due date with her second child.

She took umbrage when an emergency room physician recently suggested she take "half a Norco"—a pill akin to Vicodin, an opioid-based painkiller—for her excruciating back pain.

Smith was disdainful. "She was like, 'We know more about Norco and blah, blah, blah and what it can do to you, but we don't that much about marijuana,'" Smith said.

"I was like, 'Test me!' I was like, 'Observe me. My kid could count to 10 before she was even 2 by herself, and I smoked pot throughout my whole pregnancy. She's not stupid! There is no third eye growing.'"

---

*Originally published as Sarah Varney, "As Marijuana Laws Relax, Doctors Say Pregnant Women Shouldn't Partake," *Kaiser Health News*, January 31, 2018. Reprinted with permission of the publisher.

The number of women in the United States who use marijuana during pregnancy has been difficult to gauge, partly because some women are reluctant to tell their doctors; at least 24 states consider substance use during pregnancy a form of child abuse, so divulging such information can have serious consequences.

Still, a number of studies nationally suggest there's been a sharp jump in pot use among pregnant women. Younger mothers, especially, were reported using marijuana during pregnancy.

Andria Smith and Sauter both told their doctors of their marijuana use, and after they gave birth, their babies were tested for signs of marijuana's chief active ingredient, THC.

Because their babies tested positive, Sauter and Smith were visited at home by county social service workers, who gave the women information about the effects of marijuana use during pregnancy and breastfeeding.

Researchers say psychoactive compounds in marijuana easily cross the placenta, exposing the fetus to perhaps 10 percent of the THC—tetrahydrocannabinol—that the mother receives, and higher concentrations if the mom uses pot repeatedly.

Dr. Dana Gossett, a research obstetrician and gynecologist at the University of California–San Francisco who also treats patients, said studies have shown marijuana increases the risk of stillbirth or adversely affects how a baby's brain develops.

Gossett cited some research that suggests children exposed to marijuana while growing in the womb can have poorer performance on visual-motor coordination—tasks like catching a ball or solving visual problems like puzzles.

And studies also show, she said, these kids may have behavioral problems at higher rates than other children by age 14, and are at greater risk for initiating marijuana use.

"That is biologically plausible," Gossett said, "because the effects of THC in the brain may actually prime that child for addictive behavior, not just to marijuana but to alcohol as well."

There has been little research on the effects of THC passed to a baby via breastfeeding. But because there isn't enough evidence to determine the risk, the American College of Obstetricians and Gynecologists (ACOG) discourages marijuana use during pregnancy, and warns breastfeeding moms to avoid eating or smoking marijuana or inhaling its secondhand smoke—since some amount of THC, just like alcohol, can pass into the baby that way.

To Smith's point that her daughter, Delilah, is just as smart as her peers, studies do show that, in general, children exposed to marijuana in utero don't score worse on reading or mathematics as they get older.

Sauter said she and her friends don't smoke near their children, nor do they spend their days stoned to oblivion.

"It's not like being totally out of it," Sauter said. "I'm completely aware of my surroundings. I'm watching my kid, watching my friends' kids. I'm hanging out. You totally know what's going on."

Sauter said many parents she knows are uncertain if they can get in trouble using pot now in California. Indeed, child protection laws in most states remain at odds with liberal marijuana laws. Some moms on the Facebook page will not go to the doctor—even when they're sick.

"They don't want to get tested," Sauter said. "And that's dangerous. We should be able to be open about it. Because if something does go wrong, we've got to know."

ACOG does not endorse mandatory testing for THC in pregnant women or newborn babies—out of concern that women could be jailed or have their babies taken from them. Instead, the organization urges obstetricians to ask pregnant women about drug use during prenatal visits, counseling these patients against substance use and helping them alleviate their nausea, back pain or postpartum depression with medications deemed safe by federal drug regulators.

But with recreational cannabis now legal in at least eight states and the District of Columbia, physicians like Gossett are worried that newborns and young children, whose brains are rapidly developing, constructing billions of neural connections, will come to know the world in an altered state.

"They're learning what things look like and how things move and how to respond to the world," Gossett said. Marijuana's psychotropic effects, she added, will change "a child's ability to interpret the world around him."

Kaiser Health News *is a nonprofit news service covering health issues. It is an editorially independent program of Kaiser Family Foundation that is not affiliated with Kaiser Permanente. KHN's coverage of children's health care issues is supported in part by the Heising-Simons Foundation.*

21. Marijuana's Lasting Effects on the Brain[*]

Nora D. Volkow

A study was published in January 2013 contesting the interpretation of the large-scale marijuana study I discuss below—that heavy cannabis use begun in the teen years and continued into adulthood brings about declines in IQ scores. The contesting author used simulation models to suggest that other factors, such as socioeconomic status (SES), may account for the downward IQ trend the original authors reported. In a rebuttal letter published in the March 4, 2013, issue of *Proceedings of the National Academy of the United States of America*, the authors of the first study note that SES could not account for the findings they observed, because adolescent cannabis use was not more prevalent in populations with lower SES.

Observational studies in humans cannot account for all potentially confounding variables when addressing change in a complex trait like IQ, and future studies will be needed to further clarify exactly how much intelligence may be lost as a result of adolescent marijuana use. That such a loss does occur, however, is consistent with what we know from animal studies. Though limited in their application to the complex human brain, such studies can more definitively assess the relationship between drug exposure and various outcomes. They have shown that exposure to cannabinoids during adolescent development can cause long-lasting changes in the brain's reward system as well as the hippocampus, a brain area critical for learning and memory.

The message inherent in these and in multiple supporting studies is clear. Regular marijuana use in adolescence is part of a cluster of behaviors that can produce enduring detrimental effects and alter the trajectory of a young person's life—thwarting his or her potential. Beyond potentially lowering IQ, teen marijuana use is linked to school dropout, other drug use, mental health problems, etc. Given the current number of regular marijuana users (about 1 in 15 high school seniors) and the possibility of this number increasing with marijuana legalization, we cannot afford to divert our focus from the central point: Regular marijuana use stands to jeopardize a young person's chances of success—in school and in life.

---

[*]Originally published as Nora D. Volkow, "Marijuana's Lasting Effects on the Brain," National Institute on Drug Abuse, https://www.drugabuse.gov/about-nida/directors-page/messages-director/2012/09/marijuanas-lasting-effects-brain.

We repeatedly hear the myth that marijuana is a benign drug—that it is not addictive (which it is) or that it does not pose a threat to the user's health or brain (which it does). A major new study published last week in *Proceedings of the National Academy of Sciences* (and funded partly by NIDA and other NIH institutes) provides objective evidence that, at least for adolescents, marijuana is harmful to the brain.

The new research is part of a large-scale study of health and development conducted in New Zealand. Researchers administered IQ tests to over 1,000 individuals at age 13 (born in 1972 and 1973) and assessed their patterns of cannabis use at several points as they aged. Participants were again tested for IQ at age 38, and their two scores were compared as a function of their marijuana use. The results were striking: Participants who used cannabis heavily in their teens and continued through adulthood showed a significant drop in IQ between the ages of 13 and 38—an average of 8 points for those who met criteria for cannabis dependence. (For context, a loss of 8 IQ points could drop a person of average intelligence into the lowest third of the intelligence range.) Those who started using marijuana regularly or heavily after age 18 showed minor declines. By comparison, those who never used marijuana showed no declines in IQ.

Other studies have shown a link between prolonged marijuana use and cognitive or neural impairment. A recent report in *Brain*, for example, reveals neural-connectivity impairment in some brain regions following prolonged cannabis use initiated in adolescence or young adulthood. But the New Zealand study is the first prospective study to test young people *before* their first use of marijuana and again *after* long-term use (as much as 20+ years later). Indeed, the ruling out of a pre-existing difference in IQ makes the study particularly valuable. Also, and strikingly, those who used marijuana heavily before age 18 showed mental decline even after they quit taking the drug. This finding is consistent with the notion that drug use during adolescence—when the brain is still rewiring, pruning, and organizing itself—can have negative and long-lasting effects on the brain.

While this study cannot exclude *all* potential contributory factors (e.g., child abuse, subclinical mental illness, mild learning disabilities), the neuropsychological declines following marijuana use were present even after researchers controlled for factors like years of education, mental illness, and use of other substances. Mental impairment was evident not just in test scores but in users' daily functioning. People who knew the study participants (e.g., friends and relatives) filled out questionnaires and reported that persistent cannabis users had significantly more memory and attention problems: easily getting distracted, misplacing things, forgetting to keep appointments or return calls, and so on.

Unfortunately, the proportion of American teens who believe marijuana use is harmful has been declining for the past several years, which has corresponded to a steady rise in their use of the drug, as shown by NIDA's annual Monitoring the Future survey of 8th, 10th, and 12th graders. Since it decreases IQ, regular marijuana use stands to jeopardize a young person's chances of success in school. So as another school year begins, we all must step up our efforts to educate teens about the harms of marijuana so that we can realign their perceptions of this drug with the scientific evidence.

22. The Public Health Implications of the Legalization of Recreational Cannabis*

JULIET AKHIGBE, VASH EBBADI, KATIE HUYNH,
JAMES LECKIE, MARIA MAJOR, CARA ROBINSON,
MICHELLE SUARLY *and* DAVID WASSERSTEIN

The Ontario Public Health Association (OPHA) is a member-based, not-for-profit association that provides leadership on issues affecting the public's health and strengthens the impact of those who are active in public and community health throughout Ontario. OPHA has multiple active work groups and task forces that focus on particular public health issues.

OPHA's Cannabis Task Group has focused on developing a comprehensive analysis and literature review to inform the development of a policy position statement on the public health impacts of the upcoming legalization of cannabis in Ontario and Canada. Specific reference and considerations were paid to the context, populations, potential challenges and health equity as they relate to Ontario.

Background

Canada's Task Force on Cannabis Legislation and Legalization was first assembled in June of 2016 to consult and provide advice on the design of a new legislative and regulatory framework for legal access to cannabis, consistent with the Federal Government's commitment to "legalize, regulate, and restrict access."

A Cannabis Act has now been tabled in the House of Commons and is expected to become law in July 2018. Under this new law, Canada's provinces and territories will be responsible to license and oversee the distribution and sale of cannabis, subject to Federal conditions, and will have the power to:

---

*Originally published as Juliet Akhigbe, Vash Ebbadi, Katie Huynh, James Leckie, Maria Major, Cara Robinson, Michelle Suarly, and David Wasserstein, *The Public Health Implications of the Legalization of Recreational Cannabis: Executive Summary*, Ontario, Canada: The Ontario Public Health Association. Reprinted with permission of the publisher.

- increase the minimum age in their province or territory (but not lower it)
- lower the personal possession limit in their jurisdiction
- create additional rules for growing cannabis at home, such as lowering the number of plants per residence; and
- restrict where adults can consume cannabis, such as in public or in vehicles.

While medicinal uses for cannabis is gaining acceptance, there are public health implications associated with cannabis use. Specifically, the following are potential harms:

- risk of toxicity
- unintended exposure to children
- high mortality and morbidity attributable to cannabis, including motor vehicle accidents, lung cancer and substance use disorders
- occupational safety risks
- negative mental health outcomes
- respiratory health impacts
- impaired child and youth development
- equity implications considering differential usage rates across gender and income levels

In light of these developments and the potential harms above, OPHA calls on both the Federal and Provincial government to put health considerations at the forefront and adopt a public health approach to mitigate these harms. This would entail:

- Using public health strategies including:
  - o Health promotion to reduce the likelihood of use and problematic use;
  - o Health protection to reduce the harms associated with use;
  - o Prevention and harm reduction to reduce the likelihood of problematic use and overdose;
  - o Population health assessment to understand the extent of the situation, and the potential impact of the interventions, policies, and programs on the population (evaluation);
  - o Disease, injury and disability surveillance to understand the effect on society and to evaluate the effects of these activities; and
  - o Evidence-based services to help protect people who are at risk of developing, or have developed problems with substances.
- Applying principles of social justice, attention to human rights and equity, evidence-informed policy and practice, and addressing the underlying determinants of health

OPHA calls for a Federal and Provincial regulatory regime that advances the goals outlined in the Federal Task Force on Cannabis Legalization and Regulation's 2016 discussion paper. These include:

- Protect young Canadians by keeping marijuana out of the hands of children and youth.
- Protect public health and safety by strengthening, where appropriate, laws and enforcement measures that deter and punish more serious marijuana offences, particularly selling and distributing to children and youth, selling outside of the

regulatory framework and operating a motor vehicle while under the influence of marijuana.

- Ensure Canadians are well-informed through sustained and appropriate public health campaigns, and, for youth in particular, ensure that risks are understood.
- Establish and enforce a system of strict production, distribution and sales, taking a public health approach, with regulation of quality and safety (e.g., child-proof packaging, warning labels), restriction of access, and application of taxes, with programmatic support for addiction treatment, mental health support and education programs.
- Conduct ongoing data collection, including gathering baseline data to monitor the impact of the new framework.

Recommendations

In accordance with the objectives of Canada's Task Force on Cannabis Legalization and Regulation, OPHA proposes the following recommendations for the Ontario context. Some of these recommendations could also apply to other levels of government.

Recommendation 1: Protect Young Canadians

ACCESS

- Prohibit cannabis-containing products that could be attractive to minors (e.g., THC-infused candy or drinks), and require childproof packaging for other edible products
- Set the minimum age for purchasing and possessing cannabis at 21 years of age and have a consistent minimum age for purchasing and possessing cannabis across Canada in order to provide clear policy direction and eliminate cross-border variations, which limit the effectiveness of minimum legal age regulations to protect young people.

EDUCATION AND ENFORCEMENT

- Direct Provincial education ministries to work with public health to update and provide supports for health and physical education curriculums, embedding key evidence-based messages about risky use, especially for youth.
- Develop and implement health promotion campaigns targeted to youth describing the harms of cannabis prior to the initial sale of these products, and continue funding such campaigns through cannabis-product taxation to provide youth with on-going reliable information on the risks and harms associated with cannabis use.

Recommendation 2: Protect Public Health and Safety

IMPAIRED DRIVING

- Develop a comprehensive framework which includes prevention, education and enforcement to address and prevent marijuana-impaired driving with a focus on groups at higher risk of harm, such as youth. This includes the development and implementation of standardized roadside sobriety tests, tools and devices for use in all Canadian jurisdictions.

EXPOSURE

- Prohibit the co-location of sales of cannabis, alcohol and tobacco products.
- Adopt all relevant smoke-free bylaws for public spaces to include cannabis consumption. Including relevant workplace tobacco and alcohol consumption policies.
- Include limitations on outdoor signage, and any kind of promotional activity.
- Prohibit advertising and sponsorships associated with the sale of cannabis-containing products.

Recommendation 3: Ensure Canadians Are Well-Informed

COMMUNICATION

- Require all cannabis and cannabis-containing product labels to include evidence—informed health warnings, contraindications, harm reduction messages and information on accessing support services. In addition, subject all cannabis and cannabis-containing products to plain packaging regulations.
- Develop a comprehensive strategy to clearly communicate details of the regulations prior to implementation, so that the public and other stakeholders understand what is permitted, and so that individuals can make informed choices.

TRAINING

- Ensure training of sales staff and education of consumers at point of sale, including promotion of health risks.
- Continue with public health support for local law enforcement activities through education and awareness raising efforts on the dangers of marijuana-impaired driving.

HEALTH PROMOTION

- Develop and implement health promotion campaigns describing the harms of cannabis prior to the initial sale of these products, and continue funding such campaigns through cannabis-product taxation to provide Canadians with on-going reliable information on the risks associated with cannabis use.
- Invest in evidence-based health promotion, prevention, awareness and education, targeted at both youth and parents, with a secondary focus on other vulnerable groups (pregnant and lactating women, people with personal or family history of mental illness, and individuals experiencing issues with substance abuse) as well as harm-reduction messaging for those who choose to use marijuana.

Recommendation 4: Establish and Enforce
a System of Strict Production, Distribution and Sales

PRODUCTION

- Create and enforce legislation to ensure that cannabis products meet quality and safety standards. This includes ensuring approved fertilizers and pesticides are used, and that hazardous molds are not present in cannabis products.
- Mandate food safety training for producers of edible marijuana products.

DISTRIBUTION

- Expand regulations to include a wider variety of marijuana products (e.g., edibles, concentrates, and tinctures).
- Strengthen requirements set out in the MMPR (ACMPR as of Aug. 24, 2016) to develop a more comprehensive regulatory system, including: Development of national standards for production, packaging, storage, distribution and testing of marijuana products. This is an important strategy for public health and safety.
- Establish a government-controlled monopoly on marijuana production.

SALES

- Limit the number, density (geographic density or population density), and type of retail outlets.
- Restrict hours and days of operation and locations of retail outlets.
- Allow for broad zoning powers at the Municipal level
- Provide government resources for inspection and other accountability functions.
- Develop market information concerning the development of cannabis retail sales centres and ensure their operation by non-commercial entities. Restrict marketing, promotion and displays.
- Should a decision be made to permit storefront retail sales, establish detailed recommendations regarding their location and operation, with specific reference to the criteria established in Washington State, including limits on the distance between retail operations and areas where minors congregate (see more under subsection "Sales and Commercialization").

TAXATION

- Have governments establish (a) taxation rate(s) based on an analysis of price elasticity for these product(s).
- Establish a variable taxation rate system for all THC-containing products that is based on the concentration of THC, with higher-concentration products having a higher tax rate.
- Direct tax revenues from the sale of cannabis and related products back to support the establishment and management of the programs and activities necessary to manage its legalization and regulation and public health programs that will work to mitigate harms.
- Allocate a portion of cannabis tax revenues to strengthen the ongoing efforts of

law enforcement agencies to limit the illegal growth, production and sale of cannabis, and to ensure that officers have the necessary training to assess and prosecute those who drive under the influence of cannabis.

Recommendation 5: Conduct Ongoing Data Collection

- Invest proactively in a collaborative public health approach that prioritizes investment in a continuum of evidence-informed prevention and treatment services to prevent and respond to problematic use.

We call on all levels of government to ensure a comprehensive strategy is in place to mitigate the potential harms from the legalization and sale of recreational cannabis. An effective public health approach will require collaboration among multiple sectors (e.g., law enforcement, occupational health, education, health, municipalities, government ministries/departments) to ensure the needed supports are in place to promote and protect the health of Ontarians and Canadians.

23. Marijuana Legalization
in Two States
*A Man-Made Public Health Disaster?**

PAULA GORDON

Dwight Waldo once humorously asked the question: When was someone going to write a dissertation on common sense and administration? Common sense is in scarce supply in administration, public policy and governance, in particular as it relates to marijuana use and the law.

While Amsterdam and Switzerland have had second thoughts about the permissiveness of drug laws, the states of Colorado and Washington have legalized the recreational use of marijuana. Is this sensible public policy?

Reports indicate that marijuana use has significant consequences for mental and physical health, social and public health in general. So why would any public official or legislator want to legalize it?

Do those promoting its legalization know about widely available research its effect? Do they know that marijuana use profoundly affects brain functioning and IQ levels of those under the age of 25 because their brains are still developing? Do they know that the Tetrahydrocannabinol (THC) content of marijuana today can be 10 times more potent than the THC content of marijuana that was widely available several decades ago?

There are decades' worth of research on the harmful psychological, mental and physical effects of marijuana use, including the effects on the unborn and the offspring of users. Hundreds of references can be found in reports, articles and references at http://GordonDrugAbusePrevention.com.

Perhaps, most compelling, are recent findings outlined by Dr. Nora Volkow, director of the National Institute of Drug Abuse, in an interview with the Dalai Lama. The exchange took place November 2013 in India and focused on the effects of mood-altering substances, including marijuana, on human behavior and brain function. The video includes compelling brain scan results. Dr. Volkow discusses new information concerning the permanent harmful effects of marijuana on the developing brain. Proponents of legalizing the recreational use of marijuana may well change their views if they see that video.

---

*Originally published as Paula Gordon, "Marijuana Legalization in Two States: A Man-Made Public Health Disaster?," *PA Times*, September 19, 2014. Reprinted with permission of the publisher.

In addition, research recently published in the April 16, 2014, *Journal of Neuroscience* revealed that structural anomalies have been found in the brains of casual users; anomalies that are linked to disruptions in behavior. Most recently, long term behavioral effects, including a seven-fold increase in suicide attempts, in young users of marijuana have been reported by *The Lancet Psychiatry* in its September 9, 2014, issue.

The proponents of marijuana legalization do not seem to be paying attention to these significant research findings. They dismiss such findings as out of hand, holding fast to their view that marijuana is a "relatively" harmless substance.

In some cases, proponents may not know about the wide array of research available on the effects of marijuana and they may not have the expertise to understand the significance of those findings. The high THC potency of marijuana today is a compelling enough reason to keep its use illegal. Unfortunately, those who support legalization seem to be ill-informed. How else might their arguments in favor of marijuana legalization be characterized? The arguments are varied but ignore key facts.

Libertarian Argument: "It is my life, my mind and my body and I should be free to do what I want to with them" or "I should be free to use the intoxicant of my choice" and "My use of marijuana is not hurting anyone."

Response: Is marijuana use a victimless act if it affects the lives of all those around the user, not to mention the life and health of the user? Is marijuana use an innocuous act if it has known harmful effects on the developing brains of those who use it? Is it an innocuous act if it affects one's behavior and mental functioning? What are the consequences of a "stoned" citizenry? Can a representative democracy afford to have a dumbed down or partially stoned electorate?

Social Justice Argument: "It is unconscionable that society should disproportionately make criminals of individuals who use marijuana who are from lower socioeconomic groups."

Response: Agreed. It is a fact that more individuals from lower socioeconomic groups are negatively affected by marijuana laws. The remedy, however, is not legalization which only increases its use, including among lower socioeconomic groups. A better remedy is to use the justice system to remand users from all walks of life to drug court programs and other programs that emphasize counselling, education and treatment. Through judicial discretion, this can be done without giving individuals criminal records. The aim of drug courts and other similar programs have been to discourage use of mood and mind-altering drugs and help all individuals fulfil their potential as healthy, functioning individuals. Making marijuana use legal simply sends the false message that the marijuana has insignificant, harmless consequences to the individual and society, when in fact its use has significant harmful effects.

"Big Marijuana" Can Help the Economy: "Turning marijuana sales and distribution into a regulated business will benefit the economy. We can then regulate its use more carefully; treat it as alcohol and tobacco are treated; do away with the black or gray markets and intrusion of organized crime and cartels, and keep it out of the hands of those under the age of 21."

Response: Indeed, what is currently happening in Colorado and Washington is that many individuals are making money selling drugs in the black or gray markets, undercutting the prices that the "legal" dealers are charging. Reports indicate the numbers of users of all ages are increasing, including those who live in nearby states. According to reports, the number of individuals seeking treatment had already been growing in the years prior to the legalization of recreational use of marijuana. In addition, traffic fatalities in Colorado involving drivers testing positive for marijuana had already increased by 114 percent from 2006 to 2011. Anyone familiar with the effects of marijuana on cognition, memory, concentration, judgment, perception, sense of space and time, knows full well that users cannot safely drive or operate machinery.

States Have the Right to Legalize Marijuana: "States have the right to legalize the use of marijuana even though it is in contravention of international treaties and federal law."

Response: The president has a constitutional obligation under Article II, Sec. 3 to "take care that the laws be faithfully executed." The president is clearly not enforcing the Controlled Substance Act, which pertains to the control, distribution and use of marijuana. He is allowing the abrogation of international treaties to which the U.S. is signatory.

What are the implications for the future viability of the rule of law and the Constitution when states act in ways that are counter to international treaties and federal law? Or when the Department of Justice and the president allow states to abrogate international treaties and federal law? An article on "The Illegality of Legalizing Marijuana Use: An Open Plea to the President and Other Sworn Public Officials…" by the author at Family Security Matters focuses in further detail on these concerns.

Tax Revenue Argument: "The taxes from the sale of marijuana will have an overwhelmingly beneficial effect on state budgets."

Response: With increases in use, costs to society can be expected to grow. In Colorado where use has been on the increase for many years, there has been an increase in fatalities resulting from accidents involving individuals driving under the influence of marijuana, resulting in incalculable costs. There have also been increases in the numbers of individuals seeking emergency care at poison centers and emergency rooms; an increasing number of individuals seeking treatment for chronic use and psychological and physical addiction.

These and other public health and public safety consequences as well as consequences for work place productivity and safety should not be lessened for the sake of economic productivity or tax revenues. No amount of tax revenue would begin to equal the costs to individuals and society.

David Brooks recently made a point in his *New York Times* op-ed piece, "Been There, Done That" that law is culture. Changing the law can lead to wholesale changes in behavior, values and beliefs. Indeed, when the president (out of context, it is now said) minimized the harmfulness of marijuana, what impact did that statement have? Any parent with youngsters or teenagers knows all too well the answer to that question.

It would seem to be magical thinking (ironically, an effect of marijuana use) to assume that the use of marijuana could be widely legally sanctioned and that its use would not spread throughout society. Indeed, the authors of the 2012 Report of Organization of American States on "The Drug Problem in the Americas" discuss the profound implications of legalization: "Even with relatively restrictive regulation, the result of legalization is likely to be expanded use and dependency" (p. 94).

Proponents of legalization seem ready to jeopardize the social and public health of the nation and most significantly, the mental health, behavior, motivation and productivity of the rising generation.

Governor Jerry Brown has summed up the seriousness of the implications of marijuana legalization for the nation. In the *National Journal* (3–8–14, p. 44), he is quoted as saying: "How many people can get stoned and we still have a great state or a great nation? The world's pretty dangerous, very competitive. I think we need to stay alert, if not 24 hours a day, more than some of the potheads might be able to put together."

A governor with uncommon common sense so direly needed at this time in the nation's history....

24. Link Between Medical Marijuana and Fewer Opioid Deaths Is More Complex[*]

ROSALIE LICCARDO PACULA

The association between medical marijuana and lower levels of opioid overdose deaths—identified previously in several studies—is more complex than previously described and appears to be changing as both medical marijuana laws and the opioid crisis evolve, according to a new RAND Corporation study.

The report—the most-detailed examination of medical marijuana and opioid deaths conducted to date—found that legalizing medical marijuana was associated with lower levels of opioid deaths only in states that had provisions for dispensaries that made medical marijuana easily available to patients. Opioid death rates were not lower in states that just provided legal protections to patients and caregivers, allowing them to grow their own marijuana.

In addition, the association between medical marijuana dispensaries and fewer opioid deaths appears to have declined sharply after 2010, when states began to tighten requirements on sales by dispensaries.

"Our findings are consistent with previous studies showing an association between the legalization of medical marijuana and lower deaths from overdoses of opioids," said Rosalie Liccardo Pacula, co-author of the study and co-director of the RAND Drug Policy Research Center.

"However, our findings show that the mechanism for this was loosely regulated medical marijuana dispensaries, and that the association between these laws and opioid mortality has declined over time as state laws have more tightly regulated medical dispensaries and the opioid crisis shifted from prescription opioids to heroin and fentanyl," Pacula said. "This is a sign that medical marijuana, by itself, will not be the solution to the nation's opioid crisis today."

The study was published online by the Journal of Health Economics.

Researchers from RAND and the University of California, Irvine, analyzed infor-

*Originally published as Rosalie Liccardo Pacula, "Link Between Medical Marijuana and Fewer Opioid Deaths Is More Complex," RAND Corporation, https://www.rand.org/news/press/2018/02/06.html. Reprinted with permission of the publisher.

mation about treatment admissions for addiction to pain medications from 1999 to 2012 and state-level overdose deaths from opioids from 1999 to 2013. They also identified state laws legalizing medical marijuana, examining provisions such as whether the regulations made marijuana easily accessible to patients by allowing dispensaries.

When the researchers narrowly focused on the time period from 1999 to 2010 and replicated a model used by other researchers, they obtained results similar to those previously published, showing an approximately 20 percent decline in opioid overdose deaths associated with the passage of any state medical marijuana law. However, these general findings were driven by states that had laws allowing for loosely regulated marijuana dispensary systems.

When researchers extended their analysis through 2013, they found that the association between having any medical marijuana law and lower rates of opioid deaths completely disappeared. Moreover, the association between states with medical marijuana dispensaries and opioid mortality fell substantially as well.

The researchers provide two explanations for the decline in the association between medical marijuana dispensaries and opioid harm. First, states that more recently adopted laws with medical marijuana dispensaries more tightly regulated them, in response to a U.S. Justice Department memo saying it would not challenge state-level medical marijuana laws so long as dispensary sales were in full compliance with state regulations. Second, beginning in 2010, the primary driver of the opioid crisis and related deaths became illicit opioids, mainly heroin and then fentanyl, not prescription opioids.

The study also found no evidence that states with medical marijuana laws experience reductions in the volume of legally distributed opioid analgesics used to treat pain. Even if medical marijuana patients were substituting medical marijuana for opioids in medical marijuana states, these patients did not represent a measurable part of the medical opioid analgesic market.

"While our study finds that medical marijuana dispensaries reduce some of the harms associated with the misuse of opioids, there is little evidence that this is happening because a large number of patients suffering from pain are using marijuana instead of opioid medications," Pacula said. "Either the patients are continuing to use their opioid pain medications in addition to marijuana, or this patient group represents a small share of the overall medical opioid using population."

The RAND study was conducted before any states had begun to allow retail sales of recreational marijuana.

"Our research suggests that the overall story between medical marijuana and opioid deaths is complicated," Pacula said. "Before we embrace marijuana as a strategy to combat the opioid epidemic, we need to fully understand the mechanism through which these laws may be helping and see if that mechanism still matters in today's changing opioid crisis."

Support for the study was provided by the National Institute on Drug Abuse. Other authors of the study are David Powell of RAND and Mireille Jacobson of UC Irvine.

RAND Health is the nation's largest independent health policy research program, with a broad research portfolio that focuses on health care costs, quality and public health preparedness, among other topics.

25. Teaching Teens the Perils of Pot as Marketplace Grows*

Anna Gorman

After Yarly Raygoza attended the drug prevention program at the Boys & Girls Club in Westminster, Calif., last year, she used what she learned to talk a few friends out of using marijuana.

The 14-year-old took the class again this year but worries that counseling her friends will become more difficult.

Recreational marijuana is now legal in California, which could bring a massive boom in drug sales and advertising when stores can begin selling the drug to adults without a prescription in January.

Raygoza believes that as more people 21 and older use marijuana legally, teenagers will have trouble understanding that they shouldn't use it. Teens may also have easier access to the drug as recreational pot shops start to open, she said.

Raygoza already sees many places selling medical marijuana.

"Now that there are so many shops … kids have a better chance of getting their hands on it," she said. "And having a discussion with them like this could be a little harder."

Make no mistake: Marijuana is still illegal for youths.

Last November, voters approved Proposition 64, the Adult Use of Marijuana Act, making California one of eight states—plus the District of Columbia—to legalize the drug for recreational use. The measure immediately made it legal for those 21 and older to possess up to 1 ounce, or about 28.5 grams, of cannabis. It delayed legal pot sales from licensed stores until January 2018.

The legalization of recreational marijuana for adults in California and other states poses an added challenge for drug education and prevention programs. Teachers are trying to explain the risks of marijuana just as stores are preparing to open and marketers are planning campaigns.

Medical marijuana has been legal in California for more than 20 years, but experts say the new law on recreational marijuana could prompt more youths to believe that the drug is safe.

---

*Originally published as Anna Gorman, "Teaching Teens the Perils of Pot as Marketplace Grows," *Kaiser Health News*, November 29, 2017. Reprinted with permission of the publisher.

"That is an unintended consequence of legalization," said Pam Luna, a consultant with the Rand Corp., a nonpartisan research organization. "They think that if it's legal, it must be OK."

Luna, who trains teachers on drug prevention education, said legalization has also prompted questions and confusion among young people. They may be getting misinformation—and peer pressure—through social media, she said.

While evidence shows that medical marijuana can help ease chronic pain and other conditions, use of the drug is linked to poor respiratory health and increased car accidents. Among adolescents, marijuana use can have negative effects on their cognitive and mental health.

Recent studies show that teens who use marijuana frequently exhibit lower cognitive performance and brain function than those who don't. They also perform worse in school.

Despite that, teen perception of the harms of marijuana has dropped over time and many think it's safer than alcohol, according to Elizabeth D'Amico, a senior behavioral scientist at Rand. Currently, more than half of 10th- and 12th-graders believe that smoking marijuana isn't dangerous, according to a recent Rand report.

Adolescents in states with legal medical marijuana are less likely to believe the drug is harmful, research shows.

"The changing legal landscape has a lot to do with adolescents' changing perceptions," D'Amico said. "That's why we really need to change the conversation around this drug."

That conversation should remind young people about its potential harms and that recreational marijuana in California is still illegal for those under 21, she said.

The state Department of Public Health recently unveiled a website called "Let's Talk Cannabis" to explain the law. Youth will have to complete community service and undergo drug education or counseling if they are caught smoking, buying or possessing marijuana, the website says.

Advertising is another factor that may complicate drug prevention education for young people, said Stanton Glantz, a professor at the University of California–San Francisco School of Medicine.

Exposure to marijuana advertising is associated with the higher likelihood of using marijuana one year later, according to research.

"It's just everywhere now, and the market hasn't been fully opened," he said. "It's the same thing as alcohol and cigarette advertising. It is all directed at normalizing it and presenting it as a fun thing to do."

D'Amico said she and her children see the ongoing changes near their house in the San Fernando Valley. "It just creates a conversation pretty much every day because a new billboard pops up on our way to school," she said.

To provide most middle school students with up-to-date information about alcohol, marijuana and smoking, D'Amico developed a voluntary program called Project Choice, which is used by after-school programs like the Boys & Girls Club. In five sessions, participants role-play and discuss how to make healthful choices. They also talk about the pros and cons of marijuana and the differences between medical and recreational use.

During the first session at the Boys & Girls Club of Westminster recently, facilitator Jeovan Davila asked the group of students what percentage of eighth-graders they believed used marijuana over the past 30 days. The guesses ranged from 10 percent to 60 percent.

When Davila told them the correct answer was about 7 percent, the group looked surprised.

Davila said he doesn't lecture teens about what's right and wrong. Rather, he gives them facts to help them make their own decisions in the future. For example, if they know that most of their peers don't use marijuana, perhaps they will be less likely to use it.

With the legalization of marijuana and the discussion on social media, Davila has seen young people talking about the drug more. During the class, some said teens might want to use because they see their family members using marijuana legally.

"The kids do bring it up," he said. "We've just got to be ready, letting them know the facts."

Kaiser Health News is a nonprofit news service covering health issues. It is an editorially independent program of Kaiser Family Foundation that is not affiliated with Kaiser Permanente. KHN's coverage in California is supported in part by Blue Shield of California Foundation.

26. Challenging Marijuana Myths[*]

Nora D. Volkow

We know from abundant research that marijuana use during adolescence has the potential to set young people up for a cascade of life-altering events, impeding their success and hindering them from fulfilling their potential. Yet this reality is increasingly lost on teenagers. The annual Monitoring the Future (MTF) survey of drug use and attitudes has for several years shown a steady drop in the number of middle- and high-school students who think occasional or even regular marijuana users risk harming themselves physically or in other ways. This declining perception of risk parallels increased use. One in 15 high-school seniors now use marijuana daily. In fact, while most drug and alcohol use continues to decline or hold steady, marijuana is almost the only licit or illicit drug showing significant five-year increases in the MTF survey.

Young people's growing skepticism about marijuana's dangers is reflected in the questions I and other NIDA scientists receive from high school students every winter during our National Drug Facts Chat Day. This year's Chat Day—the biggest ever—was on January 31, and we received hundreds of questions about marijuana. Many of these students challenged our claims about the dangers of this drug, expressing their belief that it is safer than other drugs, that it is not actually addictive, or that it is even beneficial. Some teens are no doubt hearing and being influenced by marijuana's many outspoken advocates, who claim that the drug does not deserve continued Schedule I status and that decades of prevention messaging have overstated its dangers. The ongoing public conversation over medical marijuana may contribute to the impression that, since some people use marijuana therapeutically, it couldn't be that harmful.

But given that now nearly half of teens try marijuana before they graduate, some of their skepticism about the drug's dangers could also be based on their own direct personal experiences, or that of their friends. If a young person smokes marijuana once or twice and suffers no apparent ill effects, it might be natural to conclude that NIDA and other authorities are wrong—or at least stretching the truth—about the risks they face in using it.

The consequences of marijuana use indeed are somewhat different than those of

*Originally published as Nora D. Volkow, "Challenging Marijuana Myths," National Institute on Drug Abuse, https://www.drugabuse.gov/about-nida/directors-page/biography-dr-nora-volkow (February 2013).

other drugs, and they are likely to be less apparent to a casual teen user. Users of marijuana by itself are unlikely to risk a life-threatening overdose, for instance, and there is even some doubt as to whether it is as harmful to the lungs as tobacco (the jury is still out on lung cancer). Rather, marijuana use, particularly when initiated at a young age, sets the user on a downward life trajectory, one that is driven by a constellation of factors that include altered cognitive and social development. (I've discussed some of the recent evidence for this in previous messages.) Unfortunately, cognitive ability that declines over a span of months or years (as well as other, long-term effects on life and well-being) may not be the kind of harm that young people are easily able to perceive.

Given the increases we are seeing in marijuana use among this age group, it is more crucial than ever to challenge the impression many of them have that marijuana is a benign, unfairly demonized substance. We must also do more to counter their dangerous misconception that marijuana is not addictive. Research suggests that about 9 percent of all users become addicted and that, among those who start young, the percentage is closer to 17 percent—or one in six. A quarter to a half of those who use marijuana daily are addicted to the drug. Thus many of the nearly 7 percent of high-school seniors who say they smoke marijuana on a daily or near-daily basis are already addicted or are well on their way—besides functioning at a sub-optimal level all of the time.

We clearly face an uphill battle getting this message across. With recreational marijuana use recently legalized in two states and increasing public pressure to ease restrictions on the drug nationwide, the availability of this drug is bound to increase. Only time will tell how these factors influence teens' perception of marijuana's safety or lack thereof. The key may be to do a better job of educating America's youth about the value of their brains, and how utterly important it is not to engage in behaviors that could permanently compromise that organ during a very vulnerable period in its development.

27. Drugs in the Public Workplace

*The HR Challenge**

JOE JARRET

Recently, Virginia Rep. Morgan Griffith (R) introduced a resolution in Congress designed to remove federal obstacles to the possession and prescription of medical marijuana in those states where the aforementioned is legal. H.R. 4498: Legitimate Use of Medicinal Marijuana Act, dubbed "LUMMA," is being carefully tracked by public and private entities across the United States. LUMMA provides that, among other things, the federal government assume a hands-off approach when it comes to the prescription of marijuana by a physician for medical use as well. It also covers the obtaining, possessing and transporting of medical marijuana within states permitting same, by an individual for that individual's medical use. The complete resolution is available online at www. govtrack.us/congress/bills/113/hr4498.

The legalized use of medical marijuana continues to gain momentum and popularity across the U.S. Nevertheless, public sector employers have a vested interest in testing their employees in an effort to detect drug and/or alcohol use. However, unlike their private sector counterparts, governmental employers are limited by constitutional considerations. It is well settled that drug testing by government employers constitutes a search under the Fourth Amendment to the United States Constitution. Probable cause and a search warrant are generally required for government searches, although the Supreme Court has carved out some exceptions. One such exception is the "special needs" exception to the search warrant requirement. This exception permits warrantless searches of public buildings by health and safety inspectors and other administrative searches and has also been applied to the testing of employees for drugs and alcohol. For a comprehensive examination of the law relative to employee testing and warrantless searches see: http://ctas-eli.ctas.tennessee.edu/reference/governmental-employee-drug-testing-consti tutional-issues#.

Based upon the above, public employers desirous of implementing some form of drug and/or alcohol testing must first determine who is to be tested and why it is necessary

---

*Originally published as Joe Jarret, "Drugs in the Public Workplace: The HR Challenge," *PA Times*, May 2, 2014. Reprinted with permission of the publisher.

to test each particular group. Is there a documented drug or alcohol problem in the particular workforce? Is the group performing duties that are "fraught with such risks of injury to others that even a momentary lapse of attention can have disastrous consequences," similar to train operators, nuclear power plant operators and customs agents who carry firearms and are directly involved in drug interdiction? In sum, a compelling interest must be identified. Once the interest is identified, the human resources director must insure that their entities' policies and procedures are sound and legally defensible.

Working Partners, an organization that helps public and private entities develop and maintain drug-free workplace programs, suggests that an effective drug-free workplace program consist of five elements. They are:

A Written Substance Abuse Policy

This serves as an executive summary of the substance abuse program. It sets the tone of the program, outlines the responsibilities of employer and employee, references available help and explains the program including prohibited conduct, types and circumstances of testing and the consequences for violations. For a drug-free safety program to be effective, all the parameters and procedures will have been thoughtfully developed and then articulated in a user-friendly policy statement for employees, along with detailed operational guidelines and accompanying appendices (forms) for use by management.

Employee Awareness and Education: Employees are made aware of and receive education about the policy, responsibilities, consequences, alcohol and drug information, their rights and the resources available to them through the company and community if they (or one of their family members) need help.

Supervisor Training: Supervisors need to be trained in their role within the company's substance abuse program. They should receive training about:

The company policy and procedures.
The impact of alcohol and drugs on the workplace.
How to recognize, document and confront a possible substance abuse problem.
How to refer a troubled employee to available resources and/or testing.
How to support an employee returning from treatment.

An Employee Assistance Plan of Action: An employer needs to identify a plan of action and the applicable resources for employees who seek help on their own, are referred by management for a possible problem with alcohol/drugs or have a positive alcohol/drug test. The possibilities range from a comprehensive contract with an external employee assistance program provider, to knowledge of the community service network that is subsidized with tax dollars.

Drug and Alcohol Testing (as appropriate): Systems presence testing (drug and alcohol testing) serves as the scientific, objective evidence that a certain level of substance exists within the employee's system. However, decisions about testing must balance the cost and practicalities of testing with the benefits. An employer has myriad decisions to make about their drug-free testing program. These include questions such as when they will test, who will be tested, what drugs will be tested for, what are the appropriate cutoff levels and what protocols and laboratory will be used.

Summary

As Congress and various state legislatures continue to take a fresh look at the use and possession of drugs in the workplace, public employers are encouraged to insure that their drug-testing policies, procedures and protocols are not in conflict with this ever-evolving body of law.

28. Marijuana at City Hall[*]

WILLIAM KIRCHHOFF *and* STEPHEN ZIMNEY

The legalization of marijuana has stirred hot debate on both sides of the issue. According to ProCon.org, some 20 states and the District of Columbia have currently made medical marijuana legal, and there is every indication that more will follow. Until just recently, local governments could adopt a position on its use at the workplace that held—as long as the federal government considered marijuana illegal—they need not spend time or energy trying to proactively deal with the issue. There was little to do except to maintain a zero-tolerance stand.

The game, however, has now changed. No longer will public managers be able to use previously existing case law to delay or deflect facing the medical marijuana issues head-on.

With Attorney General Eric Holder's August 2013 announcement that the federal government will no longer prosecute or incarcerate users, we coauthors submit this prediction: In those states where the use of medical marijuana is legal, managers and all government officials will be confronted with the pressing reality that employees will want, and in many cases demand, that they be allowed to treat certain medical conditions with medical marijuana, both on and off the job. It's also likely that other states will follow, given current societal trends.

The purpose of this essay is twofold. First, it will hopefully generate additional study and debate, since across-the-board conclusions are hard to draw. Be it the differences in political and cultural realities or the array of actions taken by localities in a given state against which others will be compared, we suspect that each administration will face the need to customize its thinking regarding marijuana adaptation protocols.

The second purpose is to provide local government managers with the framework that will allow them to begin dealing with this complex issue. In no way does this essay advocate for or against the use of medical marijuana. That discussion is left to physicians and scientists. But the essay does postulate that managers will have to wrestle with the practicalities, friction points, and dilemmas associated with the use of medical marijuana in the workplace. It also offers suggestions on how to practically and strategically address medical marijuana at city hall.

---

*Originally published as William Kirchhoff and Stephen Zimney, "Marijuana at City Hall," *PM Magazine*, December 2013. Reprinted with permission of the publisher.

Profound Culture Swing

According to a 2013 Brookings Institute study, *The New Politics of Marijuana Legalization: Why Public Opinion Is Changing*, public opinion has shifted dramatically toward support for the legalization of marijuana in less than a decade. Polls consistently show that substantially more than 50 percent of Americans support legalized medical marijuana. The ascendancy of the public's acceptance of it is nothing short of astonishing.

This year Colorado and Washington became the first states to legalize the recreational use of marijuana from among the 20-plus states that had already legalized marijuana for medical use when this copy was written. It is also noteworthy that the adoption of the resolution "In Support of States Setting Their Own Marijuana Policies Without Federal Interference" by the U.S. Conference of Mayors this year advises the federal government to back off and leave it up to the states and local governments as to how to regulate and manage marijuana.

A Proactive Approach

The speed of this emergent trend clearly warns us that, beyond the need to institute well-thought-out policies and practices to achieve effective management and accountability, pressure will also mount on city hall to develop new standards with a new mindset and a different business model—one that is much more adaptable to this 21st century sea change in workplace dynamics.

Tiptoeing away from medical marijuana at city hall is a mistake. Resisting on the basis of knee-jerk opinion will surely backfire. Smart managers will proactively address this change by seeking input and new ideas from employees, lawyers, physicians, insurance industry members, and others.

Failure to get ahead of the problem will result in unnecessary legal, operational, and morale costs for public entities and the taxpayers they serve. It appears that only a handful of forward leaning city managers, such as Steve Pinkerton, Davis, California, and Betsy Fretwell, Las Vegas, Nevada, are using task forces and focus groups to address the long-term ramifications of medical marijuana in the public workplace.

To put it simply, what do we do now that we know employees have a right to use legally prescribed medical marijuana?

Choices with Consequences

What seems to be a practical and appropriate first step is to think through all of the obvious day-to-day impacts that legalized medical marijuana might bring with it, including insurance and risk management issues, different testing protocols, training requirements, and other challenges.

But our research and work with focus groups tells us that there is a spider web cause-and-effect element to this, which can exponentially increase the frequency and consequences of decision making. Consider one example.

Blumberg Businessweek has reported that K-9 experts in Colorado and Washington worry that a dog trained to sniff out drugs cannot differentiate between marijuana and such other drugs as methamphetamine. And it is difficult and costly to retrain them otherwise. That means, according to the government lawyers, patrolling with K-9s currently used to sniff out drugs runs the risk of civil rights violations and lawsuits. So how do the local government manager, police chief, and K-9 supervisor handle this?

Do you simply retire and replace the animals like obsolete equipment at great cost to the operations of the police department, including the emotional reaction from the K-9 officers who view their animals as their partners? How the handlers react and what their labor organization does will require some deep thinking and controversial decision making.

Mishandled, the financial, emotional, and operational well-being of local governments currently using K-9s for marijuana detection will be stressed if the disposition of the animals is not handled satisfactorily to all interests.

This is just one of many "choices with consequences" that the legalization of marijuana for medical purposes will drop on the manager's decision-making plate.

The tension between those who believe that employees have an ethical imperative as well as the legal right to treat a legitimate medical problem with marijuana, and those who oppose such a viewpoint for any one of the many valid concerns associated with the use of legal medical marijuana, is certain to complicate matters.

While these unintended consequences will eventually be sorted out, there is a more complicated and strategic issue: How do we change the organizational culture surrounding medical marijuana?

To expect the organization as a whole to accept new policies that require some managers to suspend or eliminate deeply ingrained feelings, learning experiences, and biases without recognizing that such a change requires careful navigation between the intellectual versus the emotional side of any type of change activity is professionally wrong.

A manager can either adopt a reactive wait-and-see approach or move the organization into a proactive posture. If the wait-and-see reaction is subscribed to, then we submit that the results will be similar to such turtle-like adaptation to social changes we experienced in the past decades regarding sexual harassment, workplace discrimination, and diversity at city hall.

If managers can be open to the new thinking that medical marijuana should be treated no differently than such prescription drugs as Vicodin, Endocet, and Oxycodone, then the toll on the organization can be mitigated.

Agreement with this supposition requires the drafting of policies and the implementation of management procedures that benefit from the multiple viewpoints residing in the communities of healthcare professionals, behavioral researchers, safety experts, and a locality's own employees and union officials.

In the long run, we will need all of their input to help effectively maintain maximum organizational productivity within the parameters of court decisions, moral concerns, and practical considerations.

Strategic Approach: Establish a Framework

Some fundamental questions and conflicts around moral, ethical, and values-based issues will necessarily be raised and accordingly will demand careful debate. We suspect that this exercise will lead to the inevitable conclusion that culture change is the linchpin dynamic that spells the difference between successful versus unsuccessful adaptation to medical marijuana.

Four stages of activity are required for an effective strategic planning effort. The players need to be interdisciplinary to include senior management personnel from all major functional and departmental entities within the organization.

Stage 1. Identify the collective corporate and social values at play within and throughout the organization around the subject of medical marijuana.

1. What is the corporate "world view" around employee relations principles?
2. What are the personal values of key senior management personnel, and how do those views impact organizational orientation around the issue?
3. Where are the disconnects between implicit (often hidden) values and the explicit values imbedded in formal policy statements (that now surface because of this new debate)?
4. Which values are, or potentially will be, in conflict with each other?

Stage 2. Identify the juxtaposed realities within the organization that are/will come in conflict vis-à-vis the introduction of medical marijuana.

1. Safety concerns versus equitable personnel deployment.
2. Legal exposure versus relaxed HR policy formation.
3. Labor relations versus political imperatives.
4. External PR (image) impacts versus internal adaptation realities.

Stage 3. Convene functional areas separately in groups (adding staff as needed) to formulate an integration template for their area of responsibility in the organization, taking the output of Stages 1 and 2 as the starting-point guidelines for their efforts. Necessarily, different functional areas and departments will have different priorities and trade-offs. Each group should be encouraged to develop its scenarios without consideration of the rest of the organization, so as to get to the bottom-line implementation paradigm for their functional area.

Stage 4. Reconvene the larger organization planning group, with senior representatives of each functional area returning with the output(s) from their group's individual efforts. The goal in this stage is to complete an organization-wide integration of all plans, ironing out the conflicts and inconsistencies that will undoubtedly surface. Only with thorough and careful efforts can the unintended consequences of "policies in conflict" be minimized and hopefully avoided once the integration and its policies "go live." It goes without saying that legalization of medical marijuana places many a quandary at the doorstep of city hall. This essay is intended to help managers begin addressing all the complicated policy-making issues that will accompany this sea change in workplace dynamics.

Medical Marijuana Policy Question Checklist

Throughout the process of formulating policy, it is helpful to have a set of guidelines to keep policymakers on track. Local governments need to examine the following questions before establishing policies pertaining to medical marijuana management:

- What is the purpose of your medical marijuana management policy?
- Who will be covered?
- What behavior will be prohibited?
- Will employees be required to notify their supervisors of their use of medical marijuana? What will the consequences be if the policy is violated?
- Will there be a reeducation effort and return-to-work provision?
- How will employee rights and confidentiality be protected?
- Who will be responsible for enforcing the policy for compliance?

Proactive Decision-Making Matrix

For manager who want to take a proactive approach, a decision-making tool—the "Medical Marijuana Decision Matrix"—will help them sort out the requirements for necessary change as well as identify accompanying dilemmas.

The matrix requires that the centerpiece—the 3-by-3 grid—be filled out, with all of the organization's job positions distributed across the nine boxes based on the job performance conditions and the performance impairment impact that accordingly attends each job position.

Some position impairment categorizations are clear and simple, with others falling in the grey area. The propriety and common sense, for example, of restricting first responders and dispatchers from using medical marijuana is much clearer than when considering plan reviewer and librarian positions.

Our research and management experience points to the three large categories of employees into which all local job titles (see left side of figure) can be slotted. They are public safety employees, non-safety employees, and direct public contact employees.

Across the top of the grid are the three policy categories that can be applied to each job position. For each, the city can declare medical marijuana as clearly allowable, conditionally allowable, and clearly not allowable.

What makes this task particularly daunting are the interconnecting and often conflicting pressures that can and will emerge within and between four impacting realities that, in our chart, surround the central grid.

Organization integration requires that we anticipate and eliminate, to the extent possible, the lack of synergy between the legal implications, human resource policy and practices, and operational protocols. How, for example, are the differing perspectives and beliefs between legal, human resources, and department directors dealt with? Who decides that an employee is impaired or otherwise—a medical, human resource, or legal specialist?

Policy dilemmas will emerge from the introduction of new policy around medical marijuana use and management. Are we calling into question, for example, existing policy that no longer is compatible with our new stand? And, do we create one new policy that is incompatible with other policies that are trying to meet a different set of pressures in our organization's reality?

What do you do with police resources that were dedicated to the arrest and prosecution of medical marijuana users? Is it best to transfer the positions to other duties or eliminate positions to achieve cost savings?

Will there be a second-chance policy and if so, will it be the same for all employees, including senior management staff? Will certain positions and/or work units be subjected to more frequent and invasive drug testing for medical marijuana than others? Do testing policies for marijuana clash with existing policies for such legal pain medications as Vicodin?

How do we make such policies compatible? Will that effort call many more policies into question, as clear inequities between policies begin to emerge?

Collateral fallout that attends our efforts will include unintended dislocations, community backlash resulting in elected official conflicts that politicize policymaking efforts. How does the fire chief, for example, deal with the potential need to reassign first responders to non-field duty when current budgeting has eliminated the needed number of slots that are required to handle the new reality?

29. VA Clears the Air on Talking to Patients About Marijuana Use*

MICHELLE ANDREWS

"Don't ask, don't tell" is how many veterans have approached health care conversations about marijuana use with the doctors they see from the Department of Veterans Affairs.

Worried that owning up to using the drug could jeopardize their VA benefits—even if they're participating in a medical marijuana program approved by their state—veterans have often kept mum. That may be changing under a new directive from the Veterans Health Administration urging vets and their physicians to open up on the subject.

The new guidance directs VA clinical staff and pharmacists to discuss with veterans how their use of medical marijuana could interact with other medications or aspects of their care, including treatment for pain management or post-traumatic stress disorder.

The directive leaves in place a key prohibition: VA providers are still not permitted to refer veterans to state-approved medical marijuana programs, since the drug is illegal under federal law, with no accepted medical use.

That disconnect makes veterans wary, said Michael Krawitz, a disabled Air Force veteran in Ironto, Virginia, who takes oxycodone and marijuana to treat extensive injuries he suffered in a non-combat–related motorcycle accident while stationed in Guam in 1984.

"Vets are happy that there's a policy, but they're unnerved by that prohibition," he said.

Krawitz, 55, is the executive director of Veterans for Medical Cannabis Access, an advocacy group. He has always been open with his VA doctors about his medical marijuana use and hasn't suffered any negative consequences. But Krawitz said he has worked with veterans who have been kicked out of their VA pain management program after a positive drug test and told they couldn't continue until they stopped using cannabis.

Such actions are usually misunderstandings that can be corrected, he said, but he suggests that the Veterans Health Administration should provide clear guidance to its staff about the new directive so veterans aren't harmed if they admit to using marijuana.

Although the new guidance encourages communication about veterans' use of marijuana, the agency's position on the drug hasn't changed, said Curtis Cashour, a VA spokesman.

---

*Originally published as Michelle Andrews, "VA Clears the Air on Talking to Patients About Marijuana Use," *Kaiser Health News*, January 9, 2018. Reprinted with permission of the publisher.

Cashour referred to a quote from Veterans Affairs Secretary David Shulkin at a White House briefing last May, who said he thought that among "some of the states that have put in appropriate controls [on the use of medical marijuana], there may be some evidence that this is beginning to be helpful. And we're interested in looking at that and learning from that." But until federal law changes, the VA is not "able to prescribe medical marijuana."

Cashour declined to provide further information about the new directive.

Under federal law, marijuana is classified as a Schedule 1 drug, meaning it has no accepted medical use and a high potential for abuse. Heroin and LSD are other Schedule 1 drugs. Doctors aren't permitted to prescribe marijuana. Instead, in states that have legalized the use of medical marijuana, doctors may refer patients to state-approved programs that allow marijuana use in certain circumstances. (Doctors can, however, prescribe three drugs approved by the Food and Drug Administration that are made of or similar to a synthetic form of THC, a chemical in marijuana.)

Twenty-nine states and the District of Columbia have laws that allow people to use marijuana legally for medical purposes. Patients who have a disease or condition that's approved for treatment with marijuana under the law are generally registered with the state and receive marijuana through state-regulated dispensaries or other facilities.

Moves by states to legalize marijuana for medical or recreational use have created a confusing landscape for patients to navigate. Attorney General Jeff Sessions announced last week he would rescind an Obama-era policy that discouraged federal prosecution for marijuana use in states where it is legal. That action has further clouded the issue.

Some consider caution a good thing. The accelerating trend of states approving marijuana for medical and recreational purposes may be getting ahead of the science to support it, they say.

A report released last January by the National Academies of Sciences, Engineering and Medicine examined more than 10,000 scientific abstracts about the health effects of marijuana and its chemical compounds on conditions ranging from epilepsy to glaucoma. The experts found conclusive evidence for a relatively limited number of conditions, including relief of chronic pain, nausea and vomiting associated with chemotherapy and muscle spasms associated with multiple sclerosis.

"I believe that there are chemicals in marijuana that have medicinal properties," said Dr. Otis Brawley, chief medical officer at the American Cancer Society. "I would love to know what those are, what their medicinal properties are and what the dose should be." But, he said, studies are extremely challenging to do because of restrictions in the United States on conducting research on Schedule 1 drugs.

No matter where the research stands, getting a complete medication or drug history should be standard procedure at any medical appointment, say medical providers.

In that respect, the guidance from the VA is a positive development.

"It's absolutely critical that you know what your patients are taking, if only to be better able to assess what is going on," said Dr. J. Michael Bostwick, a psychiatrist at Mayo Clinic in Rochester, Minn., who has written on medical marijuana use.

Kaiser Health News *is a nonprofit news service covering health issues. It is an editorially independent program of Kaiser Family Foundation that is not affiliated with Kaiser Permanente.*

30. Marijuana Use and PTSD Among Veterans[*]

MARCEL O. BONN-MILLER *and*
GLENNA S. ROUSSEAU

Marijuana use for medical conditions is an issue of growing concern. Some Veterans use marijuana to relieve symptoms of PTSD and several states specifically approve the use of medical marijuana for PTSD. However, controlled studies have not been conducted to evaluate the safety or effectiveness of medical marijuana for PTSD. Thus, there is no evidence at this time that marijuana is an effective treatment for PTSD. In fact, research suggests that marijuana can be harmful to individuals with PTSD.

Epidemiology: Marijuana use has increased over the past decade. In 2013, a study found that 19.8 million people reported using marijuana in the past month, with 8.1 million using almost every day (1). Daily use has increased 60 percent in the prior decade (1). A number of factors are associated with increased risk of marijuana use, including diagnosis of PTSD (2), social anxiety disorder (3), other substance use, particularly during youth (4), and peer substance use (5).

Cannabis Use Disorder among Veterans Using VA Health Care: There has been no study of marijuana use in the overall Veteran population. What we do know comes from looking at data of Veterans using VA health care, who may not be representative of Veterans overall. When considering the subset of Veterans seen in VA health care with co-occurring PTSD and substance use disorders (SUD), cannabis use disorder has been the most diagnosed SUD since 2009. The percentage of Veterans in VA with PTSD and SUD who were diagnosed with cannabis use disorder increased from 13.0 percent in fiscal year (FY) 2002 to 22.7 percent in FY 2014. As of FY 2014, there are more than 40,000 Veterans with PTSD and SUD seen in VA diagnosed with cannabis use disorder (6).

Graph of VHA Trends in diagnoses by drug for Veterans with PTSD and SUD in VA Health Care: This graph shows the rates of SUD diagnoses (y-axis) by drug type (lines on graph: amphetamines, cannabis, cocaine, and opioids) among Veterans with PTSD treated in VA health care. Data is shown for each fiscal year (FY) from 2002 through

*Originally published as Marcel O. Bonn-Miller and Glenna S. Rousseau, "Marijuana Use and PTSD Among Veterans," U.S. Department of Veterans Affairs, May 10, 2017. https://www.ptsd.va.gov/professional/co-occurring/marijuana_use_ptsd_veterans.asp.

2014 (x-axis). Data was provided by the Veterans Health Administration, 2015. Cannabis use disorder is the most diagnosed SUD among Veterans with PTSD in VA health care in FY14. Rates of cannabis use disorder diagnoses grew from 13.0 percent in FY02 to 22.7 percent in FY14. Cocaine use disorder was the most diagnosed SUD among Veterans with PTSD in FY02, at 18.9 percent. In FY09, cocaine became less common than cannabis use disorder (15.4 percent and 15.9 percent respectively), and as of FY14, cocaine use disorder is the second most common SUD diagnosis among Veterans with PTSD, at 14.8 percent. Among this subset of Veterans, opioid use disorder was diagnosed at a rate of 9.9 percent in FY02, rising to 12.5 percent in FY14. Amphetamine use disorder was diagnosed at a rate of 2.6 percent in FY02 and rose to 4.4 percent in FY14.

Problems Associated with Marijuana Use: Marijuana use is associated with medical and psychiatric problems. These problems may be caused by using, but they also may reflect the characteristics of the people who use marijuana. Medical problems include chronic bronchitis, abnormal brain development among early adolescent initiators, and impairment in short-term memory, motor coordination and the ability to perform complex psychomotor tasks such as driving. Psychiatric problems include psychosis and impairment in cognitive ability. Quality of life can also be affected through poor life satisfaction, decreased educational attainment, and increased sexual risk-taking behavior (7). Chronic marijuana use also can lead to addiction, with an established and clinically significant withdrawal syndrome (8).

Active Ingredients and Route of Administration: Marijuana contains a variety of components (cannabinoids), most notably delta-9-tetrahydrocannabinol (THC) the primary psychoactive compound in the marijuana plant. There are a number of other cannabinoids, such as cannabidiol (CBD), cannabinol (CBN), and cannabigerol (CBG). Marijuana can vary in cannabinoid concentration, such as in the ratio of THC to other cannabinoids (CBD in particular). Therefore, the effects of marijuana use (e.g., experience of a high, anxiety, sleep) vary as a function of the concentration of cannabinoids (e.g., THC/CBD). In addition, the potency of cannabinoids can vary. For example, the concentration of THC in the marijuana plant can range in strength from less than 1 percent to 30 percent based upon strain and cultivation methods. In general, the potency of THC in the marijuana plant has increased as much as 10-fold over the past 40 years (9,10). Recently, cannabis extract products, such as waxes and oils, have been produced and sold in which the concentration of THC can be as high as 90 percent. Thus, an individual could unknowingly consume a very high dose of THC in one administration, which increases the risk of an adverse reaction.

Marijuana can be consumed in many different forms (e.g., flower, hash, oil, wax, food products, tinctures). Administration of these forms also can take different routes: inhalation (smoking or vaporizing), ingestion, and topical application. Given the same concentration/ratio of marijuana, smoking or vaporizing marijuana produces similar effects (11); however, ingesting the same dose results in a delayed onset and longer duration of effect (12). Not all marijuana users may be aware of the delayed effect caused by ingestion, which may result in greater consumption and a stronger effect than intended.

Neurobiology: Research has consistently demonstrated that the human endocannabinoid system plays a significant role in PTSD. People with PTSD have greater availability of cannabinoid type 1 (CB1) receptors as compared to trauma-exposed or healthy controls (13,14). As a result, marijuana use by individuals with PTSD may result in short-term reduction of PTSD symptoms. However, data suggest that continued use of marijuana among individuals with PTSD may lead to a number of negative consequences, including marijuana tolerance (via reductions in CB1 receptor density and/or efficiency) and addiction (15). Though recent work has shown that CB1 receptors may return after periods of marijuana abstinence (16), individuals with PTSD may have particular difficulty quitting (17).

Marijuana as a Treatment for PTSD: The belief that marijuana can be used to treat PTSD is limited to anecdotal reports from individuals with PTSD who say that the drug helps with their symptoms. There have been no randomized controlled trials, a necessary "gold standard" for determining efficacy. Administration of oral CBD has been shown to decrease anxiety in those with and without clinical anxiety (18). This work has led to the development and testing of CBD treatments for individuals with social anxiety (19), but not yet among individuals with PTSD. With respect to THC, one open trial of 10 participants with PTSD showed THC was safe and well tolerated and resulted in decreases in hyperarousal symptoms (20).

Treatment for Marijuana Addiction: People with PTSD have particular difficulty stopping their use of marijuana and responding to treatment for marijuana addiction. They have greater craving and withdrawal than those without PTSD (21), and greater likelihood of marijuana use during the six months following a quit attempt (17). However, these individuals can benefit from the many evidence-based treatments for marijuana addiction, including cognitive behavioral therapy, motivational enhancement, and contingency management (22). Thus, providers should still utilize these options to support reduction/abstinence.

Clinical Recommendations: Treatment providers should not ignore marijuana use in their PTSD patients. The VA/DoD PTSD Clinical Practice Guideline (2010) recommends providing evidence-based treatments for the individual disorders concurrently. PTSD providers should offer education about problems associated with long-term marijuana use and make a referral to a substance use disorder (SUD) specialist if they do not feel they have expertise in treating substance use.

Individuals with comorbid PTSD and SUD do not need to wait for a period of abstinence before addressing their PTSD. A growing number of studies demonstrate that that these patients can tolerate trauma-focused treatment and that these treatments do not worsen substance use outcomes. Therefore, providers have a range of options to help improve the lives of patients with the co-occurring disorders. For more information, see Treatment of Co-Occurring PTSD and Substance Use Disorder in VA.

REFERENCES

Abrams, D.I., Vizoso, H.P., Shade, S.B., Jay, C., Kelly, M.E. & Benowitz, N.L. (2007). Vaporization as a smokeless cannabis delivery system: A pilot study. *Clinical Pharmacology & Therapeutics*, 82, 572–578.

Bergamaschi, M.M., Queiroz, R.H.C., Hortes, M., Chagas, N., de Oliveira, C.G., De Martinis, B.S., Kapczinski, F., Quevedo, J., Roesler, R., Schröder, N., Nardi, A.E., Martín-Santos, R., Hallak, J.E.C., Zuardi, A.W. & Crippa, J.A.S. (2011). Cannabidiol reduces the anxiety induced by simulated public speaking in treatment-naïve social phobia patients. *Neuropsychopharmacology*, 36, 1219–1226.

Boden, M.T., Babson, K.A., Vujanovic, A.A., Short, N.A. & Bonn-Miller, M. (2013). Posttraumatic stress disorder and cannabis use characteristics among military Veterans with cannabis dependence. *The American Journal on Addictions*, 22, 277–284.

Bonn-Miller, M.O., Moos, R.H., Boden, M.T., Long, W.R., Kimerling, R. & Trafton, J.A. (2015). The impact of posttraumatic stress disorder on cannabis quit success. *The American Journal of Drug and Alcohol Abuse*, 41(4): 339–44.

Buckner, J.D., Schmidt, N.B., Lang, A.R., Small, J.W., Schluach, R.C. & Lewinsohn, P.M. (2008). Specificity of social anxiety disorder as a risk factor for alcohol and cannabis dependence. *Journal of Psychiatric Research*, 42, 230–239.

Budney, A.J., Hughes, J.R., Moore, B.A. & Vandrey, R. (2004). Review of the validity and significance of cannabis withdrawal syndrome. *American Journal of Psychiatry*, 161, 1967–1977.

Butterworth, P., Slade, T. & Degenhardt, L. (2014). Factors associated with the timing and onset of cannabis use and cannabis use disorder: Results from the 2007 Australian National Survey of Mental Health and Well-Being. *Drug and Alcohol Review*, 33, 555–564.

Cougle, J.R., Bonn-Miller, M.O., Vujanovic, A.A., Zvolensky, M.J. & Hawkins, K.A. (2011). Posttraumatic stress disorder and cannabis use in a nationally representative sample. *Psychology of Addictive Behaviors*, 25, 554–558.

Crippa, J.A., Zuardi, A.W., MartÃn-Santos, R., Bhattacharyya, S., Atakan, Z., McGuire, P. & Fusar-Poli, P. (2009). Cannabis and anxiety: a critical review of the evidence. *Human Psychopharmacology*, 24, 515–523.

Grotenhermen, F. (2003). Pharmacokinetics and pharmacodynamics of cannabinoids. *Clinical Pharmacokinetics*, 42, 327–360.

Hirvonen, J., Goodwin, R.S., Li, C-T., Terry, G.E., Zoghbi, S.S., Morse, C., Pike, V.W., Volkow, N.D., Huestis, M.A. & Innis, R.B. (2012). Reversible and regionally selective downregulation of brain cannabinoid CB1 receptors in chronic daily cannabis smokers. *Molecular Psychiatry*, 17, 642–649.

Kendall, D.A. & Alexander, S.P.H. (2009). *Behavioral neurobiology of the endocannabinoid system. Current topics in behavioral neurosciences.* Heidelberg: Springer-Verlag.

Mehmedic, Z., Chandra, S., Slade, D., Denham, H., Foster, S., Patel, A.S., Ross, S.A., Khan, I.A. & ElSohly, M.A. (2010). Potency trends of Δ9-THC and other cannabinoids in confiscated cannabis preparations from 1993 to 2008. *Journal of Forensic Sciences*, 55, 1209–1217.

Neumeister, A., Normandin, M.D., Pietrzak, R.H., Piomelli, D., Zheng, M.Q., Gujarro-Anton, A., Potenza, M.N., Bailey, C.R., Lin, S.F., Najafzaden, S., Ropchan, J., Henry, S., Corsi-Travali, S., Carson, R.E. & Huang, Y. (2013). Elevated brain cannabinoid CB1 receptor availability in post-traumatic stress disorder: A positron emission tomography study. *Molecular Psychiatry*, 18, 1034–1040.

Passie, T., Emrich, H.M., Brandt, S.D. & Halpern, J.H. (2012). Mitigation of post-traumatic stress symptoms by Cannabis resin: A review of the clinical and neurobiological evidence. *Drug Testing and Analysis*, 4, 649–659.

Program Evaluation and Resource Center, V.A., 2015.

Roffman, R.A. & Stephens, R.S. (2006). *Cannabis dependence: its nature, consequences, and treatment. International research monographs in the addictions.* Cambridge, UK; New York: Cambridge University Press.

Roitman, P., Mechoulam, R., Cooper-Kazaz, R. & Shalev, A. (2014). Preliminary, open-label, pilot study of add-on oral Δ9-tetrahydrocannabinol in chronic post-traumatic stress disorder. *Clinical Drug Investigation*, 34, 587–591.

SAMHSA. (2014). Results from the 2013 National Survey on Drug Use and Health: Summary of National Findings. (Vol. NSDUH Series H-48, HHS Publication No. (SMA) 13–4795). Rockville, MD: Substance Abuse and Mental Health Services Administration.

Sevigny, E.L., Pacula, R.L. & Heaton, P. (2014) The effects of medical marijuana laws on potency. *International Journal of Drug Policy*, 25, 308–319.

Volkow, N.D., Baler, R.D., Compton, W.M. & Weiss, S.R.B. (2014). Adverse health effects of marijuana use. *New England Journal of Medicine*, 370, 2219–2227.

von Sydow, K., Lieb, R., Pfister, H., Höefler, M. & Wittchen, H.U. (2002). What predicts incident use of cannabis and progression to abuse and dependence? A 4-year prospective examination of risk factors in a community sample of adolescents and young adults. *Drug and Alcohol Dependence*, 68, 49–64.

31. Opponents of Legalized Marijuana Take Aim at Stoned Driving*

ANDY METZGER

Legalization of marijuana would result in greater dangers on Massachusetts roadways, where authorities are ill-equipped to even know whether drivers are intoxicated by the leafy green drug, opponents of Question 4 said.

"If this ballot question passes we're asking police officers on the street to do an impossible task. We're asking them to determine if somebody's impaired or not," Rep. Paul Tucker, the former chief of police in Salem, said at a press conference outside the State House.

Unlike drunk driving tests where blood and breathe measurements can give a clear indication of a motorist's state of intoxication, marijuana drug tests generally measure whether someone has used the substance over a longer period of time.

Jim Borghesani, the spokesman for the campaign seeking to legalize adult marijuana usage through the ballot initiative, said studies are underway that could potentially improve enforcement, and said police can now take action when someone is driving erratically.

"Police officers have every ability to pull over somebody who's driving impaired and take them off the road," Borghesani told reporters. There will be two studies in the field next year with researchers exploring the use of "intelligent fingerprinting" and saliva to determine recent marijuana usage, he said.

Polls have shown voters leaning toward passage of Question 4, which would legalize adult possession, home-use and eventually the retail purchase of marijuana. Opponents say easier access to the drug especially in its slow-acting edible form could create a menace on streets and highways.

Mary Maguire, the director of public and legislative affairs for the American Automobile Association in Massachusetts, said marijuana consumption hampers drivers' ability to judge distance, reduces peripheral vision and coordination, and makes it more challenging to stay in a driving lane.

"Driving is the most dangerous thing that we all do, most of us, every single day.

---

*Originally published as Andy Metzger, "Opponents of Legalized Marijuana Take Aim at Stoned Driving," *Berkshire Eagle*, October 25, 2016. Reprinted with permission of the publisher.

Let's not make it even more dangerous to get behind the wheel here in Massachusetts," said Maguire, who said marijuana also impairs drivers' judgement and reaction times.

Mark Leahy, the former chief of the Northborough police who is now executive director of the Massachusetts Chiefs of Police Association, told the News Service that police can receive training to become drug recognition experts or D.R.E.s but it is expensive.

Leahy said officers can make a stoned driving arrest even without D.R.E. training but said there is a "horrific conviction rate" even for drunk driving, a crime where there is widespread public knowledge and tests that can quantify the amount of alcohol in someone's bloodstream.

Sam Cole, a spokesman for the Colorado Department of Transportation, told the News Service the state has upwards of 250 drug recognition experts but no roadside device to measure the level of marijuana in a person's system.

In Colorado, where retail marijuana sales began in 2014, drivers suspected of marijuana intoxication are asked to consent to a blood test after they are arrested, with penalties for refusal, Cole said, and the state's legislature set a limit of 5 nanograms of THC an intoxicating chemical in marijuana per milliliter. He said there is disagreement about whether that is an accurate measure.

Essex County District Attorney Jonathan Blodgett said the state is "years away" from a roadside test for marijuana intoxication that is approved by the courts.

Borghesani said Massachusetts lawmakers should have set standards to convict someone for driving while high on marijuana after voters decriminalized possession of up to an ounce of marijuana in 2008 or after voters legalized marijuana for medical purposes in 2012.

"What we do need is the ability to prove in court that somebody is impaired on marijuana. We think the Legislature should have done that after decriminalization passed in 2008 when it was the Legislature and the [district attorneys] and the sheriffs who said, 'We can't control the roads,'" Borghesani said. "Two thousand and twelve they all said the same thing: 'It's going to be carnage on the streets. We can't prove marijuana intoxication.' It passed. They did nothing."

Earlier this year Rep. Shawn Dooley, a Norfolk Republican, proposed outlawing smoking marijuana while driving—something that is not in of itself illegal in the state—but his proposal did not make it into law.

Even without full legalization, marijuana is commonly and often openly used around Massachusetts. Mothers against Drunk Driving, MADD, opposes all impaired driving but does not take a position on the legalization of recreational marijuana, according to a spokesperson.

"Drugged driving, like drunk driving, is 100 percent preventable," Becky Iannotta, a communications manager at the anti-drunk-driving group, said.

Reisa Clardy, the widow of Trooper Thomas Clardy who was killed in a car crash by an allegedly marijuana-intoxicated driver, said the proposal would lead to "more fatalities" in a video released by opponents of Question 4 on Monday. Borghesani said in a statement if the allegedly stoned driver is convicted, he should be "punished to the fullest extent of the law."

Citing an AAA study, Maguire said fatal crashes involving drivers who have recently used marijuana "nearly doubled" in Washington state which legalized marijuana around the same time as Colorado. Borghesani pointed to the study's own acknowledgment that "the data available cannot be used to assess whether a given driver was actually impaired."

Cole said the percentage of the Colorado state patrol's intoxicated driving stops for marijuana ticked up from 12 percent of driving under the influence incidents in 2013—before full legalization—to 18 percent in 2015. During the same time period, officers have become better trained to detect marijuana intoxication, he said.

"The data is very murky," Cole said, recommending states set a legal limit, train officers, gather data, and launch a public safety awareness campaign.

32. Why the Latest News on Marijuana and Car Crashes Has Some Experts Skeptical*

Daniel C. Vock

A demonstration of a car that the Colorado Department of Transportation took to 4/20 rallies and concerts to promote safe driving.

States that legalized marijuana sales have higher rates of car crashes than neighboring states that don't allow pot sales. At least, that's what researchers from the Highway Loss Data Institute, an insurance group, concluded, after scouring 2.5 million insurance claims that drivers filed over the last three years.

The group found that Colorado, Oregon and Washington all saw increases in damage reports compared to other states. That was true even after its researchers tried to take into account weather, types of vehicles, population density and other variables that might otherwise explain the increases.

"Every measurement that we took indicated that crash risk had increased," says Matt Moore, a senior vice president at the institute, which is affiliated with the Insurance Institute for Highway Safety.

The exact size of that increase is not as clear. In Colorado, for example, the institute determined that claims were 13.9 percent higher than the combined rates of neighboring states of Nebraska, Utah and Wyoming. But there were sharp differences among those states. Colorado's claims rate was 21 percent higher than Utah's, but only 3 percent higher than Wyoming's.

Researchers used state-to-state comparisons, rather than before-and-after analyses, so that the results aren't skewed by factors that are unrelated to marijuana legalization. Year-to-year changes in the economy and weather patterns, for example, can affect the numbers of crashes. By comparing different states in the same time period, the researchers can focus on the differences among states.

Still, Moore says the overall trend is evident. "We can be confident that after each of these states legalized recreational use, crash risk increased," he says. "If those who are making laws are concerned about highway safety, they need to be concerned about the increased risk associated with recreational use of marijuana."

---

*Originally published as Daniel C. Vock, "Why the Latest News on Marijuana and Car Crashes Has Some Experts Skeptical," *Governing*, June 26, 2017. Reprinted with permission of the publisher.

But that doesn't mean it's an open-and-shut case. Other experts, looking at other data, have seen no significant effect in the number of crashes since the first three states legalized marijuana sales. Some research even suggests that crashes have declined.

The Colorado State Patrol, for example, actually saw a slight decrease in the number of crashes involving impaired drivers it responded to between 2015 and 2016, from 1,582 crashes to 1,508. That category covers drivers under the influence of any substance, including alcohol, marijuana and other drugs.

Meanwhile, a team of researchers from Texas published a peer-reviewed study in the American Journal of Public Health last week that showed only a small difference in Colorado or Washington's crash rates, and they said it wasn't significant. The effect of "0.2 fatalities per billion vehicle miles traveled, would equate to approximately 77 excess crash fatalities (of 2,890 total) over nearly 38 million person-years of exposure in the three years since legalization. We do not view that as a clinically significant effect, but others might disagree," they explained.

The health researchers' work had several key differences with the study by the insurance group. They examined data from the federal government, which only includes information on fatal crashes and is collected by police officers rather than insurance agents. The health researchers also compared Colorado and Washington to a different group of control states than the insurance researchers had.

All of that makes Mason Tvert, the communications director for the Marijuana Policy Project, skeptical of the insurance industry study. The insurance study, Tvert notes, doesn't look at the causes for the increase in collisions they found. It only highlights the correlation between legal pot sales and increased insurance claims.

"They're a well-respected organization, and it's great they're taking a look at this," Tvert says. "But you need to take a holistic look at this issue. You can't look at just one study. There are as many studies showing no reason to be concerned as there are studies that might make you concerned."

The Marijuana Policy Project supports legalization of marijuana, but it also supports policies to crack down on people who drive while impaired by the drug. Even though it is legal to buy marijuana in Colorado, Oregon and Washington, it is still illegal to drive under the influence of the drug in those places.

One of the biggest problems police face in cracking down on driving under the influence of marijuana is that there is no uniformly accepted way of measuring marijuana impairment yet. Urine samples don't reliably indicate how recently someone used pot, because chemical indicators of marijuana use can stay in someone's system for days. Even blood samples, which are more reliable than urine tests, have limits. After smoking marijuana, for example, the THC blood levels will decrease much more rapidly in occasional users than it will for chronic users.

33. With Pot on the Ballot, States Weigh How to Police Stoned Drivers[*]

Stephanie O'Neill *and* Ben Markus

In five states this fall—California, Arizona, Nevada, Maine and Massachusetts—voters will be deciding whether marijuana should be legal for recreational use. And any of those states that do legalize marijuana will have to wrestle with the question of how to enforce laws against stoned drivers.

It has been legal to smoke pot for fun in Colorado since January 2014, and the state modeled its marijuana driving-under-the-influence law on the one for alcohol. If a blood test shows a certain level of THC, the mind-altering compound in marijuana, the law says you shouldn't be driving.

It sounds straightforward, but consider the case of Abby McLean, a stay-at-home-mom from the Denver suburbs.

McLean, 30, was driving home from a late dinner with a friend two years ago when she came upon a DUI roadside checkpoint.

"I hadn't drank or smoked anything, so I was like, 'Let's go through the checkpoint,'" she recalled.

McLean is a regular marijuana user but she insists she never drives while high.

Still, the officer at the checkpoint told her he smelled marijuana and that her eyes were bloodshot. Eventually he whipped out handcuffs, and McLean said she started to panic: "Like, massive panic attack. And, 'Oh, my God, I have babies at home. I need to get home. I can't go to jail!'"

She didn't go to jail that night, but she got home hours late. A blood test later revealed McLean had five times the legal limit of THC allowed in Colorado, which is five nanograms of THC per milliliter of blood.

It may sound like an open and shut case that could have resulted in any number of penalties. But McLean's attorney, Nadav Aschner, had a field day in court with Colorado's marijuana intoxication limit.

---

*Originally published as Stephanie O'Neill and Ben Markus, "With Pot on the Ballot, States Weigh How to Police Stoned Drivers," *Kaiser Health News*, September 27, 2016. Reprinted with permission of the publisher.

"Even the state's experts will say that number alone is something, but generally not enough, and we really hammered that home," he said. Aschner got a hung jury and McLean pleaded to a lesser offense.

Still, McLean's trip through the criminal justice system is emblematic of numbers that suggest a sharp increase in marijuana DUI arrests in Colorado. So far this year, State Patrol data show that total DUI citations this year rose to 398 through early July, compared with 316 in for the same period 2015.

It turns out, measuring a person's THC is actually a poor indicator of intoxication. Unlike alcohol, THC gets stored in your fat cells, and isn't water-soluble like alcohol, said Thomas Marcotte, co-director of the Center for Medicinal Cannabis Research at the University of California, San Diego.

"Unlike alcohol, which has a generally linear relationship between the amount of alcohol you consume, your breath alcohol content and driving performance, the THC route of metabolism is very different," Marcotte said.

That's why adapting drunk driving laws to marijuana makes for bad policy, said Mark Kleiman, a professor of public policy at New York University. "You can be positive for THC a week after the last time you used cannabis," he said. "Not subjectively impaired at all, not impaired at all by any objective measure, but still positive."

Still, Colorado and five other states have such laws on the books because pretty much everyone agrees that driving stoned can be dangerous, especially when combined with alcohol.

What police say they really need is a simple roadside sobriety test. Scientists at UCSD are among researchers working on several apps that could measure how impaired a driver is. One has a person follow a square moving around a tablet screen with a finger, which measures something called "critical tracking." Another app measures time distortion, because things can slow way down when a person is high.

Those tests are still experimental.

Denver District Attorney Mitch Morrissey said the uncertainty doesn't mean Colorado should throw out its THC blood test. He said it may not be perfect, but it gives juries another piece of evidence to consider at trial.

"I think that putting in a nanogram level makes sense," said Morrissey. "I can't tell you what level it should be. I don't think Colorado's is right. I don't think it should be as high as it is. I think it should be lower."

Morrissey remembers trying alcohol DUI cases as a young prosecutor. The science wasn't settled then either, the blood alcohol standard was about twice as high as it is now, and it took years for it to be lowered.

"I think that has to do with better testing better technology," which Morrissey said will improve eventually for marijuana too.

In the meantime, some regular marijuana users, like Abby McLean, are scared to drive for fear of failed blood tests.

"I haven't gone out really since then, because I'm paranoid to run into the same surprise, 'Oh oh, there's a DUI checkpoint.'"

Kaiser Health News is a nonprofit news service covering health issues. It is an editorially independent program of Kaiser Family Foundation that is not affiliated with Kaiser Permanente. This story is part of a partnership that includes Colorado Public Radio, KPCC, NPR and Kaiser Health News.

34. Legal Marijuana Means States Struggle to Address High Driving*

SARAH BREITENBACH

Washington State Patrol Sgt. Mark Crandall half-jokingly says he can tell a driver is under the influence of marijuana during a traffic stop when the motorist becomes overly familiar and is calling him "dude."

The truth in the joke, Crandall says, is that attitude and speech patterns can be effective markers for drugged driving. And, according to legalization advocates and some in law enforcement, they can be more reliable than blood tests that measure THC—the psychoactive compound in marijuana.

When it comes time to go to court, the testimony of an officer trained as a drug recognition expert is often more valuable than a THC test because of disparities in how the drug impacts driving ability, Crandall said.

"Here's the really bad driving that I saw, here's the magnified impairment that I saw on the side of the road," he said. "It's telling a good story and making sure that it's backed up with facts, and evidence, and proof, and the ability of the officer to articulate it well."

As more states make medical and recreational marijuana use legal, they increasingly are grappling with what constitutes DUID, or driving under the influence of drugs, and how to detect and prosecute it. And they're finding it is more difficult than identifying and convicting drunken drivers.

While marijuana is the substance, other than alcohol, most frequently found in drivers involved in car accidents, the rate at which it actually causes crashes is unclear.

At least 17 states, including Washington, have "per se" laws, which make it illegal to have certain levels of THC in one's body while operating a vehicle, according to the National Conference of State Legislatures (NCSL). Under these laws, no additional evidence is required to prove a driver is impaired.

Of those states, Colorado, Montana, Nevada, Ohio, Pennsylvania and Washington allow for some amount of THC to be found in a driver's blood, ranging from 1 to 5

*Originally published as Sarah Breitenbach, "Legal Marijuana Means States Struggle to Address High Driving," *Stateline*, August 21, 2015. Reprinted with permission of the publisher. © The Pew Charitable Trusts.

nanograms per milliliter (ng/ml). Other states leave no wiggle room and consider any amount of THC to be impairing and grounds for being charged with DUID.

In Colorado, where recreational marijuana became legal in 2012, drivers are assumed to be under the influence of marijuana if they have THC levels of 5 ng/ml or higher, but the law also lets defendants produce evidence that they were not impaired.

Alaska, Colorado, the District of Columbia, Oregon and Washington allow adult recreational use of marijuana, and another 18 states permit its use for medical purposes. More states are expected to permit recreational marijuana use as legalization efforts move to the ballot in Ohio this fall and Nevada in 2016.

At a recent NCSL meeting in Seattle, nearly all policymakers who attended a session on legalizing marijuana said they expected their states would soon have to debate legalization, if they haven't already. A study by the Pew Research Center released in April found that 53 percent of adults supported the legal use of marijuana. (Pew also funds Stateline).

How THC Works

State lawmakers, conditioned by the universal system of rating blood alcohol content to determine intoxication, have long wanted similar measurements to gauge a driver's impairment under the influence of THC. But that has proven elusive.

Unlike alcohol consumption, which creates impairments that are measurable by blood alcohol content, the consumption of marijuana creates physical effects that vary from person to person and THC levels can depend on how cannabis is ingested and whether the person is a long-term marijuana user, said Rebecca Hartman, a researcher with the National Institute on Drug Abuse.

People's THC levels peak quickly as they inhale marijuana smoke and then decrease rapidly in the first 30 minutes to an hour after smoking. Even though the THC levels are decreasing, users can still be impaired, Hartman said.

How the human body processes marijuana varies so much from person to person that even on different days a user might metabolize the drug at different rates, she said.

"We've shown that cannabis increases lane weaving and some studies have shown one of the big things that cannabis is known to impair is driver attention," Hartman said.

A June study on drugged driving conducted by Hartman and others suggested that people driving with THC levels of 13.1 ng/ml had a tendency to weave within lanes, similar to those who had a 0.08 blood alcohol content, the point at which drivers can be prosecuted in all states.

George Bianchi, a criminal defense attorney in Seattle, said the rule in his state (5 ng/ml) is not appropriate because studies of driver impairment vary so much. He said he thinks Hartman's study opens the door to using 13 ng/ml as a national standard for marijuana impairment.

"I think you should try to quantify it somehow," he said. "And this recent study seems to do that."

Controlling Drugged Driving

Some states see creating DUID laws as part of the marijuana legalization process, said Morgan Fox, a spokesman for the Marijuana Policy Project.

Several states considered adding or modifying per se DUID limits in 2015. Legislation that would elevate the Illinois per se standard from zero tolerance to 5 ng/ml, as amended (down from 15 ng/ml) by Republican Gov. Bruce Rauner, is awaiting final approval by the General Assembly. And a bill that would create a per se standard in New Jersey is before that legislature. Alabama, Maine and New Mexico also reviewed bills adding per se DUID limits ranging from 2 ng/ml to 5 ng/ml, though none passed.

"Considering most states already have them in place, and they are already being enforced, we don't see the need to add them," Fox said. "But we're not going to scuttle a bill that would legalize [marijuana] because of per se [laws]."

Because of the variation in users' impairment levels, critics of blood testing like Paul Armentano, deputy director for the National Organization for the Reform of Marijuana Laws, say the tests are not an appropriate measure of how well a person was driving at the time of a traffic stop or crash.

"Where is the need to go in this [direction] with cannabis when there is a consensus among experts in the field that the presence of THC in the blood in a single sample is not an accurate predictor of recent use nor is it a predictor of performance?" Armentano said.

He cites a February 2015 drug and alcohol crash risk study from the Department of Transportation that points to contradictions between previous studies about the relationship between marijuana use and motor vehicle crashes. The analysis, which looked at marijuana and other drugs, found that, when adjusted for age, gender and alcohol use, there was no significant increase in the level of crash risk associated with the use of THC.

Inappropriate Arrests

Legalization advocates said they worry that per se standards will lead to DUID convictions of people who were not impaired by marijuana when they were pulled over for a traffic violation, but might test positive for THC because they are frequent recreational users or use marijuana as medicine.

"These laws could lead to significant unintended consequences and the most significant of those is that the law prosecutes and convicts individuals of violating traffic safety laws for simply having engaged in behavior in the privacy of their own home that at no point rose to a legitimate traffic safety threat," Armentano said. In 2014 the Arizona Supreme Court overturned a lower court ruling that allowed for the prosecution of drivers under the per se law, even if there was no evidence of impairment. The previous year, the Michigan high court ruled that police must prove driver impairment to pursue DUID charges.

States began adopting THC-specific standards in the early 1990s as a consequence of highly publicized crashes and other accidents, Armentano said, contending that the laws are largely unnecessary given established protocols for determining if a driver is under the influence of a drug.

"The officer is collecting evidence from the minute he flashes his lights," he said. "Based on evidence observed at the scene, he or she is going to start making some judgment about whether [the driver] might be under the influence."

35. Uncertainties After a Year of Legalized Marijuana[*]

Deborah Sutton

More than a year has passed since Colorado's "Green Wednesday," when hundreds of people braved the New Year's Day cold to queue outside the state's 24 marijuana retail stores.

Colorado became the first jurisdiction in the world to legalize marijuana for commercial production and sale. Washington State followed six months later and Oregon and Alaska are expected to open retail shops in 2016. Other states like California, Massachusetts, Nevada and Maine, where medical marijuana and small amounts of recreational pot are legal, are expected to pass measures in next year's elections that broaden those allowances.

Meanwhile, policymakers and advocates on both sides of the legalization debate are watching closely to see if what Colorado's governor called "the greatest social experiment of the century" is worth the fiscal and social risk.

With one year past, it's too soon for policymakers and health experts to draw reliable conclusions on the costs versus benefits of marijuana legalization. Tax revenues from legal sales were $86 million less than projected and the social costs on public health and safety remain largely unknown. Despite the uncertainty, state officials and policy analysts don't anticipate the setbacks and numerous unknowns of Colorado's experiment to deter the spread of legalization to other states.

"Oregon and Alaska voted to set up commercial markets for marijuana, but the voters in Washington, D.C., passed an initiative just to allow home production. They didn't vote for a tax and regulatory system," said Beau Kilmer, co-director of the RAND Corp's Drug Policy Research Center. "If you're a jurisdiction wanting to do something else other than prohibiting marijuana, turns out you have a lot of options."

Revenue Realities

The option Colorado voters approved—to license the manufacturing, cultivation and commercial sale of marijuana—was revolutionary compared to policies legalizing pot in other countries.

---

[*]Originally published as Deborah Sutton, "Uncertainties After a Year of Legalized Marijuana," *Deseret News*, May 22, 2013. Reprinted with permission of the publisher.

For example, the Netherlands' policy doesn't allow "marijuana stores" like Colorado and Washington. Instead, limited amounts of cannabis are sold per person in select, 18-and-over coffee shops. Production, possession and selling of marijuana is still illegal, "but they have a policy of not enforcing the law against small-scale transactions," Kilmer said.

Advocates for legalizing marijuana in the United States are framing their campaign as a responsible fiscal policy, where the sale of pot will generate tax revenue that will cover the costs of regulation and then some.

If marijuana was legal in the U.S., taxpayers would "save $7.7 billion in combined state and federal (enforcement) spending, while taxation (of sales) would yield up to $6.2 billion a year in new revenues for the federal and state governments," according to the pro-legalization blog Why Legalize Marijuana?, citing a 2005 Harvard study by economist Jeffrey Miron.

The appeal of more funding for schools, stronger local governments, better social programs and perhaps, in the long-run, lower taxes likely drew many Colorado voters to the polls in 2012 to pass Amendment 64 with 55 percent voting in favor, 45 percent opposed.

Gov. John Hickenlooper's early revenue projections in February 2014 estimated that medical and retail marijuana sales combined would reap $134 million in tax revenue for the fiscal year beginning July 2014 and ending June 2015. The sale of retail marijuana alone would generate $118 million in tax revenue.

Hickenlooper's revenue forecast was more optimistic than the Colorado Legislature's $67 million projection for retail sales.

What's the reality? The 2014–15 fiscal year is half over and the most recent projection for retail marijuana tax receipts is expected to total $36.2 million. The outlook for medical and retail sales combined is $47.7 million by the end of the fiscal year.

"It's important to keep in mind that no one has ever created a legalized recreational market to the degree that we have," Skyler McKinley, the state's deputy director of marijuana policy, said explaining the potential $86 million discrepancy. "We didn't know what use patterns would be like, how people would buy marijuana, how much they would buy, and so on and so forth."

For example, many people expected the black market to disappear with legalization, but it continues to thrive. During the first few months of legalization, the state was losing revenue to the illegal market where street prices were a fraction of store prices, which include a 15 percent excise tax, a 10 percent special state tax, a 2.9 percent state sales tax and a variable local sales tax, said Katharine Neill, Glassell postdoctoral fellow on drug policy at Rice University's Baker Institute.

Some news agencies reported that retail stores sold pot for up to $450 an ounce during the first half of 2014, while the black market prices were anywhere between $160–300, according to the crowd sourcing website Price of Weed.

Another surprise to state budgeters was an unexpected rise in medical marijuana sales. State officials anticipated that some current medical marijuana users would switch over to the legal recreational market to avoid the inconvenience of state registration. But the lone 2.9 percent sales tax on medical marijuana proved a powerful incentive for marijuana newcomers to buy the one-time medical card for as low as $20 and avoid the higher priced recreational marijuana.

"We've had people who said that they walked into a dispensary and the owner said,

'Look it's a lot cheaper to buy medical (marijuana). Go around the corner, get a red card, and then come back and buy medical,'" said Diane Carlson, director of Smart Colorado, a Colorado-based interest group focused on protecting youths from marijuana.

But Neill and other observers have already seen store prices drop to closely match street prices as more legal growers and sellers entered the market throughout the year.

"To create one of these systems, it actually takes resources. To begin regulating it will take resources, so early on you're going to have to put resources into it," said Kilmer. "But then you expect over time that the tax revenue will be enough to overcome that."

What Less Money Means

With reduced tax revenue, the state has had to scale back funding programs Hickenlooper proposed in his 2014–15 budget. He proposed $111 million for a youth marijuana use prevention program, a substance abuse treatment system, regulatory oversight, law enforcement and public safety, public health and statewide coordination.

And that $111 million total didn't include another $40 million earmarked toward a school construction fund, dubbed Building Excellent Schools Today or BEST.

"Our (new) budget request reflects the lower projections," McKinley said. "We're currently operating off of a $33 million figure. We didn't (have to) cut anything (since) no money was allocated by the time we realized that the projections were going to be lower."

Right now, all revenue from the 15 percent excise tax goes toward the school construction fund. Once the fund hits $40 million, however, excise tax revenue will be designated to the general marijuana fund to support regulation and public programs.

McKinley said the state never intended marijuana sales to generate surpluses that would spill over into other state programs, despite assurances by advocates and voters' expectations.

"We've always believed that marijuana should pay its own way," said McKinley. "We didn't legalize for the tax money. Our philosophy in Colorado is that the revenue that we're bringing in from the sale of marijuana is going to be completely allocated to any costs related to legalization."

Public Safety

Time will tell how reducing the scale of the proposed youth prevention, public health and safety and substance abuse programs will affect the social costs of legalization.

On the expenses side of the ledger, a 2010 Harvard study estimated that Colorado was spending an estimated $145 million every year enforcing its marijuana laws and that legalization would save the state a large portion of those costs.

However, that assumption is difficult to prove.

The state cannot easily track law enforcement spending since "municipalities and other local entities do the lion's share of law enforcement legwork and we don't exercise any control over their budgets," McKinley said.

There have been no unusual budget increases or decreases for the statewide departments of public safety, public health and environment or corrections since legalization.

For example, the department of corrections increased its budget by more than $70 million since 2013, but the bump in spending isn't unusual and is "reflective of general increases in operational costs," like cost of living, said Adrienne Jacobson, public information officer for the Colorado Department of Corrections. "Any budget increases are in no way related to the legalization of marijuana."

And while the state doesn't have access to local budgets, officials assume that with pot seizures down the related county expenses have also declined. "In 2012, there were 12,471 marijuana seizures reported by local law enforcement agencies to the Colorado Bureau of Investigation," said McKinley. "In 2013, there were 5,828 seizures. Through Dec. 2, 2014, there were 4,387 seizures."

And so far there hasn't been a major spike in other crimes that would undermine the apparent savings from marijuana decriminalization. The statewide crime report for 2014 doesn't come out until mid–2015, but Denver's annual crime report indicates that overall reported crime rose 2.5 percent in 2014, a smaller increase from the previous year of a 7.4 percent rise.

Another Denver city crime report that focuses only on violent and property crimes reveals a 6.9 percent decrease in 2014.

Looking Forward

The uncertainties surrounding legalizing pot haven't slowed growth in Colorado's marijuana market. As of December, 308 medical and recreational stores and some 400 cultivation facilities have launched in Denver alone, according to Gina Carbone of Smart Colorado.

The rising competition has brought commercial prices down and increased sales, which bodes well for state coffers.

But the social costs of legalization will remain largely unknown for several years, at least.

In October, Hickenlooper's office released a 74-page "data gap" report on the unknown effects to the health and safety of underage youths, traffic accidents, criminal activity, the environment, violence and gun use, hospitalization and death. The report also lays out a strategy to collect and analyze new data as it rolls in.

Smart Colorado is most concerned about how legalization will "lower perceptions of harm" among youths and impact underage use, health and school performance. "We've opened up a Pandora's Box" and it will take years to analyze the impacts to society, Carlson said.

But there have been studies that estimate that the social costs of marijuana, while concerning, are less than the costs of alcohol, Neill asserts.

Both Neill and Kilmer agree that if heavy drinkers, hard drug users and prescription drug abusers switched to using just marijuana, society would benefit. But they also agree if those people combined alcohol, hard drugs or prescription drugs with marijuana, problems related to substance abuse would increase.

The numerous unknowns in Colorado are unlikely to prevent other states from following suit—albeit perhaps with a different model.

Besides Colorado's for-profit commercial model, states could limit production and sales to nonprofits. They could allow home production only, follow a Netherlands-type policy or they could have a state monopoly where the government is in charge of production and distribution, similar to alcohol regulation in states like Utah, Kilmer explained.

"It turns out that the research on this monopoly model, at least for alcohol, is much better for public health than a commercial system where you deregulate and turn it over to the private market," he said.

In the coming years, "it will be really interesting to see what happens in other states. Are people only going to focus on the for-profit alcohol model or are they going to consider these middle ground options?"

36. As the Pro-Pot Movement Gains Popularity, Reservations Remain Among Locals*

DYLAN WOOLF HARRIS

The remote outdoors can make for natural secret garden sites, such as the several marijuana groves found in northeastern Nevada the past few years.

In October 2013, police were tipped off to a marijuana farm north of Wells where drug dealers had cultivated about 2,000 plants. Two men were arrested at the scene.

Months later, Bureau of Land Management personnel and volunteers spent 12 hours cleaning up the site. They packed out 400 pounds of garbage and estimated the damage to be about $60,000.

More concerning than the damage rendered to natural resources, illegal pot farms can be dangerous.

In 2008, three biologists in Humboldt County were held at gunpoint after they stumbled upon a marijuana patch. The men were released unharmed, but the gunmen had vanished by the time law enforcement arrived to capture them.

Clandestine pot grows, such as the one discovered in the area, are a public land problem that some believe would be less common if marijuana were legalized and regulated.

"There's a reason why we don't see large-scale illegal brewery and distilling operations on public lands or in the basements of suburban homes," said Mason Tvert, director of communications for the Marijuana Policy Project.

"Alcohol is legal," he said. "Illegal actors cannot compete with the legal market, and the economic benefit of trying to compete is not worth the risk of facing the penalties if they get caught."

In the 2016 election, Nevada could add its name to the list of states that have agreed to throw out their laws banning small quantities of pot, and allow citizens to get high for recreational use. Colorado, the first state to test legalized pot, received a flood of media attention.

The Coalition to Regulate Marijuana Like Alcohol gathered about 200,000 signa-

*Originally published as Dylan Woolf Harris, "As the Pro-Pot Movement Gains Popularity, Reservations Remain Among Locals," *Elko Daily Free Press*, January 10, 2015. Reprinted with permission of the publisher.

tures, the Associated Press reported in December, almost double the number needed to get the proposal on the next ballot.

Lawmakers will put the initiative to a vote at the upcoming session. If it fails to pass through the Legislature, voters will decide whether to pass it in the next General Election.

The petition argued that marijuana should be legal to those at least 21 years old and able to be purchased from a state-licensed business. Residents would be able to possess up to an ounce of marijuana and grow up to 12 plants. Driving under the influence of pot would remain illegal.

The pot industry would take money out of the hands of drug cartels as well as street-level dealers, the argument goes, and generate taxes for the state. Among local community leaders, however, especially those heading law enforcement departments, the idea of relaxing a drug law is worrisome.

Elko's Opposition

For Police Chief Ben Reed, who spearheaded a campaign last year to ban medical pot shops in the city and county, the potential approval creates a mixed message for officers who agree to uphold not only Nevada's constitution, but the U.S. Constitution as well.

"It's poor public policy, in that they're in conflict," he said.

The federal government continues to classify marijuana as a Schedule 1 controlled substance, according to the Drug Enforcement Administration's website. Heroin and methamphetamine are also Schedule 1 drugs.

Reed said the burden to reconcile the two at-odds laws falls on Congress' shoulders.

"They either have to legalize it at both federal and state or prohibit it at federal and state for it to be in sync," he said.

In many areas of the country, holding marijuana in small quantities is a misdemeanor offense—less than an ounce in Nevada. The Silver State is also among those in the nation that have legalized marijuana for medicinal purposes.

Given one option or the other, Reed would prefer marijuana stay illegal at all levels of government.

"I've got 32 years dealing with marijuana and I've yet to see anything positive come out of it," he said. "It's a drug that is potentially mind altering and causes under-the-influence problems. We see them, as police, every single day."

Sheriff Jim Pitts, who worked for years in the area's narcotics task force, has extensive experience combating drugs and also opposes the proposal.

Assemblyman John Ellison, R–Elko, said he's heard from a few constituents who support legalized marijuana, but more so from those in opposition.

Personally, he's also against it.

"I think it's a bad choice for children," Ellison said.

Cathy McAdoo, executive director of PACE Coalition, agrees, although she acknowledged the diverse opinions regarding pot.

PACE is a nonprofit that promotes community well-being.

McAdoo said petitions circulated the state a few years ago for a similar purpose. She believes the signatures were gathered dishonestly, and that many people signed it without reading the fine print.

During that election cycle, she helped set up a press release to inform signers how to remove their names from the petition.

This year, however, she had no such luck.

McAdoo hopes any calculation that factors potential tax revenue will also consider costs to the welfare of the community. In her estimation, that cost is more children getting their hands on pot, which could lead to more bad decisions for them down the road.

"Certainly I have, and PACE has, a great concern about our young people," she said.

McAdoo said legalized pot could make it easier and more appealing to youths.

"If a young person perceives that marijuana is dangerous for them, they're less likely to do it," she said. "…Even though it won't be legal for them, under 21, it makes it more accessible in a community and in the state."

PACE Coalition focuses its efforts on prevention and helping children and teenagers make sound choices.

"I'm going to be sorely disappointed if it's passed. You do what you can do, but I worry about our kids," she said. "We are really about reducing drug use, not promoting it," she said.

This includes alcohol. Both Reed and McAdoo cited alcohol and marijuana as well as hard drugs as a contributing factor into many societal ills.

Growing Support

To supporters, the marijuana-alcohol comparison is important precisely because one is legal to adults despite associated problems.

"Marijuana is objectively far less harmful than alcohol," Tvert said. "It's less addictive, less damaging to the body and less likely to contribute to violent and reckless behavior."

Supporters compare the outlaw of marijuana to America's brief prohibition on alcohol, which is widely considered an abject failure that gave rise to criminal bootleggers.

"If adults would rather use marijuana instead of alcohol, they should not be prohibited from making that safer choice," he said.

Tvert also disputed claims that legalizing pot would make it more available to teens. Citing a survey done by Monitoring the Future, he said more than 90 percent of high school seniors say they can easily get marijuana.

"If the goal of prohibition is to keep marijuana away from teens and it's universally available to them right now, it's a failed policy," he said. "Right now marijuana is available to anyone who wants it, but those who are selling it are not asking for proof of age."

A legal system would incentivize sellers to comply with age-restriction rules or face fines and criminal charges.

The MPP argues law enforcement and the criminal justice system would be better spent targeting dangerous criminals.

"Hundreds of thousands of Americans are arrested each year for marijuana-related offenses, the vast majority of which are for simple possession," a statement from the group reads. "Meanwhile, clearance rates for many serious crimes are exceptionally low, many never result in an arrest."

At the request of the Elko *Daily Free Press*, the Elko County District Attorney's office compiled a list of charges filed in 2014 that have "as near as (the office) can tell" a "marijuana component."

Last year, 25 felony cases were filed in the county, which includes allegations of possession of more than an ounce of marijuana, as well as transporting, trafficking, or selling marijuana.

Fifteen juvenile cases involved marijuana.

But the majority of last year's marijuana charges–54 cases—were for misdemeanors.

Legal Options

The petition specifies that local governments would have the autonomy to ban pot stores. After policymakers approved a bill in 2013 that allowed for medical marijuana establishments, Elko County passed a zoning ban. The City of Elko voted on a two-year moratorium.

If passed, businesses would be allowed to ban marijuana use of its employees.

The mine sites of northeastern Nevada already adhere to a strict anti-drug policy.

The area's two largest mine employers, Barrick Gold Corp. and Newmont Mining Corp., test employees before hiring, after an accident and randomly.

Lou Schack, communications director for Barrick, said the initiative wouldn't change mine practices.

Newmont's Director of External Relations Mary Korpi echoed the same sentiment.

"If marijuana was legalized in Nevada, it would still be illegal under federal law and Newmont would continue to prohibit the use or being under the influence of marijuana in the workplace," Korpi wrote in an email.

"A safe working environment requires an uncompromising commitment of all of our people to demonstrate leadership in safety through a drug- and alcohol-free workplace," she added.

37. Colorado's Pot Legalization Creates Challenges*

Diane Raver

Several states have legalized marijuana, and legislators in others are considering it. But what effect has this had on the citizens and cities where the drug is readily available for purchase?

Chelsey Clarke, Rocky Mountain High Intensity Drug Trafficking Area strategic intelligence analyst, shared information on this topic when she was in Batesville in the fall.

She explained, "The RMHIDTA is a federally-funded grant program that covers four states (Colorado, Montana, Utah and Wyoming). We receive funding from Congress each year … (and) we bring down the biggest, baddest drug runners."

"The term war on drugs is a terrible term because we're never going to completely eliminate it…. The purpose of our nation's drug policy is to limit the number of people using drugs." The group documented the impact of marijuana for medical and recreational use in Colorado in "The Legalization of Marijuana in Colorado: The Impact— Volume 4," which was published in September 2016.

"Why do we care about drug use? Because it's not a victimless crime. It not only affects the user, but also family and friends, victims of crimes (that the user may commit while under the influence) and taxpayers."

She revealed three drug-related deaths: "College student Levy Thamba Pongi, 19, ate some marijuana-infused cookies and then ate some more. Then he jumped off a six-story building.

Kristine Kirk, 44, was shot and killed by her husband after he ate some marijuana candy with prescription medicine. He started hallucinating and killed his wife. Luke Goodman, 23, tried edibles. He had no suicidal tendencies prior to this, but he started hallucinating and shot and killed himself…. These were all the result of the marijuana industry."

Prior to the drug being legalized in the Centennial State, supporters said it would eliminate arrests for possession and sale; free up law enforcement resources; reduce traffic fatalities; there would be no increase in use, even among youth; there would be added

*Originally published as Diane Raver, "Colorado's Pot Legalization Creates Challenges," *The Herald-Tribune*, January 4, 2017. Reprinted with permission of the publisher.

revenue generated through taxation; and it would reduce profits for the drug cartels trafficking marijuana.

Those who argued against legalization said there would be increases in marijuana-related traffic fatalities, use among youth and adults, people in drug treatment, diversion for unintended purposes and impacts and costs for public health and safety, Clarke revealed.

To put the legalization impact into perspective, she said as of January 2016, Colorado had 202 McDonald's, 322 Starbucks, 424 recreational marijuana shops (it has since grown to 500) and 516 medical marijuana dispensaries. "In just two years, look how quickly it (places to purchase the drug) has exploded all over our state."

To make it legal, "voters supported an amendment to our (state) constitution, saying we have a constitutional right to use marijuana and grow it in our houses. If it ever changes, it has to go to popular vote…. City (officials) can decide whether the recreation shops can operate within their borders. Not all cities are on board. About 75 percent of cities and towns have banned them. It's cities like Denver and Boulder that support them.

Impaired Driving

The speaker noted that the number of statewide traffic deaths "was decreasing (from a high of 554 in 2007 to a low of 447 in 2011) … now with the legalization, the numbers are increasing again." In addition, traffic deaths related to marijuana have increased from 71 in 2013 to 115 in 2015. Not all of these are caused by those operating vehicles. "We've had some cases where bicyclists or pedestrians have walked into the path of a car."

In 2015, of those vehicle operators who tested positive for marijuana, 33 percent only had this drug in their system. Data also showed that 30 percent had both marijuana and alcohol; 24 percent, marijuana and other drugs (no alcohol); and 13 percent, marijuana, other drugs and alcohol, she reported.

Youth Marijuana Use

"We were told use among youth would not increase because it was such a restrictive environment…. While media headlines said 'Marijuana use remains flat among Colorado teens, survey finds' and 'Colorado's good news on teen pot use,' indicated one result, the data showed something else.

"According to the Healthy Kids Colorado Survey, there was an 8 percent increase in all high school grades from 2013 to 2015 with a 14 percent increase in seniors and a 19 percent increase in juniors; one out of three Denver junior and seniors are marijuana users; and in Colorado mountain towns, there was a 90 percent increase in seniors using the drug….

"Colorado was ranked first in the nation for current marijuana use among youth (according to the 2013 and 2014 National Survey on Drug Use and Health), which is 74 percent higher than the national average. Colorado youth use increased 20 percent (2013–14 compared to 2011–12), where nationally, youth use declined 4 percent."

According to data from the Colorado Department of Education for the 2015–16 school year, of the 337 expulsions, 58 percent were marijuana violations; of the 1,143 referrals to law enforcement, 73 percent were due to this drug; and of the 4,236 suspensions, 63 percent involved marijuana, Clarke said.

The predominant marijuana violations included student under the influence during school hours, 45 percent; student in possession of the drug, 43 percent; student in possession of marijuana infused edibles, 7 percent; student selling marijuana to other students and student sharing the drug with other students, 2 percent each. "There were some cases of elementary school students bringing marijuana-infused brownies or cookies to sell."

How was the drug obtained? Sources included: friend who obtained it legally, 45 percent; black market, 24 percent; parents, 22 percent; medical marijuana dispensaries, 6 percent; retail marijuana stores, 2 percent; and medical marijuana card holders, 1 percent.

"If kids see their parents using marijuana every day, it becomes second nature, and they'll do it too.

Other Challenges

"One of the biggest problems in Colorado is edible products. These come in gummy bears, Swedish fish…. They're made to look exactly like candy. This is a huge problem, especially for our young population," Clarke pointed out.

"Another problem is for our pets. Prior to legalization, there were one or two cases of animals presenting with marijuana issues every several months. Now it's about seven every day due to edible products."

Colorado Info

- 2000–08—Early Medical Marijuana Era, 1,000–4,800 card holders and zero known dispensaries
- 2009–12—Medical Marijuana Commercialization and Expansion Era, 108,000 card holders and 532 licensed dispensaries
- 2013–present—Medical Marijuana Commercialization and Recreational Marijuana Era

Other Statistics

- 2013–14 current marijuana use for college-age adults ages 18–25: Colorado average, 31.24 percent; national average, 19.32 percent; the state was ranked first in the nation for current use among this group, 62 percent higher than the national average
- 2013–14 current marijuana use for adults ages 26 and older: Colorado was ranked first the nation for this group. It was 104 percent higher than the national average. Adult use increased 63 percent compared to prelegalization years 2011–12.

- The number of hospitalizations related to this drug increased from 6,715 in 2012 to 8,272 in 2013 when it was legalized. In rose again to 11,439 in 2014.
- The number of adolescents ages 6–17 who had marijuana-related exposures increased by 112 percent from 2009–12 to 2013–15 from 25 to 53. The number of children ages 5 and below who had marijuana-related exposures increased by 169 percent from that same set of years from 13 to 35.

38. Licensing Medical Marijuana Stirs Up Trouble for States[*]

Rebecca Beitsch

The seven lucky balls that popped out of the Arizona Department of Health Services lottery machine in October produced big winners—not in the state's Powerball game, but in the competition to make money in the medical marijuana industry.

The prize winners were granted licenses to open a medical marijuana dispensary in a state where patients with prescriptions to treat conditions such as glaucoma and cancer spent $215 million last year on marijuana products. Arizona's public health officials awarded most licenses based on rules designed to place new dispensaries within range of the greatest number of medical-marijuana patients. But when it wasn't clear which applicant was in the most patient-dense area, they used a lottery to randomly select the winners, hoping to sidestep conflict.

States have struggled with how to give out potentially lucrative medical marijuana licenses—trying to balance public health concerns against an entrepreneurial spirit and avoid a bevy of lawsuits. Many want to ensure the businesses are well run and are supplying quality products. But even in states like Arizona where dispensaries are required to be nonprofits, competition for licenses can lead to a gold rush mentality and lawsuits as entrepreneurs eye a medical marijuana industry with $4.2 billion in sales in 2014.

"There's a lot of cash that goes through these businesses," said Kris Krane with 4Front Ventures, a medical marijuana consulting firm. "As [marijuana] becomes more legitimate and more legal, it's only going to be a growth industry. People are looking to get in now because as the industry grows and expands they're positioned to be market leaders."

Medical marijuana businesses often have between $1 million and $5 million in sales annually, Krane said, though he's seen some that do more than $20 million.

Twenty-eight states have medical marijuana programs, but Arizona is rare in that it awards some licenses by a lottery. About a dozen states have strict merit-based systems that award a small set of licenses to businesses viewed as the most qualified. Several have no limit on the number of licenses they give out and review companies through a rolling application process. Others are still developing their programs or have combined the licensing of medical marijuana with that of recreational marijuana businesses.

---

*Originally published as Rebecca Beitsch, "Licensing Medical Marijuana Stirs Up Trouble for States," *Stateline*, December 23, 2016. Reprinted with permission of the publisher. © The Pew Charitable Trusts.

Those involved in the cannabis industry, including legalization advocates and business consultants, say there's no perfect system for deciding who gets a license. States that grant them based on applicants' business proposals produce intense competition and often bring cries of cronyism. Lawsuits pending in Maryland contend the system there unfairly factored in geography as part of its qualifications.

Massachusetts switched from granting a few medical marijuana licenses to granting an unlimited number of licenses in 2015, but found its requirement that applicants get support from local leaders to open an outlet was leading to pricy contracts between businesses and the towns.

Arizona has mostly avoided lawsuits by turning to the lottery to choose between applicants, but critics say infighting often begins among license winners with poorly vetted business plans.

Luck of the Draw

States have encountered many headaches in creating a legal, state-sanctioned business from what was the underground trafficking of a drug the federal government still considers illegal. When Florida first proposed awarding medical marijuana licenses through a lottery, in 2014, the state was sued.

"This ensures only that the luckiest eligible applicant, not best qualified eligible applicant, is approved," wrote Costa Farms, a nursery that grows marijuana, in its suit against the state. The suit prompted Florida to scrap its lottery and evaluate applications based on their businesses qualifications.

But Arizona figured that using a lottery to dole out licenses was a way to avoid lawsuits, and it has used the system both times it has awarded licenses.

The number of potential patients served by a business location wasn't a factor when the state began its medical marijuana program, in 2012, and that year more than 90 licenses were awarded by lottery. In both years, the application process has required potential dispensary owners to have basic qualifications, such as showing they can provide inventory tracking and security, but Arizona doesn't analyze business proposals the way other states do.

"We stress that we're not doing a merit-based process. We're doing it by chance," said Tom Salow, who is in charge of licensing for the state health department, which oversees medical marijuana.

Taylor West with the National Cannabis Industry Association said lotteries have some benefits. They make the decision less subjective and help allay concerns of political influence. But, she said, "The problem with the lottery is it doesn't always get you your best results."

The businesses "have to all be meeting minimum requirements, but there's certainly an argument for trying to get the best," West said. "A lottery doesn't reward the really diligent actors who give a lot of thought to the application and have done a lot of planning ahead of time and focused on building the best business possible."

Ryan Hurley, a lawyer with the Rose Law Group who has represented several marijuana businesses in Arizona, said the lotteries have been successful in largely insulating the state from lawsuits. But, he said, they don't guarantee that businesses are ready to operate smoothly. He said he's seen conflict between partners once they get a license.

Many applicants don't take the time to figure out and document their venture, Hurley said, and questions arise afterward over the investment, the order in which people will get paid, and even who's in control of decision-making.

"They rush, but then don't think what will happen if they actually won," he said. "They've got dollar signs in their eyes. Then they get a license and think they're millionaires and start fighting over who gets what."

Krane, the industry consultant, said a "qualified lottery" system, such as the one the state of Washington used when it legalized recreational marijuana sales in 2014, lets states screen businesses before choosing the qualified candidates through a lottery. Though more subjective, the qualified lottery gives states a chance to closely review security plans, operational procedures and owners' backgrounds.

On the Merits

Though many in the marijuana industry, such as West of the Cannabis Association, see a competitive, merit-based application process as a better selection method, trying to evaluate and pick the best businesses brings its own complications.

West said factors that allow states to look at the nuances of applications, such as judging business and security plans, also can expose states to complaints that personal connections have dictated some decisions. States such as Maryland have faced lawsuits challenging the criteria for judging applicants or how they were applied.

Although states typically have tried to make the selections anonymous, West said, it's not always possible and makes it harder to find the most-qualified applicants. "If part of the judgment is whether you have experienced people on your team, you can't do that anonymously," she said. "But it does interject personalities and conflicts and the potential for political influence."

Maryland tasked Towson University with ranking anonymous applications for growing marijuana on factors such as financing and plans for storing data and providing security. But the system ran into trouble when the state's medical marijuana commission chose some lower-ranked companies to have better geographic diversity.

Edward Weidenfeld, a partner with Maryland Cultivation and Processing, one of the companies suing the commission, said the state's system is good in that applications are ranked by a disinterested but knowledgeable third party. But he said the state erred in giving the commission too much power to ignore the rankings. Commissioners, he said, should only step in to ensure the identifying information from an application doesn't disqualify a business, such as including someone with a criminal record.

How an application is designed can have unintended consequences. In Massachusetts, for example, the state required medical marijuana dispensaries to form as nonprofits and get letters of support from the towns where they were hoping to open. In some cases, the nonprofits, which don't pay property taxes under state law, agreed to make payments to the towns or turn over a percentage of sales to help cover a town's costs, such as extra policing.

Those agreements became expensive for some businesses. According to reporting by the Boston Globe, a dispensary in Worcester agreed to pay $450,000 over three years, and another in Salem agreed to pay more than $82,000 the first year. A dispensary in Southborough agreed to pay a portion of its sales and contribute $50,000 annually toward substance abuse and mental health programs.

"Word got out fairly quickly," among mayors and city councilmen, industry consultant Krane said. "They all started trying to outdo each other in terms of how much they could get in hosting agreements. It's where some people have been crying extortion."

Massachusetts voters also recently approved recreational marijuana in a ballot measure that many elected officials said was flawed. A new commission created by the measure is directed to give licenses to companies with "the most experience operating medical marijuana treatment centers and then by lottery among qualified applicants."

Limited Licenses

The number of licenses states choose to award can change the way businesses pursue them.

States that don't limit their licenses may give out hundreds of them to businesses the state views as qualified. Krane said these states regulate marijuana more like a pharmacy, making sure applicants meet strict standards before they are allowed to open. Colorado has given medical marijuana licenses to more than 500 centers and nearly 800 growers, which are licensed separately from those in the recreational market. States with a cap on licenses often give out fewer than 10 in a highly competitive process.

"It creates these incentives for organizations to spend more time drumming up capital and political influence so that they can corner these licenses that give them this huge market share, rather than developing the best business or best model for taking care of patients," West of the Cannabis Association said. "In other states, it's a little less clear that any one license is a golden ticket worth bending the rules to get."

Costa Farms, the company that sued over Florida's plan for a lottery, later became one of the companies on a panel designed to help write Florida's medical marijuana regulations. According to the Miami Herald, a last-minute addition to a House bill requiring that licensees be in business since 1984—the earliest year Costa Farms has documentation of being a registered nursery—would have made it difficult for other companies to get a license. Pedro Freyre with Costa Farms said the company did not lobby for the provision.

Industry advocates say the most important thing is just having enough licenses that patients don't have to travel far to get the medicine they need.

Florida initially planned to have five licenses, though more are being added as nurseries sue the state. Krane said just a few licenses for a state can make sense when prescriptions are limited to noneuphoric marijuana for a small set of diseases, as is the case there.

But Freyre said such restrictions also help ensure the program stays strictly medical.

"Policymakers' approach has been, 'We don't want recreational by another name,' which is what has happened in other states with sort of a wink, wink, nudge, nudge," he said.

39. Legal Cultivation Challenges and California[*]

PATRICK MURPHY, HENRY MCCANN
and VAN BUSTIC

California voters passed Proposition 64 in the fall of 2016. One year later, the state of California, its counties, and many of its cities and towns are engaged in the hard work of building a legal market for cannabis. With recreational sales slated to start January 2018, government officials are trying to sort out a host of details that will determine the who, what, where, and when of cannabis transactions. It's not an easy task. It is likely to evolve over time. And, don't expect the illegal market to disappear any time soon.

The cannabis market will have many parts: sales, distribution, manufacturing, and cultivation. To illustrate the challenge, we will focus here just on cultivation—the growing of the plants. But, it is worth keeping in mind that regulating the other elements of the market is no simple task.

Marijuana growers who plan on growing cannabis on private lands next season will encounter new state requirements—including provisions that address the crop's impacts on California's creeks and streams. Last year, CalCannabis, a cultivation licensing system, began as a new program by the California Department of Food and Agriculture (CDFA) for permitting legal grows on private lands. The State Water Board recently adopted interim policies that will inform the water-related requirements of CDFA's cultivation license, including checks on a grower's water rights, restrictions on the diversion of water for irrigating cannabis crops, and site-specific requirements to control runoff into local streams from grow operations. Many elements of the new statewide requirements are based on pioneering regional efforts to regulate cannabis cultivation in the North Coast.

The regulations are quite specific. For example, as a prerequisite for the cultivation license, growers relying on water from local tributaries must have valid water rights or apply for a new surface water right that allows them to divert and store water. This requirement is critical to the State Water Board's new policies that compel growers to divert surface water to storage in winter (when flows are high) for irrigating cannabis during the dry months when streams are low. Diversions are allowed to resume in winter once a stream's minimum flow target is met.

---

*Published with permission of the authors.

The new statewide requirements also seek to reduce the risk of contamination to tributaries from farm runoff. For example, licensed growers across the state will be required to provide adequate distance between cultivation operations and streams and wetlands. The requirements also establish rules for reducing erosion from access roads, increasing irrigation efficiency, minimizing runoff, and safe handling of fertilizers, pesticides, and herbicides.

Compliance with the regulations will come with a hefty price tag for growers who want to join the legal market. Growers will need to obtain necessary permits and capital for constructing on-site water storage. Water measuring and recording requirements will also compel growers to install devices to track their stream diversions and usage.

Some of these costs will be one-time investments. Others will be on-going expenses. These new requirements will result in additional costs to many growers looking to enter the legal market, on top of new compliance costs, and taxes. Cannabis cultivators, like any business, will have to factor the impact that these expenditures will have on their bottom line. And, it is worth noting that the increase in costs will come at a time when the legal market causes prices—and in turn, revenue—to drop.

Many growers will decide to comply, but we suspect that a significant number will not, at least in the near to medium term. For some, the costs may not pencil out, with the compliance spending washing out profits. Other growers may want to make the investment, but the nature of their business limits their access to capital. Some growers may simply decide that compliance takes too big a bite out of their earnings and decide to continue to operate in the illegal market. Finally, other growers may forego permitting and the associated documentation out of fear of retaliation from federal authorities, for whom cannabis production is still illegal.

What happens to the growers who don't comply? In theory, inspectors and law enforcement will be free to step in and penalize these *bad actors*. Paying a fine, or worse, spending time in jail, imposes a cost too. So surely, all of the growers will choose the legal versus the illegal path? Not necessarily. The costs of compliance—following the legal path—are significant and certain. The costs of non-compliance are also significant, but far less certain. In short, it may come down to whether illegal growers think they are likely to be caught.

We cannot predict how aggressive enforcement of the new cultivation regulations will be, but we suspect it will be some time before compliance enforcement becomes much of a deterrent. If recent state arrest figures are any indication, the risk of facing a criminal marijuana charge has been falling dramatically.

While criminal enforcement declines, the amount of area being cultivated appears to be increasing. In the time leading up to January 2018, growers will be making a risk-and-reward calculation. Given that compliance will not be cheap, a significant number of growers will opt for the illegal market. Indeed, a report prepared for the California Department of Agriculture estimated that legal medical and recreational consumption will account for less than 20 percent of the state's total cannabis production in the first year.

It is unlikely that the state will be willing to tolerate such a large illegal market in the long run. Instead, regulators and law enforcement will have to work together to make adjustments over time. They will have two levers to use. On the one hand, they could decide to lower the cost of compliance, therefore encouraging more growers to join the ranks of the good actors. Such a step, however, raises difficult public policy questions.

For example, how do regulators reduce the cost of compliance while continuing to protect water quality and the environment? The state also could increase the costs of non-compliance by aggressively pursuing enforcement and increase the likelihood of punishment for bad actors. Determining the right mix will require some basic data about cultivation and consumption and getting that mix right will take some time.

When Proposition 64 passed a year ago, there was a sense that, having moved cannabis out of the shadows, all of the problems would go away. It is far too early to say whether legalizing recreational marijuana will decrease the amount cultivated as part of the black market. But, we know two things. First, growers will face a complicated cost-benefit calculation when deciding whether to enter the legal market. Second, the size of the challenge facing regulators is getting larger, not smaller, as full implementation of the proposition gets nearer.

40. The Adult-Use Marijuana Act

Issues and Impacts

Mickey P. McGee

This essay provides examples of some of the challenges facing California local governments today as they implement the new Adult-Use Marijuana Act (AUMA). These issues include concern for the local health of its population, the economic impact and crime. This essay includes a review of how elected and non-elected municipal leaders are implementing the complex and intricate new cannabis law in in their cities. The views of commercial cannabis business owners are provided on what they consider the key concerns for this new business. Small growers and marijuana dispensaries have been important outlets for individuals needing medical marijuana to treat their medical concerns. A medicinal marijuana grower and seller was interviewed for this essay and provides her thoughts on the impact of the AUMA on small growers.

Background

In 1996, Proposition 215, also known as the Medical Use of Marijuana Initiative or the Compassionate Use Act, was approved by voters and legalized the use of medicinal cannabis in California.

In 2015, three California bills—AB 243, AB 266 and SB 643—were combined and resulted in legislation known as the Medical Cannabis Regulation and Safety Act (MSRSA). The regulation created a framework for the state licensing and enforcement of cultivation, manufacturing, retail sale, transportation, storage, delivery and testing of medicinal cannabis in California.

On November 8, 2016, voters passed Proposition 64, the legalization of recreational marijuana. California became one of eight states (Oregon, Washington, Alaska, Colorado, Nevada, Massachusetts, Maine and Washington D.C.) where marijuana is legal for recreational use. Proposition 64, also known as the Adult Use of Marijuana Act (AUMA), allows adults 21 years and older to legally grow, possess and use cannabis for non-medicinal purposes with certain restrictions. As of January 1, 2018, AUMA made it legal to sell and distribute cannabis through a regulated business.

Senate Bill 94, the Medicinal and Adult-Use Cannabis Regulation and Safety Act (MAUCRSA) was signed into law by Governor Jerry Brown on June 27, 2017. The

MAUCRSA basically repealed the MSRSA, incorporated certain provisions of the AUMA and integrated a single regulatory system to govern the medical and adult use cannabis industry in California.

The California Bureau of Cannabis Control (BCC) has been created for businesses that wish to cultivate, distribute or sell recreational marijuana on a commercial scale. The Bureau of Cannabis Control (BCC) is the lead agency in developing regulations for medical and adult-use cannabis in California. The BCC is responsible for licensing retailers, distributors, testing labs and microbusinesses. A state taxation system has been established to manage the cultivation and commercially distributed marijuana. Businesses are required to obtain a local business license and are subject to local regulations.

In Monterey County, considered one of the traditional agricultural centers of the world, perfect growing conditions exist to make it the center of the "Garden of Eden" for growing marijuana. Converted flower, fruit and vegetable plant growing facilities and greenhouses exist and can be used in large-scale cannabis growing farms. As the process moves forward, there remain many unanswered questions from the public in what the impact of this industry will be for Monterey County.

Tale of Two Cities

Blueberry Pie, Golden Pineapple, Black Mamba, Liquid Sunshine, and Green Crack are not paint colors from Home Depot. They are names of cannabis products offered today in some of the legalized adult-use and medicinal marijuana dispensaries in Monterey County. Since January 1, 2018, many new cannabis dispensaries have opened in Monterey County cities. In the City of Salinas, cannabis dispensary East of Eden (a homage to the city's favorite son, John Steinbeck), has received a state license to sell recreational marijuana to anyone 21 year or age or older. Other licensees in Monterey County include: Monterey Bay Alternative Medicine in Del Rey Oaks, Higher Level Care in Castroville, Big Sur Cannabotanicals in Carmel and Purple Trilogy in Salinas.

City of Del Rey Oaks

On October 24, 2017, the City Council of the City of Del Rey Oaks, California passed "Ordinance Number 289, A Cannabis Ordinance" allowing commercial cannabis operations in the city, establishing commercial cannabis business regulatory permits, regulating the personal use and cultivation of cannabis. The purpose of the ordinance was to regulate commercial and personal cultivation, retail sales, manufacturing, testing, distribution, delivery, and transportation of medicinal and nonmedicinal adult use cannabis, including cannabis products and edible cannabis products, within the City of Del Rey Oaks.

The city established that commercial cannabis businesses can operate in the city in a safe and limited manner, subject to review and approval of a regulatory and conditional use permit. The ordinance established that cannabis businesses operate in accordance with State Law and requires all commercial cannabis businesses to obtain licensing from the State Bureau of Cannabis Control.

The ordinance provided that no more than the following quantity and types of regulatory Commercial Cannabis Business (CCB) Permits shall be issued: one (1) retail sale permit; (4) manufacturing permits; and four (4) distribution permits. Permits were issued on a first come, first serve basis and existing CCBs in good standing and currently operating in the City were to be given priority. Permits would not be issued for commercial cultivation of cannabis.

CCBs are required to provide the following financial information in their application for a regulatory permit:

1. a list of funds belonging to the CCB held in savings, checking, or other accounts maintained by a financial institution;
2. a list of loans made to CCB;
3. a list of investments made into the CCB.

Other information required in the CCB's permit application include:

1. a copy of the applicant's completed application for electronic fingerprint images submitted to the Department of Justice and the Federal Bureau of Investigation;
2. a list of each applicant's misdemeanor and felony convictions, if any;
3. a complete and detailed diagram of the proposed premises showing the boundaries of the property and the proposed premises to be permitted;
4. a detailed security plan;
5. an odor control plan;
6. a comprehensive business operations plan.

In terms of personal use and cultivation, the ordinance provided that:

1. use of cannabis is prohibited on all City properly, including parks;
2. smoking cannabis is subject to all state and local regulations;
3. smoking or use of cannabis is prohibited within 1,000 feet of a school or childcare facility;
4. no more than six (6) cannabis plants may be cultivated for personal use indoors at any one residence;
5. use of volatile solvents as defined by State Codes, are prohibited for indoor and outdoor cultivation at a private residence;
6. indoor cultivation must have adequate ventilation;
7. six (6) or fewer cannabis plants may be cultivated outdoors for personal use at any single-family residence, regardless of the number of occupants;
8. no cannabis plant shall exceed the height of fence surrounding a property and in no case grow to more than six (6) feet.

Two officials from the City of Del Rey Oaks, Mayor Jerry Edelen and City Manager Dino Pick, provided insights on the city's Cannabis Ordinance. Mayor Edelen felt that the legalization of recreational and medicinal marijuana would provide an increase in revenue for cities. Edelen expressed that retail sales and business taxes collected from CCBs would help to provide money to fund city services. The Cannabis Ordinance provides the structure and regulatory framework to implement California's approved ballot measure Proposition 64.

City Manager Dino Pick stated that medicinal marijuana has been legal in Del Rey Oaks for the past two years and the city's one dispensary has been operating successfully. Pick echoed Mayor Edelen's belief that the City's budget would grow as the number of

CCBs, especially medical marijuana dispensaries, increased. The CCB business tax rate of 5 percent of the business' annual gross receipts for the first three years is expected to generate approximately $500,000 and will help support the City's infrastructure, i.e., fix roads, improve parks, etc. Pick noted that the city's Cannabis Ordinance established the permitting process to support legalized sale of cannabis. Current and future areas of concern for him include zoning, security, on-site monitoring, distribution, parking, and cultivation issues and were addressed by the Ordinance. Pick admits that the "all cash business" creates a financial management challenge for CBBs and will require law enforcement attention.

Susan, a plant horticulturist and long-time resident of Del Rey Oaks, related that she provides medical cannabis to many people in the Monterey County community, especially those with serious illnesses and diseases including cancer. She grows and manufactures cannabis oils and believes that it saves lives. She sells other products like Liquid Sunshine, a cannabis tincture for treating anxiety and inflammation. Prior to 2018, she did not need a permit to grow or sell medicinal cannabis. Today, the City of Del Rey Oaks has new requirements regarding number of plants and square footage needed to grow, security, licensing and testing. She no longer is able to get a permit with these new requirements. Sales taxes of over 15 percent and other taxes make the cost of doing business too expensive and she will not be able to sell products. Susan believes that only the large producers like Taylor Farms (a multi-billion-dollar agriculture company in Monterey County) who can pay the $500,000 dollars in production costs, will be able to comply with the security, state of the art manufacturing and lab testing requirements. Small growers are considered artisanal while large cannabis growers are able to vertically integrate (grow, manufacture, test, transport, distribute) its business. The new law will drive small growers into the black market.

Over half of the U.S. states have adopted "medical marijuana" laws (MMLs), and 58 percent of Americans now favor recreational marijuana legalization. Despite public support, federal law continues to prohibit the use and sale of marijuana due to public health concerns of increased dependence and abuse, youth access, and drugged driving. As marijuana is still illegal on at the federal level and banks are federally chartered, Commercial Cannabis Businesses (CCB) will find it difficult to get a loan. It is likely that legalization of marijuana will shift from small grower operations to large greenhouses/warehouse with state of the art energy and water systems.

City of Salinas

According to Salinas Mayor Joe Gunter, public safety is his primary concern in amending restrictions to the availability of medicinal marijuana products to residents of the City of Salinas. According to Gunter, the primary restriction would be to keep medicinal marijuana dispensaries away from schools, parks, churches and places where people meet. The city's Cannabis Ordinance provides for a 1,000-foot buffer between cannabis business and schools, parks and other sensitive locations.

Matt Pressey, City Finance Director, projected that the cannabis industry in Salinas is expected to generate tax revenue of $500,000 in 2017/18, about $1 to $2 million in 2018/19 and as much as $3 million in subsequent years. The City of Salinas fee and regulatory framework for the commercial cannabis industry was developed based on the costs the city would incur for regulating the industry and are provided below:

- Work permit application—$161.75
- Work permit renewal—$129.75
- Work permit transfer—$129.75
- Administrative permit—$102.70
- Monitoring fee—police—$7,714.69
- Monitoring fee—administration—$2,053.97
- Monitoring fee—city attorney—$674.03

Salinas CCBs responded both positively and negatively to the fee structure. Some CCB owners thought that the application and regulatory processes emplaced was needed for this new industry. Additionally, they felt that the general public will have more of a sense and understanding of the industry. Clearly, the tax revenues not captured in earlier underground/black market operations would now be available to the cities. On the other hand, some CCB owners felt that the fee structure is not cost effective and will drive out independent growers who will not be able to meet the regulatory costs.

The City of Salinas Economic Development Office administers the permit process and is the lead agency for regulating the process by issuing permits, identification cards and regular monitoring including reviews of inspections and videos. In July 2017, the City of Salinas issued nine permits to five cannabis companies and in December 2017, approved 20 businesses to do business in both adult-use and medicinal cannabis within the City of Salinas. Businesses included manufacturing, cultivation, dispensary delivery categories.

Conclusion

As the cities in Monterey County issue marijuana permits, public concerns surface about the commercial cannabis law. Issues surrounding health have surfaced regarding the impact of potential toxins and odors related to manufacturing and public safety. Especially of high concern for business owners is the impact of the AUMA on property value, the potential increase in insurance rates and the negative perception should their business be located near a commercial cannabis business. One source said that "In an industrial business park every business owner is concerned about property value. If you say I am next to a marijuana candy manufacturing plant automatically the perception is that isn't a place I want to be."

Call to Action

The approval of Proposition 64 changes the way municipal governments view adult-use and medicinal marijuana. Legalization will likely displace illicit markets potentially impacting neighborhood criminal activities. There are direct implications for public finance through increased tax revenue and decreased enforcement costs. City and county officials will need to address government, business and citizen issues related to increased use and decreased costs of cannabis and its effects on local health, economic issues, crime and safety. restrictions, legally grow a limited amount of marijuana.

41. Managing Marijuana

*The Role of Data-Driven Regulation**

STEPHEN GOLDSMITH

When Colorado voters approved a ballot measure to legalize the sale of recreational marijuana in 2014, state officials knew they would have to quickly develop a robust system to safely and securely control the flow of the drug across the state, and they managed to do just that with the help of advanced tracking and data analytics. What Colorado is doing provides an impressive example of an emerging, more effective regulation model.

To deal with the consequences of marijuana's legalization, Gov. John Hickenlooper appointed Andrew Freedman as director of marijuana coordination, and the legislature created the Marijuana Enforcement Division (MED) in the state's Department of Revenue. MED drew on the state's experience with its preexisting medical marijuana regulations, examining what had worked previously to regulate and inventory controlled substances.

The widespread legal availability of marijuana and marijuana-infused products, however, presented a host of new concerns for Colorado, with those surrounding public health and safety first and foremost. The state established a comprehensive set of goals surrounding health and safety concerns, analyzed the gaps in its existing data, and devised a plan to better track and regulate marijuana.

To begin with, the state needed a way to track plants from seed to sale. MED contracted with Franwell, a Florida-based company, to create a Colorado-specific version of its Marijuana Enforcement Tracking Reporting Compliance (Metrc) system. The state requires growers to track each plant with a unique radio frequency identification tag. The RFID tags allow the plants to be inventoried more quickly without direct contact, and they create data at each step of the supply chain as plants move from growers to shippers to final packaging.

The RFID tags, like the sensors that are becoming ubiquitous in the emerging economy of connected devices, build regulatory intelligence directly into the regulated object, streamlining enforcement across the board. The tracking system, for example, can automatically flag facilities that are producing substantially less marijuana than expected based on the outputs of comparable growers, which allows state employees to more easily identify potential illegal diversion. And because the state is able to track the origins of

*Originally published as Stephen Goldsmith, "Managing Marijuana: The Role of Data-Driven Regulation," *Governing*, August 17, 2016. Reprinted with permission of the publisher.

any product, it can easily issue public recalls for specific batches or growers if regulators discover traces of potentially harmful pesticides.

This system of constant, real-time tracking allowed Colorado to shift away from an older regulatory model in which governments must depend on slow bureaucratic procedures for permitting and licensing. Rather than simply hoping that procedural factors would prevent noncompliance, the state can respond to problems as they arise, which increases accountability and allows for better-informed enforcement.

The Colorado Department of Public Health and Environment, for example, analyzed hospital-visit data and found that marijuana-related visits had tripled after commercialization and that poison control calls had doubled. Around the same time, MED noticed that marijuana-infused edibles were comprising significantly more of the market than expected—fully 50 percent, according to Freeman. As MED discovered, the two were correlated: Many of the hospital visits and poison-control calls stemmed from a lack of dosing information or packaging safeguards.

MED quickly intervened, adopting new requirements that included childproofing edibles and clearly marking doses on the edibles' packaging. These changes have helped lower the instances of unintentional exposure to edible marijuana products. Colorado has hired a full-time analyst dedicated to deriving similar insights from these new flows of marijuana data.

Whatever one might think of the advisability of legalizing marijuana, there's much to be learned from Colorado's experience in data-driven regulation. While many of the practices Colorado is pioneering can be adopted by other states that may be considering legalizing marijuana, they also could help to broadly improve regulatory systems across all levels of government. Colorado is demonstrating how data-driven regulatory models can enable governments to quickly understand the realities of a market and hold businesses accountable—ultimately resulting in stronger, more effective consumer protections.

42. Medical Marijuana

*Do States Know How to Regulate It?**

DYLAN SCOTT

"This could get you 10 years in prison," Norton Arbelaez quips as he opens a 50-gram bag of Jack Frost, one of the highly potent strains of cannabis in storage at River-Rock, the Denver medical marijuana dispensary that Arbelaez co-founded. The stench from the bag wafts through RiverRock's inventory room, where black plastic tubs filled with marijuana are stacked in cabinets to the ceiling. Back through the inventory room's locked door is the front retail area, where a long glass counter holds jars of the dispensary's colorfully named strains: Sour Tsunami, Bruce Banner, Hindu Banana Cheese. Dispensary customers—patients who have each received a "red card," a doctor referral for medicinal marijuana—browse through the jars, sometimes stopping to take a whiff, while RiverRock staff members explain the strains' various effects. One staffer, outfitted in blue surgical gloves, describes a strain's chemical properties and genetic history with the same calm, clinical tone of a doctor addressing a patient.

In many ways, the entire operation at RiverRock, a warehouse indistinguishable from the other industrial buildings in its central Denver neighborhood, feels like any retail establishment in the city. But there are a few minute details, a handful of reminders that the whole place is, technically, illegal—according to the federal government, anyway. For starters: Security cameras behind black domes watch every corner of every room, covering every inch of the 60,000-square-foot facility. As required under the complex regulatory scheme that state policymakers have crafted, the cameras' feeds are transmitted to video screens at the offices of the Colorado Medical Marijuana Enforcement Division a few miles away. No part of RiverRock's cultivation and distribution escapes the eyes of state regulators. Each of the hundreds of plants growing in the dispensary is tagged with a radio frequency identification chip. Employees must sign in every time they enter the inventory room. The route that the company's trucks take to its other Denver retail location has been precisely outlined and approved by the enforcement division. Even the size of the font on signs posted on the dispensary's doors is dictated by state law.

These meticulous regulations are the result of Colorado's decade-long debate over how to manage medical marijuana. When voters approved Amendment 20 in 2000, res-

---

*Originally published Dylan Scott, "Medical Marijuana: Do States Know How to Regulate It?" *Governing*, August 2012. Reprinted with permission of the publisher.

idents gained the right to possess cannabis for therapeutic use. But the distribution system was only loosely conceived. "Caregivers" were allowed to grow and provide marijuana for up to five people, but many patients still resorted to purchasing from the black market. A series of court battles ensued after the Colorado Department of Public Health and Environment loosened the caregiver restrictions in June 2009 (seeming to pave the way for dispensaries), only to reverse its decision four months later and then reverse it again following a state Supreme Court ruling a month after that.

Finally, the Colorado General Assembly convened in 2010 to develop a more organized regulatory model. As a result of its work, a 77-page green binder sits on Arbelaez's desk at RiverRock, filled with requirements that he and his staff must follow to the letter. "We've recognized that this is a business, and our voters have said that they want patients to have access to this medicine," says state Sen. Pat Steadman, who was intimately involved in drafting the legislation that set the rules for medical marijuana dispensaries. "We want to make sure there is a legitimate industry to serve this population, so we've created a tight chain of control from seed to sale."

Colorado's evolution reflects the broader lessons states have learned in the decade and a half since California became the first state to approve medical cannabis in 1996. In that time, California has gained a reputation as something of the Wild West for weed: no state regulatory model, notoriously lax enforcement and an undefined set of prescription criteria that makes obtaining a medical marijuana card little more than a wink-wink formality. But as more states have legalized medical marijuana—today it's legal to some degree in 17 states plus the District of Columbia—a more tightly controlled approach seems to be emerging. Ten states and D.C. have set up a system of authorized dispensaries, and 16 states have outlined specific conditions for which medical marijuana can be used. Even California has considered reining things in: Lawmakers moved this summer to develop the state's first comprehensive licensing and permitting structure.

But no matter how controlled a state's medical marijuana policy may be, federal law still bans the cultivation, distribution and possession of marijuana for any purpose. The Obama administration has stated that it will not prosecute patients, but growers and distributors in medical marijuana states have still been targeted by multiple federal agencies, including the Justice Department and Internal Revenue Service (IRS). Medical marijuana businesses continue to operate in a legal gray zone. "In any other business, if you fail, you file for bankruptcy and move on. If you fail in this business, you go to jail," says Arbelaez, a patient himself and a former attorney who moved to Denver from New Orleans in 2009. "The one thing I can hold onto is complete compliance. The Colorado legal code is our only line of defense. It's the only way to show regulation is better than prohibition."

When Colorado lawmakers in 2010 decided to set up a regulatory system for dispensing marijuana, they didn't have many models to follow. So they turned to Matthew Cook, then the state's senior director of enforcement at the Department of Revenue for its gaming, alcohol and tobacco industries. Cook's credentials included his years as a special agent at the U.S. Air Force Office of Special Investigations in the late 1970s and another 30 years in alcohol enforcement for the city of Colorado Springs and the state of Colorado.

"I understood the culture," Cook says. "You have to communicate with the people you regulate. They need to know where you are." Cook convened a workgroup of 32 people—district attorneys, law enforcement agencies and individuals already selling marijuana—that met twice monthly for eight hours. Each side shared its concerns. Public justice advocates wanted to eradicate illicit dealing; distributors were worried that overly aggressive enforcement would neuter their ability to run a sustainable business. Compromises were made. One rule required dispensaries to be 1,000 feet from schools. Another allowed growers to continue tending their plants even if their license was under review, thus preventing lost revenue if the ruling turned out to be in their favor.

Out of those meetings came 21 specific rule-making mandates, which state lawmakers formalized and passed and Gov. Bill Ritter signed into law in June 2010. In the two years since, nearly 600 medical marijuana centers have been licensed, serving more than 100,000 patients. The experiment hasn't been flawless. Localities are authorized to issue their own moratoriums on commercial centers, and 105 have done so. As a result, fewer dispensaries have opened than originally projected, and the state enforcement office, which is partly funded through licensing fees paid by dispensaries, has had less money than expected. A bill introduced this year sought to close a $5.7 million shortfall for the office.

Colorado still has by far the most licensed distributors in the country (California has more dispensaries, but many remain unauthorized and unregulated), and other states are learning from the relative success of its system. Cook has left public employment and started a consulting business, advising states such as Arizona and Connecticut as they've developed policies in the last two years. "The Colorado approach is probably the model approach at this point," says Robert Mikos, a law professor at Vanderbilt University who has analyzed medical marijuana laws. "They have much more control of the industry. Other states can look at that, and they can learn from Colorado's experience."

They have. The California Assembly this May passed a bill to create a statewide structure for regulation and bring the state closer in line with its peers. The bill faltered in the state Senate in June, but supportive lawmakers expect it will keep resurfacing until it passes. "It's a little late out of the gate," says state Assemblyman Tom Ammiano, who introduced the legislation. "It's going to make our system viable and credible in the long term. Some of us could have told you 15 years ago that this is what we would need."

Connecticut, which in June became the most recent state to pass legislation, has crafted what some analysts say is the most tightly regulated medical marijuana system yet—and state officials credit the lessons they learned from states like Colorado and New Mexico. Connecticut lawmakers set a strict list of conditions for which medical cannabis could be used, including a cap on the amount of marijuana that patients could possess and a limited number of licensed pharmacists who could distribute the drug. "What's emerged here is something that will work," says Michael Lawlor, Connecticut's undersecretary for criminal justice policy and planning, who helped draft the law. "Attitudes toward marijuana generally are evolving. People think of it less as a crime and more of a health issue—that this is something that police and prosecutors should not be involved in."

That perspective—that marijuana use is a health issue—is not shared by the federal government. Under the Controlled Substances Act of 1970, marijuana is considered a Schedule I narcotic, which means it has no medicinal value under federal law. "It's illegal. That's it," says Mark Kleiman, a public policy professor at the University of California in Los Angeles who has studied marijuana policy. But because the act prevents research universities, for example, from undertaking studies to verify marijuana's therapeutic value, Kleiman says he considers the law "legally incoherent." Thanks in part to the lack of a fully developed body of research, marijuana's medicinal value is still the subject of some debate—although a 1999 Institute of Medicine of the National Academies report, often cited by advocates, concluded that marijuana's active ingredient, THC, could potentially treat appetite loss and nausea, despite reservations about the health risks of smoking cannabis.

After years of drug enforcement raids under the George W. Bush administration, many advocates and policymakers expected a shift in federal enforcement when President Obama took office in 2009. A now infamous White House memo issued on Oct. 19, 2009, seemed to affirm that assumption. U.S. Deputy Attorney General David Ogden told federal prosecutors that they "should not focus federal resources in your states on individuals whose actions are in clear and unambiguous compliance with existing state laws providing for the medical use of marijuana."

As states began to take more action—at least 10 states have passed or updated their policies since October 2009—the federal government started to walk back on the Ogden memo. U.S. district attorneys have since sent letters to officials in 11 states, clarifying that the federal government "remains firmly committed to enforcing the [Controlled Substances Act] in all states."

The letters have even, in some instances, appeared to imply that state employees could face criminal charges for enforcing state medical marijuana policies. In an April 2011 letter to Washington Gov. Christine Gregoire, for example, U.S. District Attorneys Jenny Durkan and Michael Ormsby wrote that "[s]tate employees who conducted activities mandated by the Washington legislative proposals would not be immune from liability." Gregoire vetoed the majority of a bill establishing a regulated dispensary system after receiving the letter.

A court ruling this January muddied the waters even further: Spurred by concerns about the legal risks to public workers if her state passed a medical marijuana policy, Arizona Gov. Jan Brewer sought a judgment on whether state employees administering the programs could be prosecuted. A U.S. district judge dismissed the suit as premature because no "genuine threat of imminent prosecution exists." The U.S. Justice Department supported the ruling.

A Justice spokesperson explains that the department is focused "on investigating and prosecuting significant drug traffickers, not state and local employees. However, as a matter of law, the Controlled Substances Act does not exempt state and local employees from potential enforcement action, and the department's communications with the states have appropriately noted that reality."

Other federal agencies have enforced anti-marijuana policy through less obvious channels. The IRS, for instance, has audited dozens of dispensaries in recent years, relying on a section of the federal tax code that prohibits companies from deducting expenses related to drug trafficking. The IRS has alleged that some California businesses owe millions of dollars in back taxes. "No business in America could survive if all of its expense deductions were disallowed," says Steve DeAngelo, owner of Oakland's Harborside Health Center, a marijuana dispensary that serves more than 100,000 customers, and from whom the feds are trying to reclaim $2.4 million. "This is not an attempt to tax us. It's an attempt to tax us out of existence."

Reports have also circulated that the U.S. Treasury Department is applying pressure to major banking institutions, such as Bank of America and Wells Fargo, to close the accounts of medical marijuana businesses. In response to Colorado dispensaries' banking struggles, state Sen. Steadman introduced a bill this year that would have allowed medical marijuana businesses to form their own credit union, but it was rejected by the Senate Finance Committee.

"We have an opportunity in a federalist system to let states try different approaches," says Steadman. "There are times when I'd prefer the federal government stay out of our way. Something needs to give here, and that something is federal law."

As medical marijuana supporters like to point out, nearly half of the U.S. population already lives in a state where medicinal cannabis is legal. (Three more states—Arkansas, Massachusetts and North Dakota—could place medical marijuana initiatives on their ballots in November.) In opinion polls, Americans overwhelmingly support allowing marijuana for medical use; a November 2011 CBS News poll showed that 77 percent of people believe it should be allowed. Some recent research also suggests that legalizing medical marijuana hasn't affected overall drug use. A May study by the University of Colorado found that marijuana use among teens has remained steady or dropped slightly since 2000.

Against that backdrop, some advocates say it may be time for yet another shift in marijuana policy: outright legalization. A Gallup poll last fall showed for the first time that 50 percent of Americans support legalizing marijuana use. California's Proposition 19, which would have decriminalized possession of marijuana for personal use, failed in 2010, but it garnered 47 percent of the vote. Some observers think that California has essentially become a quasi-legalized system anyway. In a forthcoming book, four academics, including Kleiman, estimate that fewer than 5 percent of medical marijuana recommendations in California are issued to treat serious diseases.

Residents in Colorado and Washington state will vote on full legalization this fall, and advocacy groups in Colorado say their internal polling shows initial support around 60 percent. "The genie is out of the bottle," Steadman says.

Somewhere between legalization and prohibition is the concept of decriminalization, which reduces criminal penalties for possession to small administrative sanctions and prevents those caught with small amounts of marijuana from being arrested or jailed. So far, 16 states have decriminalized marijuana possession, along with some major cities (the Chicago City Council passed a policy in June). New York Gov. Andrew Cuomo made headlines this summer when he stated his support for decriminalization. Although his proposal stalled in the state Legislature, many advocates saw an endorsement from the governor of the second-biggest state in the union as an important symbolic gesture.

While medical marijuana interest groups are, of course, aware of the push for broader decriminalization and legalization, they generally concentrate on the therapeutic sliver of the marijuana debate. The focus is on better regulation, which they hope will convince skeptics that a system like Colorado's can work. "We are in favor of strict regulation," says RiverRock's Arbelaez, "because that is the only way to show legitimacy."

"Cannabis doesn't need to be fully legalized to legitimize itself," says Michael Elliott of the Medical Marijuana Industry Group, which represents about 50 Colorado dispensaries. "It's not a stepping stone for patients. This is a medicine."

That medicine is now fueling hundreds of tightly controlled, multimillion-dollar businesses just like RiverRock. At Arbelaez's operation, the feeling is a blend of upstart commerce and the communal kumbayah of cannabis culture. His greenhouses churn out marijuana with industrial efficiency, and Arbelaez and his partners have invested hundreds of thousands of dollars in their business. (He declines to say exactly how much.) But as he walks among the patients in the front retail room, shaking hands and greeting them by name, it's clear that he's familiar with their individual stories and how they came to use marijuana for therapy. "It all goes back to the medicine for us," he says. "We think of ourselves as social entrepreneurs."

43. Managing Medical Marijuana*

WILLIAM KIRCHHOFF

Marijuana has been glorified, vilified, and medicalized. With 23-plus states and the District of Columbia having legalized medical marijuana, it is now a cascading event that is becoming a new social norm. In 2014, the House of Representatives passed a bill that if approved by the Senate, would remove marijuana from the federal government's Controlled Substance Act Schedule I.

Thus far, most of the efforts by local government officials in states that have legalized medical marijuana have focused on enforcement, zoning, licensing, sales monitoring, distribution control, and revenue collection. But when there are no longer legal restraints against its use, it could emerge as a unique workplace problem for local government management to cope with, including legal, ethical, operational, and organizational culture issues.

Local governments in those states that have legalized medical marijuana will be pressed by employees to treat the use of medical marijuana no differently than other legally prescribed medicines like Vicodin or Percocet, which can impair judgment. This could bring about a variety of challenges, with some having costly unintended consequences that managers will have to adjust to.

Protecting City Hall's Interests

The protection of local government employees is the intent of this essay, which is a follow-up to one I coauthored on medical marijuana in the December 2013 issue of *PM*. This essay addresses some of the issues that managers might have to deal with because of the ease with which marijuana can be obtained and the growing acceptance of its use—both medically and recreationally.

Cities in Colorado, Washington, and other states where medical marijuana has been legalized have been dealing effectively with such external challenges as dispensary location, taxing mechanisms, and permit requirements. Communities that I am familiar with, however, don't seem to be thinking through the workplace implications that will arise if marijuana is removed from Schedule 1 and the consequences of it emerging as a unique public workplace problem.

---

*Originally published as William Kirchhoff, "Managing Medical Marijuana," *PM Magazine,* January/February 2015. Reprinted with permission of the publisher.

Legitimate Challenges

The challenge now is whether sensible and systematic policy changes will be implemented, or will inaction leave employees unclear of their rights and status? Most current local government drug and alcohol policies I have studied are not sufficiently comprehensive to effectively control the use of medical marijuana.

In fact, most of the policies leave an organization with considerable exposure to the threat of employment law litigation, workplace confusion, unnecessary labor strife, and loss of community confidence.

Current policies, for example, use such drug policy terms as testing site, testing facility, and drug test without the specificity needed to assure the accuracy and reliability of the techniques, equipment, and laboratory facilities used in the testing. Another example is the term safety-sensitive, which is used to establish which employees are subject to drug testing.

Often this general term is not specific in a job description or designation. To most people, emergency responders, truck drivers, and equipment operators are understandably safety-sensitive positions. But what about water plant operators, recreational leaders, mechanics, and code enforcement personnel for whom the safety of others is their responsibility?

A tough-to-deal-with furball of legal, operational, and labor-related challenges is possible if a local government's written drug policy is ambivalent and lacking in specifics.

Up to now, management has focused almost exclusively on the minority group of employees who are illegally using marijuana while at work—the abusers. The legal right to use medical marijuana, however, will affect two other employee groups—the legitimate users and the innocents. Legitimate users will medicate in accordance with the law and their physician's advice, and they will adhere to workplace policies.

Managers will also have to deal with the innocents—those employees who have not used any marijuana but are affected by simply being in the workplace and might test out false-positive in a random drug test. Such edibles as poppy seeds can cause a false-positive test outcome. Prescription drugs like Marinol that are used for anorexia, HIV, and cancer patients can test false-positive for marijuana.

I believe it's the responsibility of the employer to protect these workers from the embarrassment, stigma, and possible discipline attached to testing positive for marijuana as a result of using other medications or eating a common food.

Modernizing Drug Policies

My research indicates that local government policies pertaining to drug use might need to be tightened up with respect to marijuana. Should, for example, a medical marijuana prescription that's written by any physician suffice?

In California, for example, it is remarkably easy to obtain a medical prescription called a recommendation to use medical marijuana. Would it be more responsible to require such prescriptions to be reviewed by the organization's medical review officer (MRO), usually a contract physician specializing in pharmacology and toxicology?

An already weak drug policy that does not take legalized marijuana into account is detrimental to the organization, which might result in two inevitable outcomes. One is the almost incalculable number of legal, operational, financial, and political consequences that will arise.

The other is that organized labor will seek to protect their memberships regarding testing protocols, second-chance opportunities, confidentiality, random testing procedures, and so forth. The discussions I have had with public sector labor officials make it evident that they are ahead of local government management and are currently developing negotiating strategies to protect the rights of their membership as it pertains to medical marijuana.

Evolving societal and legislative norms, court rulings, and potential legal consequences mandate that whatever changes made to a government organization's drug policies be done with first-rate attention from legal staff, human resources professionals, and operational managers.

Workplace "What Ifs"

One purpose of this essay is to use the "What If" decision-making model as a mechanism to brainstorm the unintended consequences of medical marijuana. By using this approach, managers, attorneys, human resource specialists, and department directors will be able to anticipate some of the unintended consequences.

Cannabinoids affect sensory, psychomotor, and cognitive function. According to the U.S. Chamber of Commerce, studies reveal that a worker using marijuana is two times more likely to request time off, three times more likely to injure themselves or another employee, and five times more likely to file a worker's compensation claim.

There are two considerations that frame the new marijuana challenge for local government. The first is the necessity of identifying the preferred outcomes of those in charge. The second consideration should be the seamless and positive acceptance of marijuana as a drug that can be used legitimately by employees once the legal barriers vaporize.

While the list can seem endless, here are some examples of the "What Ifs" that public officials will have to contend with.

What if:

- An employee who has been prescribed topical marijuana for joint pain tests positive without having inhaled or ingested marijuana? Will he or she face disciplinary action?
- An employee fails to notify his or her supervisor as is required for the use of other judgment-impairing prescriptions? Will the marijuana-using employee be treated the same as employees who have not reported their use of hydrocodone, antidepressants, cold medicines, sleep inhibitors, and the like?
- An employee is suspected of being in an impaired mental or physical state because of marijuana use? Will the regulatory protocols be identical to other prescribed judgment-impairing medications commonly used by employees?
- An employee's legal counsel asks, "How many other employees of record have officially advised their employer that they are using prescription medications that might impair their judgment?" Experience as a former manager warns me that only a few employees will share this information with their employers.

- A supervisor who has not been adequately trained to observe "marijuana behavior" in the workplace selects an employee who is not under the influence of marijuana or judgment-impairing prescription medication for testing? What are the legal implications and liabilities?
- An employee's physician certifies that the prescribed amount of marijuana does not impair judgment? Is she or he required to report the use of medical marijuana?
- An employee uses medical marijuana during off-duty hours and tests positive to random testing but exhibits no judgment impairment?
- The union demands that the testing process, frequency of testing, or review process that is used for medical marijuana must be identical to the standards applied to other prescription medications that may impair judgment?
- Labor initiates contract negotiations to protect its employees' rights regarding the use of medical marijuana? Will the government's negotiators have the adequate expertise to protect its interests and the civil rights of its workforce?
- A supervisor discriminates because she or he can't get past the stigma associated with marijuana?
- Unionized employees demand that the use of medical marijuana by employees be prohibited?
- An employee using medical marijuana is injured on the job because of impaired judgment?

Emerging Questions

The "What Ifs" lead to these questions, among others, that must be addressed:

- How does the employer protect the professional reputation of employees who choose to use medical marijuana legitimately?
- How does the employer establish testing thresholds that will meet reasonable legal standards?
- What process will the employer use for a third-party medical review of marijuana prescriptions issued to employees?
- What methods will be used to determine the acceptable length of time medical marijuana can be in an employee's system before it is not considered judgment impairing?
- What are the employer/employee options if an employee is prescribed medical marijuana for a chronic problem—light duty, medical leave, disability retirement, and so forth?
- What are the testing levels that qualify an employee as being judgment impaired if he or she is using prescription marijuana?
- What if the union demands that whatever testing process, frequency of testing, or review process that is used for medical marijuana be identical to the existing standards applied to other prescription medications that might impair judgment?

Checklist for Drug Policy Revision

The fundamental rule here is that the drug policies developed by local governments should be specific, comprehensive, and understandable. General suggestions regarding "tighter" drug policy revisions are found in the checklist outlined below.

The checklist is organized into three categories. Category 1 pertains to policy and legal nuisances. Category 2 relates to testing procedures and protocols. Category 3 addresses the likely management challenges local governments will face.

Category 1: Policies and Procedures

- Review the current policies pertaining to controlled substances—such drugs as hydrocodone, antidepressants, cold medicines, and sleep inhibitors. Failing to differentiate the use of medical marijuana from other prescription drugs that are commonly used without oversight will invite labor challenges and litigation.
- Require medical marijuana prescription holders to be examined by the employer's contract medical review officer (MRO). The duties and responsibilities of this position should be specifically defined by the employer. Without this policy requirement that even a small city can contract for, any licensed physician can prescribe marijuana in those states that have approved medical marijuana.
- Make sure the policies are not in conflict with state antidiscrimination statutes. While federal courts have held that the Americans with Disabilities Act (ADA) does not require employers to permit marijuana use to accommodate a disability, state law may do so.
- Clarify whether or not physician-prescribed topical applicants, capsules, suppositories, food, and beverages containing cannabis can be used in the workplace. Can smokeless electronic devices or inhalers be used? Should there be a designated area for such use?
- Require employees to notify human resources in writing that they have been prescribed medical marijuana and how they intend to use it. Human resources (HR) should review usage policies with the applicant, refer the applicant to the organization's MRO, and notify the chain-of-command with complete confidentiality. The employee's use of medical marijuana and workplace behavior should be monitored and reviewed formally on a clearly established schedule.
- Establish the protocols for random testing, the type(s) of test to be used, and facilities for the testing event. Employee confidentially and privacy during testing are important elements of the policy and process. Define the testing levels that qualify an employee as being judgment impaired and the review process for appeal.
- List the positions considered safety-sensitive by your organization and specify the employee pools for random testing. The random process needs to be unequivocally fair and absent of any bias. The U.S. Department of Transportation (USDOT) is the best source of information regarding the subject of random testing safety sensitive positions (www.dot.gov/dapc).
- Impose specific disciplinary and second-chance rules that can be applied to the workforce. Unduly strict policies can result in the termination of a solid

employee who casually smoked or ingested marijuana off duty days before a random test.

- Consider polices to prevent the increased recreational use of recreational marijuana. The ease with which recreational users can use these products (e.g., smokeless inhalers, edibles, topicals, and beverages) undetected in the workplace has increased significantly. This group of employees, the abusers, will use medical marijuana to game the system.

Category 2: Mandate Specific Testing Guidelines

Developing a legally defendable testing protocol is critical. Detection time differs with the type of testing. Hair follicle testing, for example, can trace marijuana usage as far back as 90 days, with urine testing for a single-use event testing positive for 48 to 72 hours. Currently, there is no way a test can determine when marijuana was used.

USDOT testing thresholds are the best general reference for testing guidelines.

Category 3: Management Challenges

- Train supervisors to detect the use of unauthorized marijuana. Without an acceptable training curriculum, supervisors will not be able to identify drug use behavior, nor will they be able to withstand challenges from the opposing employment law counsel.
- Require management protocol training for all supervisors. Such sensitive employee information as drug-test results and requests for special needs to accommodate the use of prescribed marijuana, need to be treated confidentially.
- Address how off-duty recreational use of marijuana is treated if its use is permitted by law. Organizations can prohibit the use of alcohol four hours before reporting for duty. What prohibitions are legal and sensible for the use of recreational marijuana off-duty, which can test positive for up to 90 days after its use?
- Recognize organized labor's interest. It is important to recognize that labor could resist additional oversight policies that will be necessary to manage the employee's use of medical marijuana. A first-to-the-table strategy by management is a recommended approach for labor negotiations.
- The scope of HR's oversight involvement will need expansion. Confidential recordkeeping, chain-of-evidence management, management of testing protocols, and disciplinary actions and appeals are but a few of the challenges most HR departments will face, particularly those of smaller jurisdictions.

Managing marijuana in the local government workplace will certainly become more complicated when the federal government drops it from the Controlled Substance Acts Schedule 1 and as states continue to approve the use of medical and recreational marijuana. The core challenge will be getting ahead of the curve by drafting comprehensive drug policies so that the worker and the workplace are protected.

Drug and Alcohol Policy Red Flags

The evolution of marijuana as a legitimate medicine requires careful review of public sector drug and alcohol policies. The good news is that the policy modifications necessary to deal with the changing laws associated with medical marijuana are relatively simple.

The bad news is that many of the policies used by local government organizations require extensive recalibration to reduce the threats of adverse litigation, organizational confusion, administrative embarrassment, unfavorable publicity, unnecessary labor-management conflict, and a loss of community confidence.

One way to quickly determine if your organization's existing drug and alcohol policy may need modification is if the answers to any of these questions is "no."

- Is the policy in compliance with USDOT regulations? USDOT is the gold standard for testing thresholds and processes. Information regarding USDOT regulations can be found at www.dot.gov/dapc.
- Are the drug-testing procedures clearly defined? Such commonly used policy terms as testing site, testing facility, and drug test lack the specificity needed to assure the accuracy and reliability of the techniques, equipment, and laboratory facilities used in the testing.
- Does the existing policy specifically identify the types of drugs to be tested? Policies use such ambiguous references as illegal drugs, non-prescribed controlled substances, and mind-altering substances rather than specific identification, including marijuana, cocaine, opiates, and propoxyphene.
- Does the policy specifically define what the unacceptable test thresholds are? Such terms as testing positive and positive laboratory results may leave the decision of what is acceptable or unacceptable outside the organization's control.
- Does the policy identify what positions are safety sensitive? A core requirement of any drug and alcohol program is the identification of those positions the organization identifies as safety sensitive.
- Is the definition of reasonable suspicion consistent with applicable law? Reasonable suspicion is when a trained supervisor has a distinct belief based on specific, contemporaneous, and articulable observations of an employee, that he or she poses a threat to themselves or safety of other because of drugs. The definition of reasonable suspicion must support the legal requirements for further investigation on some factual foundation.
- Are random testing guidelines clear and specific enough to stand legal challenge? Pool size for random testing, what positions are in the pool, frequency of testing, and the random selection process necessary for total objectivity are some of the elements of policy inclusion.

If the answer to these red flag questions is "no," then the drug and alcohol policy needs to be tightened up. My reading of more than 100 current municipal drug policies leads me to conclude that if the above issues aren't sufficiently specific and comprehensive, then there are most likely additional deficiencies of import that are problematic and risk inducing.

Is there, for example, a clear definition of what constitutes a failure to submit to a mandated drug test, and what official is responsible for recordkeeping confidentiality and the chain of evidence? What about off-duty use? What are the return-to-work options and requirements and fitness-for-duty testing? How often and when can follow-up testing occur?

44. Marijuana Management

What's Happening Now[*]

MICHELE FRISBY

At the 2014 ICMA Annual Conference, experts discussed the impact of marijuana legalization on local governments.

In September 2014, in conjunction with its 100th annual conference in Charlotte/Mecklenburg County, NC, ICMA hosted a telephonic news event during which a group of local government advisors and managers representing jurisdictions at the forefront of marijuana legalization efforts, shared their perspectives on what legalization has and will mean for local governments and their communities. The panel examined the challenges local jurisdictions will face when what appears to be an inevitable and major shift in the longstanding criminal status and public policy regarding marijuana takes place.

Today, in addition to the 19 states and the District of Columbia that have legalized pot for medicinal reasons, the use of marijuana for recreation is now legal in Alaska, Colorado, Oregon, and Washington, D.C.[1] Colorado marked the first-year anniversary of recreational marijuana sales in January 2015,[2] and in 2016, an additional five states are expected to vote on legalization.[3]

New Meaning to the Words "Marijuana Management"

A new development in the evolution of one of the most complex social experiments since prohibition is the establishment of the country's first government-owned pot store. The Cannabis Corner, owned and operated by the city of North Bonneville, Washington (pop. 1,000), is located along the Columbia River just 40 miles from Portland, Oregon. According to Governing.com, the store is run out of a renovated storage barn by a team of 10 government employees and offers customers small baggies of marijuana for $12 to $20 each.

The Cannabis Corner's business model, reports Governing.com, is a public devel-

[*]Originally published Michele Frisby, "Marijuana Management: What's Happening Now," International City/County Management Association, June 25, 2015. https://icma.org/articles/marijuana-management-what%E2%80%99s-happening-now. Reprinted with permission of the publisher.

opment authority similar to the one that runs Seattle's Pike Place Market. A five-member board makes all the business decisions, and the store's profits will fund community projects. Because it is run by the government, unlike its competitors, The Cannabis Corner is free from any federal tax responsibility.

Present and Future Tax Revenues

The Council for State Governments reports that as more states consider adding marijuana and industrial hemp to their agricultural industries, the costs and benefits to those states and the local jurisdictions within them are becoming clearer.[4]

Legal medical marijuana sales in California alone totaled just over one billion dollars in 2014.[5] During its first year as a legal recreational drug, marijuana generated tax revenues totaling $63.4 million for the state of Colorado. Yet, experts say it's too early to predict what this means for future marijuana revenues and cite the need for more historical data.[6]

Despite the tight timeframe between voter approval in November 2012, the creation two months later of statutory regulations, and the sale of retail licenses and opening of the first stores in January 2014, Colorado's move to recreational marijuana use was made relatively smooth because of the state's previous history with medical marijuana[7]—an advantage cited repeatedly by the panelists who participated in the ICMA media event.

The state of Washington, which opened its initial retail stores in July 2014, did not have the same prior-knowledge advantage as Colorado[8] but managed to generate $120 million in sales of recreational marijuana as of March 2015, with nearly $30 million in revenue generated during so far this fiscal year.[9]

Banking Challenges

What happens to all the revenues generated as part of the marijuana commerce industry? Because marijuana is still classified by the federal government as an illegal, Schedule 1 controlled substance, most banks refuse to accept pot-based businesses, whether medical or retail, as customers for fear of violating laws against money laundering.[10]

The result is a potentially unsafe, inefficient, cash-only business that is highly susceptible to "robbery, burglary, or assault … or tax evasion, fraud, and skimming," according to a July 2015 PM magazine article.[11]

The situation changed dramatically in February 2014 when the Obama administration allowed the banking industry to conduct business with legal marijuana sellers. Today these individuals can establish checking and savings accounts in which to deposit revenues,[12] a development which signals that marijuana commerce is about to come "out of the shadows and into the mainstream financial system."[13]

New Local Government Workplace Realities

Employee workforce issues promise to become a key local government marijuana-management challenge. The question soon will become what local governments will do when federal law no longer prohibits the medical use of marijuana, which many believe is inevitable,[14] and cities, towns, and counties will need to shift virtually overnight from treating marijuana as a criminal issue to supporting it as a medical product that many employees feel they have the right to use.

A free, 20-page e-book, Managing Medical Marijuana in Local Government: An Integrated Action Plan, can help communities navigate this potentially thorny issue. The book provides local government managers and human resources directors with an action plan—which involves policy rewriting and value alignment—to cope with the likely removal of marijuana from the federal government's Schedule 1 list of toxic substances.

Additional information on the topic of marijuana-related workplace issues is available through two *PM* magazine resources: "Marijuana at City Hall: It's Medicine Now" (December 2013) and "Managing Medical Marijuana" (January/February 2015).

Notes

1. "Legality of cannabis by U.S. jurisdiction" (n.d.). https://en.wikipedia.org/wiki/Legality_of_cannabis_by_U.S._jurisdiction; and "State Marijuana Laws Map" (n.d.). Governing.com. http://www.governing.com/gov-data/state-marijuana-laws-map-medical-recreational.html

2. Abner, Carrie. "Budding Growth." Capitol Ideas (March-April 2015). Council of State Governments. http://www.csg.org/pubs/capitolideas/2015_may_june/budding_growth.aspx?utm_source=The+Current+State+%2321&utm_campaign=Current+State+%2321%2C+6.22.15&utm_medium=email

3. Daigneau, Elizabeth. "America's First Government-Owned Marijuana Store" (June 2015). Governing.com. http://www.governing.com/topics/mgmt/gov-cannabis-corner-portland.html

4. Daigneau, Elizabeth. Ibid.

5. Ferner, Matt. "Legal Marijuana Is the Fastest-Growing Industry in the U.S.: Report." Huffington Post. January 26, 2015. http://huffingtonpost.com/2015/01/26/marijuana-industry-fastest-growing_n_6540166.html

6. Ferner, Matt. Ibid.

7. Ferner, Matt. Ibid.

8. Ferner, Matt. Ibid.

9. Ferner, Matt. Ibid.

10. "Local Government Leaders and Experts Discuss Marijuana Management." http://icma.org/en/Article/105027/Local_Government_Leaders_and_Experts_Discuss_Marijuana_Management; and Harper, Kevin. "Medical Marijuana Emerges from the Shadows and into the Mainstream Financial System." *Public Management* (PM). July 2015, p. 21.

11. Harper, Kevin. Ibid.

12. Harper, Kevin. Ibid

13. Harper, Kevin. Ibid.

14. "Local Government Leaders and Experts Discuss Marijuana Management." http://icma.org/en/Article/105027/Local_Government_Leaders_and_Experts_Discuss_Marijuana_Management

45. Advertising Marijuana[*]

Seth Poe *and* Alan R. Roper

Recreational marijuana will be sold in outlets to consumers by business owners intent on making a profit. As with any retail business, proper online and media marketing is necessary to drive the customer to the seller. Without advertising and promotion, the recreational marijuana retail store or outlet will rarely achieve a high level of exposure needed for a successful business.

This raises some questions about how legalized marijuana will be advertised, and what kind of regulation may be imposed to safeguard the public. As with any product limited to customers over the age of 21, advertising should not target minors. In 1997, the Federal Trade Commission charged the R.J. Reynolds Tobacco Company with illegally aiming tobacco advertising at minors with the *Joe Camel* campaign. This caused a shift in tobacco product advertising, and may be viewed as cautionary to marijuana advertisers who may otherwise test the limits of acceptable targeted advertising.

While retailers are restricted from directly advertising to minors, any form of advertising can be inherently persuasive. Studies have shown any exposure to pro marijuana advertising can lower the perceptions of danger and increases the likelihood of use in minors. States have established regulations on advertising that include print, broadcast, televised and digital media. Colorado and Washington modeled their regulations on advertising legalized marijuana after the existing tobacco and alcohol regulations. The Colorado Department of Revenue, Marijuana Enforcement Division regulations explain: "Voluntary standards adopted by the alcohol industry direct the industry to refrain from advertising where more than approximately 30 percent of the audience is reasonably expected to be under the age of 21" (Colorado Department of Revenue, 2018).

This essay will look at the risks of marijuana advertising on minors, and what regulatory actions have been taken to restrict targeted advertising. Additionally, this essay will look at the effectiveness of anti-marijuana advertising. It is not practical to think minors will be prevented from seeing cannabis ads. However, it is important to consider the ethical use of advertising in a way that does not encourage or promote marijuana usage among minors.

---

[*]Published with permission of the authors.

Current Regulation on Advertising Marijuana in California

California's Proposition 64, which legalizes adult use of marijuana provides guidelines on how marijuana can be advertised. In the interest of not advertising to minors, Chapter 15 of the State law describes advertising and marketing restrictions as follows:

> Section (b) Any advertising or marketing placed in broadcast, cable, radio, print and digital communications shall only be displayed where at least 71. 6 percent of the audience is reasonably expected to be 21 years of age or older, as determined by reliable, up-to-date audience composition data (CA.Gov, Legislative Information (2017).

So why can't we just leave it up to State regulators to ensure that marijuana advertising will not cause an increase in use by underage consumers? The federal and state regulations are not able to prevent marijuana advertisements from being publicly viewable for people of all ages. In San Francisco last year, a growers' collaborative bought ads on dozens of city buses and billboards promoting their "small batch" crops. The tagline: "That's cannabis, the California Way" (Adams, 2017). If you drive north from San Francisco up through Oregon and Washington, you're bound to spot numerous billboard advertisements for dispensaries and cannabis products. Marijuana advertising is excluded from online advertisements on major social media platforms and television, but the digital ads on websites and outlet locator applications are difficult to regulate.

Effects of Marijuana Advertising on Minors

The legalized sale of recreational marijuana is in its infancy in California, but medical marijuana sales and advertising have been around for over twenty years. A recent study was conducted on marijuana advertising by D'Amico, Miles, & Tucker (2015) called *Gateway to Curiosity: Medical Marijuana Ads and Intention and Use During Middle School U.S.* This study focused on the advertisement of medical marijuana and its impact on changing attitudes or promoting marijuana use to sixth- to eighth-grade youth. Results of the study indicate a link between accessibility and changing tolerations of marijuana among adults, resulting in a perception by adolescents as it being more beneficial and less harmful. "Exposure to medical marijuana advertising may be an important influence on adolescents' perceptions about marijuana and marijuana use" (D'Amico, et al., 2015).

The results showed, 22 percent of adolescents in 2010 and 30 percent in 2011, reported seeing at least one advertisement for medical marijuana on billboards or in magazines within three months. Concluding, "Youth who reported seeing any ads for medical marijuana were twice as likely as youth who reported never seeing an ad to use marijuana and to report higher intentions to use marijuana 1 year later" (D'Amico, et al., 2015). Concluding recommendations of the study state: "Regulations should be put in place on medical marijuana and recreational marijuana advertising, similar to regulations that are in place for the advertising of alcohol and tobacco products" (D'Amico, et al., 2015).

Many Marijuana advertisers are turning to digital media/social media marketing platforms such as Twitter, Facebook, YouTube, Instagram, Cannabis websites, & smart phone applications. While these digital mediums are regulated by states like Colorado, it's difficult to detect and enforce age restrictions among them. In the study *Marijuana*

Advertising Exposure Among Current Marijuana Users in the U.S., 742 people ranging 18–34 years old responded to anonymous online surveys. The study concluded 66 percent of the young adults viewed or heard marijuana advertisements in 30 days (Krauss, Sowles, Sehi, Spitznagel, Berg, Bierut & Cavazos-Rehg, 2017). Sixty-seven percent of those advertisements came from digital media social sites like, Facebook, Instagram, Twitter and traditional websites.

Social media sites may take action against the advertising of marijuana. Facebook previously shut down pages promoting marijuana dispensaries (Krauss, et al., 2017). Regulation of web content and social media is difficult to enforce by states, and may require websites to participate through age restricting software. An example of this is the website *Weedmaps*, a popular marijuana dispensary locator that does not have age restriction in place (Krauss, et al., 2017). This research concludes that although their study did not specifically target younger youths, "the prevalence of young adult users who see such advertisements online and on social media sites where youth are known to spend a lot of time highlights the need for increased monitoring as well as research into better methods to regulate online advertising" (Krauss, et al., 2017).

Another recent study on the effect of digital and social media marijuana advertising on young people was conducted by Hongying Dai (2017). This study also focused on exposure to marijuana advertisements and the relationship with marijuana use among U.S. adolescents in grades 8, 10, and 12. The study found that 13.8 percent of the underage population reported marijuana use in the past 30 days. From this study, exposure to marijuana advertisements was prevalent among adolescents, with 52.8 percent reporting exposure from internet advertisements, 32.1 percent from television advertisements, 24.1 percent from magazine or newspaper advertisements, 19.7 percent from radio advertisements, 19.0 percent from advertisements on storefronts, and 16.6 percent from billboards (Dai, 2017).

Despite attempts to regulate marijuana advertising as to not expose young people, there may be limited capability in doing so. Current studies indicate a connection between young people viewing marijuana advertising and marijuana curiosity and use. "Exposure to advertising for medical marijuana, marijuana intentions, and marijuana use showed a reciprocal association of advertising exposure with marijuana use and intentions during middle school" (D'Amico, et al., 2015).

The Evolution of Digital Marijuana Advertising

Digital advertising has become the most prevalent form of marketing marijuana. The regulations regarding digital advertising vary. For example, Colorado requires that 30 percent of the audience be reasonably expected to be 21, and that age affirming software must be present on sites containing marijuana advertising (Colorado Department of Revenue, 2018). However, these software-based safeguards rely on self-reporting of the viewer/consumer.

The popular marijuana retail locater website, Weedmapswww was examined in a recent study to determine effectiveness of age verification. In the study of the advertising content, and age verification practices on *Weedmaps* and the websites it sponsors (146 retailers that are listed on *Weedmaps* from Colorado [89] and Washington [57]), findings showed that among the independent retailers listed, 41 percent (31/76) in Colorado, and

35 percent (13/37) in Washington lacked any form of restriction to verify the user's age before entering the website (Bierut, Krauss, Sowles, Cavazos-Rehg, 2016).

The *Weedmaps* website provides links to the following social media sites: Facebook, Twitter, Instagram, LinkedIn, Google+, YouTube, and Vine. *Weedmaps* had the greatest number of followers on Facebook (over 130,000) and YouTube (nearly 150,000), followed by Twitter (58,000)," with 15 percent being under the age of 20" (Bierut, et al., 2016).

Regulating internet content and the age of those who access it may be difficult at best. Age verification was not present in 44 out of 113 Colorado, and Washington retailers listed from this one online resource, and with the anticipated growth in the marijuana industry, new innovations in digital advertising will likely emerge.

Success of Anti-Marijuana Advertising on Minors

At this point, you may reasonably assume that if viewing pro marijuana advertisements by minors increases likelihood of use, then viewing anti-marijuana advertisements by minors will have the reverse effect. A study from 2001, *Television campaigns and adolescent marijuana use: Tests of sensation seeking targeting* assessed television viewing and exposure to public service announcements, attitudes toward and use of marijuana and other substances. The findings concluded that carefully targeted campaigns that achieve high levels of reach and frequency, and with messages designed specifically for the target audience can play an important role in future drug abuse prevention efforts (Palmgreen, Donohew, Lorch, Hoyle, & Stephenson, 2001).

In a subsequent study, *Adolescents' Attitudes Towards Anti-Marijuana Ads, Usage Intentions, and Actual Marijuana Usage,* the anti-marijuana television ads used in the National Youth Anti-drug Media Campaign were assessed for effectiveness. The research collected survey data from nearly 3,000 respondents ages 12 to 18 years old. The study evaluated over a dozen ads featuring, "celebrity testimonials, refusal skills, alternatives to drugs, physical harms of use, and so forth" (Johnson, & Nakawaki, 2013). Findings demonstrated that the early interventional advertisements introduced to potential users can be effective in curtailing use, but overall impact on those who have used marijuana had little to no effect on their potential continued use.

As with all advertising, some ads will be more effective than others. A recent study evaluated the "My Anti-Drug" and "Above the Influence" anti-drug video Public Service Announcements. "My Anti-Drug" (MAD) was developed using the help of advertising agencies and behavior experts and ran from 1999 to 2004. Being mostly a fear based advertising campaign that, "Emphasized the negative consequences" of drug use (Comello, 2013). MAD was deemed a failure and was overhauled in 2005, replaced by the "Above the Influence" (ATI) campaign, which concentrated on more positive actions for avoiding marijuana. Comello (2013) states, "Increased personal autonomy and other positive consequences of avoiding substances, such as being able to pursue career goals or exciting activities." Although differences emerged for emotional tone and perceived risk, there were no differences observed for attitude toward campaign or mean attitude toward ad" (Comello, 2013). Findings identified a problem with the fundamental message of anti-marijuana advertisements stating, "[a]lthough billions of taxpayer dollars have funded televised national campaigns to prevent youth substance use, most of these efforts have had null or even adverse effects" (Comello, 2013).

Despite the reasonable assumption that viewing anti-marijuana advertisements by minors will counterbalance the effects of legalized marijuana advertising, this may not be true. Anti-marijuana campaigns have had only a limited success at curbing drug use in the past. Fear-based anti-marijuana advertising is not as effective as emotional goal oriented campaigns (Comello, 2013). Carefully targeted anti-marijuana advertising may be effective. However, these campaigns have not evolved technologically, or at the same rate legal marijuana advertising has.

State Research on Marijuana Advertising Effects on Minors

As early adopters of legalized marijuana laws, both Colorado and Washington State have sponsored studies to determine if youth marijuana use has increased after legalization. This resulted in the 2015, *Healthy Kids Colorado Survey*, and the 2016, *Washington State Healthy Youth Survey*. The surveys in both states concluded that marijuana use rates among teens have remained steady despite the legalization and sale of recreational marijuana. The data in both states determined that the perceived risk of regular marijuana use is declining, with Colorado seeing a drop from 54 percent in 2013, to 48 percent in 2015 (Healthy Kids Colorado Survey, 2015). While Washington saw a drop from 53 percent, to 48 percent in 8th graders that perceive marijuana use as risky, and emphasizing "Decreases in perceived risk are often followed by increased use" (Washington State Healthy Youth Survey, 2016).

Oregon also conducted a similar study, *Exposure to Marijuana Marketing After Legalization of Retail Sales: Oregonians' Experiences, 2015–2016*. The objective of the study was to "assess exposure to marijuana advertising in Oregon after the start of retail marijuana sales in October 2015" (Fiala, Dilley, Firth & Maher, 2018). Surveying over four thousand adults over 18 in 2015 and again in 2016, the findings report that 54.8 percent or half of the adults saw marijuana advertising in the past month, with over 50 percent of that advertising coming from storefront, street side and billboards (Fiala, et al., 2018). The authors note that exposure was not limited to only users. "People who do not use marijuana and those in the 18 to 24 age group were as exposed to advertising as other groups" (Fiala, et al., 2018).

Moving Toward Responsible Marijuana Advertising

Local governments in California can still exercise some controls on marijuana advertising. In order to apply for a temporary or permanent cannabis business license in the potential marijuana entrepreneur must receive permission from their local city or, if they're outside an incorporated city, the county. Economics can also play a role in the balance of pro-marijuana and anti-marijuana advertisements. The advertising capabilities of a multi-billion-dollar marijuana industry may outpace those of public service announcements aimed at dissuading minors from trying or using cannabis.

Retailers are banned from targeting marijuana advertising to minors. However, with the prevalence of Internet advertising, along with peer-to-peer interaction on social media, minors will be exposed to this advertising. Retailers may have already increased this attraction by offering marijuana edibles which use popular candy name brands and package designs such as *Fruity Pebbles, Plum Gummy,* and *Citrus Deamsicle Caramel.* This branding may also contribute to minors' curiosity in seeking out advertisements.

Both Colorado Washington State surveys concluded that marijuana use rates among teens have remained steady despite the legalization of recreational marijuana. Interestingly both states did both see a drop in perceived risk of regular marijuana use in minors surveyed, which can lead to a potential increase of use among those minors. The only way to ensure minors will not be exposed to any type of marijuana advertising is to prohibit it entirely. California is just getting started with legalized recreational marijuana for adult use. They have yet to conduct research on advertisement prevalence and exposure to minors. Further research into cannabis marketing regulation will be essential in developing guidelines that prevent harmful effects of young people viewing marijuana advertisements.

REFERENCES

Adams, D. (2017), For Marijuana Advertisers, Options Are Limited. *Boston Globe*, Business. Retrieved from https://www.bostonglobe.com/business/2017/03/01/for-marijuana-advertisers-options-are-limited/bNLDg38KHaqRvP4lwFggJN/story.html.
Alvaro, E.M., Crano, W.D., Siegel, J.T., Hohman, Z., Johnson, I., & Nakawaki, B. (2013). Adolescents' Attitudes Toward Antimarijuana Ads, Usage Intentions, and Actual Marijuana Usage. *Psychology of Addictive Behaviors,* Vol. 27, No. 4, 1027–1035. doi: 10.1037/a0031960.
Barcott, B. (2017, September 06). First Cannabis Ad Runs on CNN, Fox News, and MSNBC. Retrieved February 18, 2018, from https://www.leafly.com/news/politics/first-cannabis-ad-runs-on-cnn-fox-news-and-msnbc.
Bierut, T., Krauss, M.J., Sowles, S.J., Cavazos-Rehg, P.A. (2016). Exploring Marijuana Advertising on Weedmaps, a Popular Online Directory. *Society for Prevention Research*, No. 18, 183–192. doi 10.1007/s11121-016-0702-z.
California Code of Regulations, Bureau of Cannabis Control, Title 16, Division 42. Article 4 & 5040. (2018). Retrieved January 20, 2018, from https://govt.westlaw.com/calregs/Document/I683039CDC2054CC9A41CBFE647BB91AD?viewType=FullText&originationContext=documenttoc&transitionType=CategoryPageItem&contextData=(sc.Default).
Code Section Group. (n.d.). Retrieved March 01, 2018, from http://leginfo.legislature.ca.gov/faces/codes_displayText.xhtml?lawCode=BPC&division=10.&title=&part=&chapter=15.&article.
Colorado Department of Revenue, Marijuana Enforcement Division, 1 CCR 212–2, R 1104. (2013, September 9). Retrieved January 20, 2018, from https://www.colorado.gov/pacific/sites/default/files/Retail%20Marijuana%20Rules,%20Adopted%20090913,%20Effective%20101513%5B1%5D_0.pdf.
Comello, M.G. (2013). Comparing Effects of "My Anti-Drug" and "Above the Influence" On Campaign Evaluations and Marijuana-Related Perceptions. *Health Marketing Quarterly*, 30(1), 35–46. doi-10.1080/07359683.2013.758014.
Dai, H. (2017) Exposure to Advertisements and Marijuana Use Among U.S. Adolescents, National Center for Chronic Disease Prevention and Health Promotion. Retrieved from: https://www.cdc.gov/pcd/issues/2017/17_0253.htm.
D'Amico, E.L., Miles, J.N.V., & Tucker, J.S. (2015). Gateway to Curiosity: Medical Marijuana Ads and Intention and Use During Middle School. *Psychology of Addictive Behaviors,* Vol. 29, No. 3, 613–619. doi: http://dx.doi.org/10.1037/adb0000094.
Fiala, S. C., Dilley, J. A., Firth, C. L., & Maher, J. E. (2018). Exposure to Marijuana Marketing After Legalization of Retail Sales—Oregonians' Experiences, 2015–2016. *American Journal of Public Health*, 108(1), 120–127. doi-10.2105/AJPH.2017.304136.
Hanson, K. (2018, February 15). State Medical Marijuana Laws. Retrieved February 18, 2018, from http://www.ncsl.org/research/health/state-medical-marijuana-laws.aspx.
Krauss, M.J., Sowles, S.J., Sehi, A., Spitznagel, E.L., Berg, C.J., Bierut L.J., & Cavazos-Rehg, P.A. (2017). *Marijuana Advertising Exposure Among Current Marijuana Users in the U.S. Drug and Alcohol Dependence*, No. 174, 192–200. doi.org/10.1016/j.drugalcdep.2017.01.017.
Marijuana Use Among Youth in Colorado, Healthy Kids Colorado Survey (Rep.). (2016). Retrieved February 18, 2018, from Department of Public Health and Environment website: https://www.colorado.gov/pacific/sites/default/files/PF_Youth_HKCS_MJ-Infographic-Digital.pdf.
Palmgreen, P., Donohew, L., Lorch, E.P., Hoyle, R.H., Stephenson, M.T. (2001). Television Campaigns and Adolescent Marijuana Use: Tests of Sensation Seeking Targeting. *American Journal of Public Health*,

Washington, Vol. 91, Iss. 2, 292–6. Retrieved from https://0-search.proquest.com.library.ggu.edu/doc view/215118021?pq-origsite=summon.

Robinson, M. (2018, January 23). Here's Where You Can Legally Smoke Weed in 2018. Retrieved February 18, 2018, from http://www.businessinsider.com/where-can-you-can-legally-smoke-weed-2018-1/#alaska-1.

Washington State Healthy Youth Survey, 2016 Analytic Report (Rep.). (2017, June). Retrieved February 18, 2018, from Looking Glass Analytics, Inc. website: https://www.doh.wa.gov/Portals/1/Documents/Pubs/160-193-HYS-AnalyticReport2016.pdf.

46. A Framework for Regulating Legal Marijuana*

PATRICK MURPHY *and* JOHN CARNEVALE

Despite the federal prohibition against marijuana, state-level recreational use appears to be moving forward. Public opinion is shifting. Following well-publicized state-legalization in Washington and Colorado, states across the U.S. have begun considering similar measures. This essay does not consider whether states should legalize marijuana nor does it weigh all regulatory options available to states. Instead, it outlines a *practical* framework to regulate recreational marijuana, particularly in a climate of federal uncertainty where marijuana remains illegal.

To develop that framework, we draw primarily on lessons from Colorado and Washington—and to a lesser degree the early experience of other states. The analysis is based on the assumption is that most states will adopt similar regulatory models to oversee commercial, for-profit supply firms and regulate use. Considering both the variety of goals that states could adopt and how they interact, we offer recommendations in five areas: cultivation, production, and processing; sale, consumption, and possession; taxes and finance; public health and safety; and governance.

The Murky Federal-State Relationship

Twenty-nine states and the District of Columbia have legalized medical marijuana, and over 63 percent of the nation's population lives in a state that permits medical marijuana. In addition, many states have increasingly moved towards decriminalizing the possession of small amounts of marijuana for personal use. Accounting for over 21 percent of the U.S. population, Washington, Colorado, Oregon, Alaska, California, Maine, Massachusetts, Nevada, and the District of Columbia have gone one step further—legalizing recreational marijuana under state law. And, most recently, Vermont legalized the possession of marijuana (but did not legalize sales). These changes have occurred while marijuana remains illegal under federal law, categorized as Schedule I under the U.S. Controlled Substances Act of 1970 (CSA).

The initial moves by Colorado and Washington to permit recreational use may have

---

*Published with permission of the authors.

been viewed as "experiments" that authorities could learn from (Caulkins et al., 2012). Even if legal recreational use is still considered an "experiment" by some, no one can deny its scale. This moves the task of regulating the new industry to the forefront of the policy agenda. And it raises the issue of whether the federal government should combat the movement or respect the wishes of states and their constituents. Moreover, it raises unique challenges for states that may seek to create legal regulatory frameworks for a drug that remains illegal under federal law.

The CSA is the "elephant in the room" for state-level legalization in the U.S. Any person or entity engaged in a state-legal marijuana enterprise (arguably, including regulators employed by U.S. states) is in violation of the CSA. As a practical matter, the CSA has been modulated by policy memoranda in the United States for many years. Although the CSA's prohibition remains in force, the Obama Administration's Justice Department issued memoranda characterizing enforcement of federal marijuana prohibitions as low priority—first for the medical market and then more broadly (Ogden, 2009; Cole, 2013). This guidance identified eight areas where it was implied that the federal government would step in should states laws and enforcement efforts not offer adequate protection: (1) preventing marijuana distribution to minors; (2) preventing revenue from marijuana sales going to criminal enterprises, gangs, or cartels; (3) preventing diversion of marijuana to states where it is not legal under state law; (4) preventing state-authorized marijuana activity from being used as a cover or pretext for other illegal activity; (5) preventing violence and the use of firearms within the marijuana trade; (6) preventing drugged driving and the exacerbation of other adverse public health consequences associated with marijuana use; (7) preventing the growing of marijuana on public lands and the public safety/environmental dangers to those lands; and (8) preventing marijuana possession on federal property (Cole, 2013). But policy memoranda do not carry the force of law, and the DOJ memoranda did not alter the CSA. In January 2018, the Trump Administration shifted the policy simply by repealing the memoranda, leaving the question of federal prosecution open (Sessions, 2018).

This murky state of affairs confounds any state's efforts to regulate their state-legal marijuana markets. We cannot address the future of the federal enforcement or, indeed, the future of U.S. federal marijuana policy in general. From a practical perspective, the lack of clarity presents a crucial practical concern for any U.S. state implementing legalization.

Developing a Framework: Regulation and Goals

State policymakers must design a regulatory regime to monitor and manage a new state-legal marijuana industry. Marijuana regulations will cut across many areas, including health, public safety, agriculture, environment, revenue collection, parks and recreation, education, and workplace rules. Authorities must define a set of objectives aligned with the public's desire for reform, state policy preferences (e.g., prioritizing public health or tax revenue), and federal instructions to ensure non-interference (assuming future administrations maintain current policies). To that end, states can pursue several objectives in regulating recreational marijuana (Pacula et al., 2014). But how can the value of different objectives be measured? And what if pursuing one objective works at cross-purposes with another?

For the sake of simplicity, we group regulatory objectives in five general policy areas, though the boundaries overlap. Different policy goals are associated with each of these areas as state regulators seek to balance explicit state preferences and implicit federal concerns.

1. Cultivation, production, and processing
Goal: Manage cultivation; limit supply; product standardization; quality control; eliminate diversion; protect the environment.
Regulatory examples: Licensure; canopy limits; location (e.g., distance from schools); plant tracking; use of pesticides; employee age and criminal history; flower/trim tracking; concentrates/extracts standards; waste management; THC/CBD restrictions; packaging; employee age and criminal history; owner/employee residency requirements; product labeling; warning labels.

2. Sale, consumption, and possession
Goal: Limit access by youth; reduce arrests; eliminate diversion.
Regulatory examples: Age restrictions; product sale limits; inventory control; age of seller and employee restrictions; outlet types and density restrictions; product pricing; advertising; nonresident sale/use; hours of operation; advertising; gifting; home grows; use in public; personal possession of amounts above state limits.

3. Taxes and finance
Goal: Limit abuse and dependence; raise revenue; limit illegal markets; prevent diversion.
Regulatory examples: Excise taxes; licensure fees; use of proceeds, i.e., general fund and/or earmarking of marijuana tax revenue for prevention, treatment, regulatory enforcement, and research.

4. Public health and safety
Goal: Limit abuse and dependence; quality control; prevent impaired driving.
Regulatory examples: Use and driving; workplace use; prevention and treatment programs; use/consequences monitoring and evaluation.

5. Governance
Goal: Oversee and ensure compliance; mount public information campaign focused on legalization costs and benefits.
Regulatory examples: State regulatory oversight; regulatory enforcement; marijuana policy outcome monitoring; regulatory flexibility.

Constructing a Coherent Regulatory Regime and Tradeoffs

How does a state move from such a complex collection of policy areas and goals to develop a coherent regulatory model? The first step is to establish the key priorities of the state. These priorities form the basis used to evaluate regulatory tradeoffs and make decisions. Rather than walking through the different tradeoffs associated with each of the regulatory areas, for the sake of brevity, we articulate our normative preferences, and then offer an example of what such a system would look like.

Based on our research, a practical regulatory model would embrace a for-profit commercial model (as opposed to one where government monopolizes the market) while minimizing the harms to the public's health. From a practical perspective, any state regime also must incorporate the considerations contained in the U.S Department of Justice's policy memoranda. Finally, effective regulations are transparent and enforceable, but anticipate the need to adapt in the future. An application of these principles to the areas and goals described earlier is presented here.

1. Cultivation and production

Recommendation: Limited number of licenses and size of cultivations; seed-to-sale tracking; strict environmental and water use requirements.

Future flexibility: Expandable license availability; technology used to improve tracking systems.

2. Sales, use, and consumption

Recommendation: Sales limited to individuals 21 and older; retail outlets restricted to marijuana-only stores; home grows prohibited.

Future flexibility: Expansion of the number of outlets; legalization of home growing.

3. Taxes and finance

Recommendation: A sales and/or excise tax as a percentage of selling price.

Future flexibility: Tax rates raised or lowered as market performance and social impact indicate.

4. Public health and safety

Recommendation: Aggressive prevention/education campaign aimed at youth; funded research to develop an impairment standard; substance abuse treatment for the uninsured.

Future flexibility: New research-based impairment standards and prevention efforts.

5. Governance

Recommendation: A single regulatory system that requires reporting and data collection across many indicators; built in reporting and impact assessment.

Future flexibility: Adjustable data and reporting systems; determination of whether exceptions needed for medical consumers.

The regulatory model that grows out of these principles requires a relatively restrictive approach that limits access at the beginning. This should make marijuana laws easier to enforce, help reduce diversion, and satisfy federal guidance. States can build in the capacity to ease regulations in the future, as they learn from experience. For example, home grows—marijuana cultivation for personal use—present a "wild card" for regulators. The states that allow personal cultivation limit the number of plants an individual may grow. Nonetheless, allowing home grows creates a loophole in cultivation and consumption regulations. Individuals found with marijuana that cannot be traced in the tracking system, is unlabeled, or exceeds quantity limits can claim to have grown it at home. To maintain tight control over the market, Washington prohibits home grows. We believe other states should consider doing the same.

Consistent with the priorities stated above, we recommend that states create a single regulatory market for recreational and medical marijuana. Combining medical and recreational markets is particularly important for states with large existing medical markets. An integrated market is most consistent with our approach because it maximizes simplicity, transparency, and ease of enforcement. For similar reasons, our model would favor a single point of taxation based upon a percentage of the retail sales price.

We also suggest robust data collection and performance monitoring that supports a thorough evaluation. This should allow states to "learn as they go"—a must, given the uncertainty surrounding marijuana. Very little is known about most state's illegal marijuana markets, and the same is often true for existing medical markets. Building in strong oversight and data collection will help ensure that future changes are based on research and analysis. Of course, states with tightly regulated medical marijuana markets should use any available data a starting point.

Ultimately, given the novelty and unique legal situation of the U.S. state-legal marijuana industry and the uncertainty about its impact, we believe most states would be well served to err on the side of more-restrictive regulation. Keeping the market smaller and well-controlled will make it easier to regulate, reduce the enforcement burden, and reduce the likelihood of diversion. Of course, a tightly regulated approach will have drawbacks—including a significant illegal market. But the arguments for a relatively restricted market outweigh those for a more lightly regulated one. Politically, states will be better off loosening a tight market than attempting to tighten a loose one.

The model we propose is based on the priorities we feel are the most important. States have, and will continue to construct regulatory models that are different than the one proposed here, often because they begin with a different combination of priorities. What doesn't change, however, is that states must grapple with a complex collection of rules that cut across a number of different policy areas, and present a challenging set of tradeoffs.

REFERENCES

Caulkins, Jonathan, Angela Hawkens, Beau Kilmer, Mark Kleiman. 2012. Marijuana Legalization: What Everyone Needs to Know. Oxford University Press.
Cole, James M. 2013. "Memorandum to All U.S. Attorneys: Guidance Regarding Marijuana Enforcement." U.S. Department of Justice. (August 29).
Ogden, David. 2009. Investigations and Prosecutions in States Authorizing the Medical Use of Marijuana. Memorandum for Selected United States Attorneys. (October 19).
Sessions, Jefferson B. 2018. "Marijuana Enforcement." U.S. Department of Justice. (January 4).

47. Medical Marijuana Law Enforcement

Lessons from District Attorneys*

GARY A. CRAFT *and* MICKEY P. McGEE

This essay delves into lessons from the experiences of District Attorneys from Monterey County, California. Data was collected from a focus group of twenty-four (24) Chief District Attorney Investigators/Inspectors from 24 of the 58 counties in California. Two questions were addressed by the focus group: (1) What do authorities need to arrest an individual for a marijuana violation of the law? (2) What proof is needed to convict an individual of a crime in a court of law? For law enforcement officers to arrest an individual for cultivation of marijuana, possession, possession for sale, or transportation or distribution law enforcement personnel need probable cause, i.e., a reasonable, prudent belief that the person committed the crime under investigation. The probable cause burden is low. However, in a court of law, to prove the case and convict a person of a crime, the burden of proof is much higher, i.e., beyond a reasonable doubt. The medical marijuana programs often create the reasonable doubt necessary to acquit in cases such as those referenced above—at least at the state level. People within the medical marijuana limits are usually safe from arrest and prosecution as they follow state law.

Focus Group Findings

Nevada County Chief DA Investigator Randall Billingsley referenced a case in their county which resulted in acquittal, *People v. Ronald Hansen*. Ronald Hansen was a Nevada County man accused of selling medical marijuana on "Craigslist" and was ultimately found not guilty at his jury trial. Hansen was acquitted of three marijuana charges, i.e. (1) possession for sale, (2) cultivation, and (3) sales/transportation of marijuana. The investigation of the case involved an undercover buy of marijuana, which was purchased by undercover Nevada County law enforcement personnel. The undercover buy led to a search of Hansen's home where dozens of marijuana plants where located. The street

---

*Published with permission of the authors.

value of the marijuana was estimated at over $100,000.00. The medical marijuana defense worked in this case.

Santa Cruz Chief District Attorney Inspector Mike Roe shared an undercover operation his department conducted because of large numbers of young students and young adults allegedly obtaining medical marijuana cards from a local doctor without any apparent legitimate medical ailments. Chief Roe said he sent one of his undercover district attorney investigators into the doctor's office to see how easy it would be to obtain a medical marijuana card. Chief Roe said within an 11-minute period, his undercover District Attorney Investigator (DAI) had obtained a medical marijuana card with no physical examination and was directed to a marijuana dispensary with a recommendation to obtain his marijuana.

In a debrief of the undercover DAI, it was learned that the recommending doctor didn't review the medical records which the undercover DAI provided. That the undercover DAI had the records with him was sufficient enough documentation for the doctor to recommend the marijuana and issue him a medical marijuana card. At the debriefing, the DAI mentioned that the waiting room at this doctor's office was filled with young adults between the ages of 18 and 25 years. Chief Roe also said the undercover DAI went to the Santa Cruz County Health Department to obtain another medical marijuana card, which took him about 15 minutes—no examination or medical records were required (Roe, 2013, personal communication).

Other Chiefs at the focus group voiced concerns about how easy one can obtain a medical marijuana card without serious medical conditions to be a qualified as a patient. The concern is the medical marijuana program creates a defense mechanism in many criminal cases where the defendants possess large quantities of marijuana, far and beyond a reasonable personal use limits.

The trends since the CUA was enacted have changed the way many counties are doing business dealing with marijuana violators. Many chiefs at the focus group reported that long time growers and dealers are using the medical marijuana law very successfully in the criminal defense of charges of possession for sale. To combat this, many counties are teaming up with federal task forces (federal agents) to overcome the burden of proof needed, which might otherwise slip through the cracks of the court system at the state level—bringing those cases into federal court.

El Dorado County Chief DA Investigator Bob Cosley spoke about the changing trends in his county. Chief Cosley stated that he had assigned one of his investigators to serve on federal task forces to combat marijuana and other drugs.

Others in the focus group indicated that the CUA and MMPA have provided too much of a gap between arresting and/or just walking away from the cannabis grow. Butte County attendees stated that they are now looking beyond the marijuana grow to the land grading and other code violations to hold the perpetrators responsible for their actions. Monterey County Sheriff's Department (MCSD) is also looking at code violations as well as Fish & Game (F&G) Code violations regarding the grading and movement of land. MCSD Sergeant Matthew Luther said the United States Forest Service is looking for the same violations on federal property. Sgt. Luther said that "the feds have shifted their focus from eradication [marijuana] to reclamation," i.e., the conversion of land, streams, water sources, or other wasteland into land suitable for cultivation. They focus on illegal camps and destruction of federal property caused by bringing in plastic waterlines and other structures into the U.S. National Forests, crimes which carry a heavier fine than growing marijuana.

Sgt. Luther said their department doesn't have a medical marijuana policy; they typically follow DEA guidelines looking for the large marijuana grows (drug cartels) and making sure when they do find medical marijuana gardens, they check for certification (medical marijuana cards) and the doctor's recommendation so that the amounts grown match the legal limits. Sgt. Luther says they interview the marijuana growers when they are well over their limits. In some cases, the growers admit to selling a little. "When they do admit to selling, whether medical marijuana or otherwise, they're toast [arrested], because there are no legal provisions to sell marijuana in California law." It should be noted, however, that dispensaries and their customers "sell" marijuana because they claim they are part of a cooperative or collective. The legality of such sales is not clear. Sgt. Luther said their department has walked into a marijuana grow with a white flag hanging with a red cross in the garden. Also, in the garden were the posted names of collectives and qualified patients and caregivers. Sgt. Luther said they (MCSD) have had to walk out of a marijuana garden when the collectives' names and number of plants were consistent with the limits of the law at the time.

San Francisco (SF) County Chief DA Inspector James Kerrigan advised that many of the San Francisco marijuana dispensaries have closed or downsized for many reasons. Chief Kerrigan said, "We have had the illegal dispensaries which have probably increased mostly due to lack of enforcement." Chief Kerrigan attributes this to San Francisco law enforcement resources focusing more on other types of drug related activity. Chief Kerrigan said "a couple of years ago there were a couple of real proactive people with Pacific Gas & Electric, who worked with the Narcotics Units identifying a lot of indoor growing operations and shutting them down. We are not as aggressive with the enforcement due to the lack of resources to investigate."

According to Chief Kerrigan, the newer marijuana dispensaries are downsizing and receiving a lot more opposition from the community; especially, when they are close to a school. San Francisco remains progressive when it comes to medical marijuana and the MMPA. San Francisco's policy allows qualified patients and caregivers in San Francisco to possess 24 cannabis plants and no more than eight ounces of dried marijuana. The policy restricts a marijuana growing area to be no greater than twenty-five square feet (similarly to Nevada County DA's policy).

Conclusions

Federal law: (1) it is illegal to grow/cultivate marijuana (2) it is illegal to possess marijuana; (3) it is illegal to sell marijuana; (4) it is illegal to transport marijuana; and (5) it is illegal to furnish marijuana. Federal law states there is no medical use for marijuana and it remains a Schedule I Drug under the Controlled Substance Act. California State laws include a provision in the law which makes marijuana legal to the qualified patient and caregiver with a recommendation from a doctor—under Federal law patient, caregiver and doctor could be arrested and charged.

District Attorney Chief Inspectors and Chief DA Investigators throughout the state observe that criminals who are growing marijuana for profit and are successfully using the medical marijuana program as a credible means for their large-scale marijuana grow operations, i.e., they are using the process to further their profit selling marijuana to the black market. Many of the large dealers and growers are using the medical marijuana defense to protect themselves from arrests and prosecution, and in many cases, it is working.

The key to the success of these marijuana investigations is to get the federal authorities involved in the beginning of the investigation so they can identify whether the case merits a federal investigation and prosecution. These federal task forces are not targeting legitimate medical marijuana qualified patients; however, in many cases, the large-scale marijuana growers and dealers are obtaining medical marijuana certification to shield themselves from prosecution so they may profit from their illegal growing and selling operations. With the federal agencies involved, authorities can successfully arrest and convict the perpetrators—particularly those who have medical marijuana credentials, who are dealing in large scale marijuana operations for profit.

48. Medical Marijuana Law Enforcement

Lessons from Police Chiefs*

GARY A. CRAFT *and* MICKEY P. MCGEE

This essay examines, from the enforcement experiences of Monterey County police chiefs, the California law which permits the cultivation, transportation, possession and furnishing of marijuana for medical purposes. The *California Health & Safety Code* (*H&S*) allows the qualified patient and qualified caregiver to possess eight ounces of marijuana per patient and/or to cultivate six mature or 12 immature cannabis plants per patient, and transportation of the same pursuant to *H&S §11362.77, subsection (a)* (p. 2011). There are provisions in the *California H&S Code* that provide for additional amounts of marijuana to be possessed that exceed these standards with a doctor's recommendation pursuant to *H&S §11362.77, subsection (b)* (p. 2011). The *California H&S Code* also authorizes counties and cities to retain or enact medical marijuana guidelines allowing qualified patients or primary caregivers to maintain or exceed the state's limits set forth in *H&S §11362.77 (c)* (p. 2011). The problem with all of this is—that under Federal law nothing in this paragraph is legal. Hence the State and Federal laws both align and misalign.

Under federal law marijuana is illegal to grow, possess, and smoke. Marijuana is categorized under federal guidelines as a "Schedule I" drug under the Controlled Substance Act—having no accepted medical use or treatment in the United States. However, under "California Law" marijuana is quasi-legal to grow, possess, and use pursuant to the Compassionate Use Act (*California Health & Safety Code § 11362.77, subdivision (a)* through *subsection (d)*). However, in California in 1996, the voters passed Proposition 215 called the Compassionate Use Act (CUA). This proposition made it legal to possess and use marijuana if a "critically ill" patient had the recommendation from a physician.

In 2004, the legislature passed, and the governor signed into law SB 420 called the Medical Marijuana Program Act (MMPA). One goal of this legislation was to provide patients with a means of acquiring their medical marijuana. The MMPA placed the main emphasis on "primary caregivers" defined as persons who consistently assumed responsibility for the care of the qualified patient. Even before the passage of the MMPA, medical marijuana dispensaries had sprung up all over California and continue to do so today

---

*Published with permission of the authors.

in many jurisdictions. These dispensaries sell marijuana to people who have doctor's recommendations. The California Supreme Court has since ruled that dispensaries are not primary caregivers under the law. Therefore, even under California law the system of retail retribution of marijuana currently in place in California may not be legal. Clearly this entire system and any possession of marijuana is illegal under federal guidelines pursuant to the Controlled Substance Act (CSA) *Title 21 U.S.C. §§ 801–812 (b) (1), et seq.*

Monterey County law enforcement agencies typically follow and enforce State Laws pursuant to various California Codes—such as the *California Penal Code and the California Vehicle Code*, and the *California Health and Safety Code*. The laws pertaining to marijuana possession are found in the California *Health & Safety Code* (2013) as to how the *qualified patient* and/or *qualified caregiver* may possess marijuana under California Law (H&S *§11362.77*, p. 2011). Although possession of marijuana (including the growing of cannabis) is permitted pursuant to this section—there is a strict number limit of cannabis plants associated with the cultivation aspects and a strict weight limit associated with dried processed marijuana one qualified patient or caregiver may possess. Any amounts over these limits require a doctor's recommendation, although the California Supreme Court has ruled the limits don't apply to possession and a doctor's recommendation with the CUA.

Interview Findings

Police Chiefs from Monterey County were collected in 2014, pre–Proposition 46 approval by the voters of California. Below are their thoughts.

The former City of Gonzales Chief of Police Paul Miller, 2012 Chair of the Monterey County Law Chief's Associations, stated that the Gonzales Police Department had a medical marijuana policy (MMP) dealing with medical marijuana for qualified patients and caregivers. Chief Miller said their policy was provided to them by "Lexipol LLC" a law firm that specializes in writing policies for law enforcement agencies (Police & Sheriff) throughout the State of California. According to Chief Miller, most police agencies in Monterey County have Lexipol policy # 452 and/or a similar MMP policy. The policy guidelines for amounts a patient or caregiver could grow or possess were consistent with the guidelines set for in the *California Health & Safety Code § 11362.77 (a) & (b)*. The Gonzales Police Department's Medical Marijuana Policy #452 was and is consistent with other police chiefs' policies. Police Chiefs from the Cities of Salinas, Greenfield, Soledad, Monterey, Seaside, Pacific Grove and the City of Carmel also have and use the same Lexipol policy.

The former Monterey Police Chief Phil Penko said their department looks for a medical marijuana card and/or a doctor's recommendation and then try to exercise common sense in the investigation of their cases. If the amounts don't match up, an arrest is made, and the case is then sent over to the District Attorney's Office for a filing decision. Chief Penko said many high school students have medical marijuana cards and that cards have been issued for treating minor medical conditions such as insomnia and anxiety. Although Chief Penko believes the CUA law is being abused for recreational purposes in one sense, he sees a purpose for it in another. Chief Penko explained how a former Monterey Police Sergeant's son was dying from leukemia and in his final stages of dying smoked marijuana for pain relief. Chief Penko said the police sergeant was adamantly against marijuana use altogether, and was a former narcotics officer; however, he acquired another view of marijuana when he saw how it relieved his son's pain and suffering.

Police Chief Earl Lawson, California State University at Monterey Bay Police Department, 2013 Chair of the Monterey County Law Chief's Association, indicated his department didn't have a medical marijuana policy. Chief Lawson said if his officers encounter a person with a medical marijuana card, they usually walk away from the contact without citing or arresting the person. Other chiefs with Lexipol use the common-sense approach to enforcement, i.e., if the doctor's recommendation doesn't match the possession, and it is over the limit, appropriate action is taken. That could range from seizing the marijuana and citing the person to a misdemeanor or felony arrest.

Most chiefs reported that their respective counties were still arresting and prosecuting people for cultivation/growing marijuana and possessing marijuana for use and sale. The problem most counties were encountering was that most suspects in these marijuana cases were people in possession of large quantities of marijuana who all possessed medical marijuana cards. These arrests resulted in people using the CUA and medical marijuana laws as their criminal defense.

Conclusions

Federal law: (1) it is illegal to grow/cultivate marijuana (2) it is illegal to possess marijuana; (3) it is illegal to sell marijuana; (4) it is illegal to transport marijuana; and (5) it is illegal to furnish marijuana. Federal law states there is no medical use for marijuana and it remains a Schedule I Drug under the Controlled Substance Act. California State laws include a provision in the law which makes marijuana legal to the qualified patient and caregiver with a recommendation from a doctor—under Federal law patient, caregiver and doctor could be arrested and charged.

Data collected from Monterey County Police Chiefs indicate that various departments were still adjusting to the enforcement of marijuana laws as they relate to medical marijuana. State laws were not clear. Although on the one hand, marijuana is illegal to grow, possess, sell, possess for sale, transport, and furnish, on the other hand medical marijuana laws authorize the qualified patients, collectives and cooperatives to grow, possess, transport and presumably distribute marijuana. However, the qualified patient and caregiver cannot sell marijuana for "profit"—if they do, they go to jail. But there are many non-profit enterprises in California that compensate their CEOs and employees with lucrative salaries.

The chief of police interviews also revealed that the medical marijuana card provision is being abused and cards are being issued to many young adults who clearly do not have a serious medical condition; the medical marijuana cards appear to be obtained for recreational purposes, opposed to their intended purpose—compassionate use. The majority of police interactions are with the undesirable majority of the minority of people who are abusing the medical marijuana system; or crimes in general—they (police) do not always see the legitimate majority of people who are complying with the law and/or the medical marijuana program. And there is no need for law enforcement to come in to contact with these people, who are not violating statutory law.

49. A Tale of Two Memos

Joaquin Jay Gonzalez III

In this essay, we invite you to examine the two memos below. Memo #1 is from Obama Administration Deputy Attorney General James M. Cole issued August 29, 2013, while Memo #2 is from Trump Administration Attorney General Jefferson B. Sessions released January 4, 2018.

From my reading, while both memos are unified in the position of the federal government grounded on the Controlled Substances Act, that "marijuana is a dangerous drug and that the illegal distribution and sale of marijuana is a serious crime," they vary in terms of enforcement guidance to states and cities.

What do you think?

How do they vary?

How do you think state interpret(ed) their enforcement?

How do you think cities interpret(ed) their enforcement?

Judge for yourself:

Memo #1

August 29, 2013

MEMORANDUM FOR ALL UNITED STATES ATTORNEYS

FROM: James M. Cole, Deputy Attorney General

SUBJECT: Guidance Regarding Marijuana Enforcement

In October 2009 and June 2011, the Department issued guidance to federal prosecutors concerning marijuana enforcement under the Controlled Substances Act (CSA). This memorandum updates that guidance in light of state ballot initiatives that legalize under state law the possession of small amounts of marijuana and provide for the regulation of marijuana production, processing, and sale. The guidance set forth herein applies to all federal enforcement activity, including civil enforcement and criminal investigations and prosecutions, concerning marijuana in all states.

As the Department noted in its previous guidance, Congress has determined that marijuana is a dangerous drug and that the illegal distribution and sale of marijuana is a serious crime that provides a significant source of revenue to large-scale criminal enterprises, gangs, and cartels. The Department of Justice is committed to enforcement of the

CSA consistent with those determinations. The Department is also committed to using its limited investigative and prosecutorial resources to address the most significant threats in the most effective, consistent, and rational way. In furtherance of those objectives, as several states enacted laws relating to the use of marijuana for medical purposes, the Department in recent years has focused its efforts on certain enforcement priorities that are particularly important to the federal government:

- Preventing the distribution of marijuana to minors;
- Preventing revenue from the sale of marijuana from going to criminal enterprises, gangs, and cartels;
- Preventing the diversion of marijuana from states where it is legal under state law in some form to other states;
- Preventing state-authorized marijuana activity from being used as a cover or pretext for the trafficking of other illegal drugs or other illegal activity;
- Preventing violence and the use of firearms in the cultivation and distribution of marijuana;
- Preventing drugged driving and the exacerbation of other adverse public health consequences associated with marijuana use;
- Preventing the growing of marijuana on public lands and the attendant public safety and environmental dangers posed by marijuana production on public lands; and
- Preventing marijuana possession or use on federal property.

These priorities will continue to guide the Department's enforcement of the CSA against marijuana-related conduct. Thus, this memorandum serves as guidance to Department attorneys and law enforcement to focus their enforcement resources and efforts, including prosecution, on persons or organizations whose conduct interferes with any one or more of these priorities, regardless of state law.[1]

Outside of these enforcement priorities, the federal government has traditionally relied on states and local law enforcement agencies to address marijuana activity through enforcement of their own narcotics laws. For example, the Department of Justice has not historically devoted resources to prosecuting individuals whose conduct is limited to possession of small amounts of marijuana for personal use on private property. Instead, the Department has left such lower-level or localized activity to state and local authorities and has stepped in to enforce the CSA only when the use, possession, cultivation, or distribution of marijuana has threatened to cause one of the harms identified above.

The enactment of state laws that endeavor to authorize marijuana production, distribution, and possession by establishing a regulatory scheme for these purposes affects this traditional joint federal-state approach to narcotics enforcement. The Department's guidance in this memorandum rests on its expectation that states and local governments that have enacted laws authorizing marijuana-related conduct will implement strong and effective regulatory and enforcement systems that will address the threat those state laws could pose to public safety, public health, and other law enforcement interests. A system adequate to that task must not only contain robust controls and procedures on paper; it must also be effective in practice. Jurisdictions that have implemented systems that provide for regulation of marijuana activity must provide the necessary resources and demonstrate the willingness to enforce their laws and regulations in a manner that ensures they do not undermine federal enforcement priorities.

In jurisdictions that have enacted laws legalizing marijuana in some form and that have also implemented strong and effective regulatory and enforcement systems to control the cultivation, distribution, sale, and possession of marijuana, conduct in compliance with those laws and regulations is less likely to threaten the federal priorities set forth above. Indeed, a robust system may affirmatively address those priorities by, for example, implementing effective measures to prevent diversion of marijuana outside of the regulated system and to other states, prohibiting access to marijuana by minors, and replacing an illicit marijuana trade that funds criminal enterprises with a tightly regulated market in which revenues are tracked and accounted for. In those circumstances, consistent with the traditional allocation of federal-state efforts in this area, enforcement of state law by state and local law enforcement and regulatory bodies should remain the primary means of addressing marijuana-related activity. If state enforcement efforts are not sufficiently robust to protect against the harms set forth above, the federal government may seek to challenge the regulatory structure itself in addition to continuing to bring individual enforcement actions, including criminal prosecutions, focused on those harms.

The Department's previous memoranda specifically addressed the exercise of prosecutorial discretion in states with laws authorizing marijuana cultivation and distribution for medical use. In those contexts, the Department advised that it likely was not an efficient use of federal resources to focus enforcement efforts on seriously ill individuals, or on their individual caregivers. In doing so, the previous guidance drew a distinction between the seriously ill and their caregivers, on the one hand, and large-scale, for-profit commercial enterprises, on the other, and advised that the latter continued to be appropriate targets for federal enforcement and prosecution. In drawing this distinction, the Department relied on the common-sense judgment that the size of a marijuana operation was a reasonable proxy for assessing whether marijuana trafficking implicates the federal enforcement priorities set forth above.

As explained above, however, both the existence of a strong and effective state regulatory system, and an operation's compliance with such a system, may allay the threat that an operation's size poses to federal enforcement interests. Accordingly, in exercising prosecutorial discretion, prosecutors should not consider the size or commercial nature of a marijuana operation alone as a proxy for assessing whether marijuana trafficking implicates the Department's enforcement priorities listed above. Rather, prosecutors should continue to review marijuana cases on a case-by-case basis and weigh all available information and evidence, including, but not limited to, whether the operation is demonstrably in compliance with a strong and effective state regulatory system. A marijuana operation's large scale or for-profit nature may be a relevant consideration for assessing the extent to which it undermines a particular federal enforcement priority. The primary question in all cases—and in all jurisdictions—should be whether the conduct at issue implicates one or more of the enforcement priorities listed above.

As with the Department's previous statements on this subject, this memorandum is intended solely as a guide to the exercise of investigative and prosecutorial discretion. This memorandum does not alter in any way the Department's authority to enforce federal law, including federal laws relating to marijuana, regardless of state law. Neither the guidance herein nor any state or local law provides a legal defense to a violation of federal law, including any civil or criminal violation of the CSA. Even in jurisdictions with strong and effective regulatory systems, evidence that particular conduct threatens federal priorities will subject that person or entity to federal enforcement action, based on the circumstances. This memorandum is not intended to, does not, and may not be relied upon to create any rights, substantive or procedural, enforceable at law by any party in any matter civil or criminal. It applies prospectively to the exercise of prosecutorial discretion in future cases and does not provide defendants or subjects of enforcement action with a basis for reconsideration of any pending civil action or criminal prosecution. Finally, nothing herein precludes investigation or prosecution, even in the absence of any one of the factors listed above, in particular circumstances where investigation and prosecution otherwise serves an important federal interest.

Memo #2

January 4, 2018

MEMORANDUM FOR ALL UNITED STATES ATTORNEYS

FROM: Jefferson B. Sessions, Attorney General

SUBJECT: Marijuana Enforcement

In the Controlled Substances Act, Congress has generally prohibited the cultivation, distribution, and possession of marijuana. 21 U.S.C. § 801 et seq. It has established significant penalties for these crimes. 21 U.S.C. § 841 el seq. These activities also may serve as the basis for the prosecution of other crimes, such as those prohibited by the money laundering statutes, the unlicensed money transmitter statute, and the Bank Secrecy Act. 18 U.S.C. §§ 1956–57, 1960; 31 U.S.C. § 53 18. These statutes reflect Congress' determination that marijuana is a dangerous drug and that marijuana activity is a serious crime.

In deciding which marijuana activities to prosecute under these laws with the Department's finite resources, prosecutors should follow the well-established principles that govern all federal prosecutions. Attorney General Benjamin Civiletti originally set forth these principles in 1980, and they have been refined over time, as reflected in chapter 9–27 .000 of the U.S. Attorneys' Manual. These principles require federal prosecutors deciding which cases to prosecute to weigh all relevant considerations, including federal law enforcement priorities set by the Attorney General, the seriousness of the crime, the deterrent effect of criminal prosecution, and the cumulative impact of particular crimes on the community.

Given the Department's well-established general principles, previous nationwide guidance specific to marijuana enforcement is unnecessary and is rescinded, effective immediately. This memorandum is intended solely as a guide to the exercise of investigative and prosecutorial discretion in accordance with all applicable laws, regulations, and appropriations. It is not intended to, does not, and may not be relied upon to create any rights, substantive or procedural, enforceable at law by any party in any matter civil or criminal.

NOTE

1. These enforcement priorities are listed in general terms; each encompasses a variety of conduct that may merit civil or criminal enforcement of the CSA. By way of example only, the Department[apost]s interest in preventing the distribution of marijuana to minors would call for enforcement not just when an individual or entity sells or transfers marijuana to a minor, but also when marijuana trafficking takes place near an area associated with minors; when marijuana or marijuana-infused products are marketed in a manner to appeal to minors; or when marijuana is being diverted, directly or indirectly, and purposefully or otherwise, to minors.

50. Berkeley's Medical and Recreational Cannabis Policy[*]

Jim Hynes

The City of Berkeley is a relatively small city in the San Francisco Bay Area that has a liberal reputation that goes far beyond California and the U.S. While this is due historically in large part to the presence of the flagship campus of the University of California, it is also a center for many progressive and socially challenging causes, such as the free speech movement in the 1960s, and it continues to a be a leader in forging a path forward on controversial issues of the day. This includes, and is the subject of this essay, cannabis policy, administrative and land use regulations governing access to cannabis, and enforcement of municipal codes governing the operating conditions on medical and recreational cannabis dispensaries so as to allow reasonable and healthy access to cannabis, promote public safety and prevent negative community impacts.

Background

Like many progressive initiatives in the City of Berkeley, liberalization of cannabis originated through a combination of local citizen activists, and at times concurrent state-level legislative actions and ballot initiatives. The City of Berkeley's earliest efforts aimed at cannabis started at the ballot box in 1979 when Berkeley voters overwhelmingly voted to decriminalize cannabis. The ballot measure directed police to treat cannabis as a low priority, and prohibited arrests for the sale, possession and cultivation of cannabis. Since police swear an oath to support enforcement of all laws, and thus the 1979 ballot measure was largely symbolic, it nevertheless communicated a message of tolerance and acceptability that in fact did affect police behavior.

Medical Cannabis: The Berkeley Story

Preceding any state-wide efforts, the City of Berkeley passed three ballot measures between 2008 and 2010 permitting dispensaries and cultivation, and establishing taxation.

---

*Published with permission of the author.

These actions also lead to the establishment of the Cannabis Commission, with each member appointed by a city council member to advise the City Council on cannabis policy and conduct an open government public process to develop recommendations for the Berkeley City Council to consider in allowing the establishment of cannabis dispensaries. (Cannabis Commission Mission Statement "To ensure that cannabis provision in Berkeley is conducted in a safe and orderly manner to protect the welfare of Qualified Patients and the community. The commission shall consist of nine members. At least one commissioner shall be a member of a medical cannabis dispensary, one shall be a member of a collective that is not a dispensary, and one shall be a cultivator who is not primarily associated with a single dispensary and provides medical cannabis to more than one dispensary.")

In July 2014, after several years of public debate, public process and citizen input, the Berkeley City Council approved regulations over medical dispensaries in term of total number permitted, allowable locations across the City, operating conditions, including hours of operation, and provisions for security personnel, anti-theft and burglary deterrents etc. Three were already council approved prior to 2004 but by 2018 six were permitted. The selection process for an additional dispensary (a fourth) started as a result of the 2014 legislation but during the selection process the City Council voted to allow two additional dispensaries resulting in six dispensaries.

Most significant in the July 2014 legislation was a testing and cannabis quality assurance requirement (more on this below) developed in the absence of any State or Federal direction, and a "compassionate care" requirement for dispensaries to provide 2 percent of cannabis sold for free to low-income patients. Both of these were pioneering, cutting edge requirements. Simultaneously, and interestingly, between 2011 and 2015 the Berkeley City Council also dealt with 3 illegal dispensaries, Greenleaf Wellness Group, 40 Acres, and Perfect Plants Patients Group, which apparently perceived the City's permissive historical policy stance on cannabis as a basis of legitimacy to set up illegal cannabis dispensary operations, but were successfully ordered to cease and desist through the nuisance abatement procedures by the City's Code Enforcement Unit.

It is important to note that the impetus for abatement derived almost entirely from the complaints of neighborhood residents, who perceived the presence of illegal operations as not just a "NIMBY" issue, but an issue that created a significant negative and demonstrable impact on the surrounding quality of life. It is also significant to note that such abatement efforts were occurring simultaneously to the creation of public policy on cannabis dispensaries and the rogue-like ambitions and abatement responses by the City provided a real-time example of how the city needed to position itself to be proactive against such problems. That is, while "unintended consequences" are the bane of public policy making, these rogue operators gave the policy makers, city attorneys, managers and enforcers a "gift," a preview of problems they might not otherwise have considered without the illegal initiatives of such rogue operators.

The public policy discussion in the aftermath of city council approval to permit medical cannabis dispensaries was dominated by a variety of different concerns. The majority of the discussion focused on the selection process of new dispensaries, what criterion would be used, the importance and weight of the criterion, geographic location amongst the most important, and how and where locations would complement other related city policy initiatives.

These other policy considerations played a significant role. For example, since the city of Berkeley around the same time that it had discussed and approved medical cannabis dispensaries also embarked on an initiative to develop one of the country's first city-based climate action plans to reduce greenhouse gasses and global warming, it was imperative for the sake of coordinated policy development that the two policy initiatives relate to each other. Hence, policy discussions on medical cannabis regulations also included rules to reduce and/or eliminate dispensaries' carbon footprints. Shortly after the city of Berkeley adopted its climate action plan, separate from the dispensary ordinance in 2014 (Berkeley Municipal Code 12.27), in 2017 the Berkeley City Council approved regulations over carbon emissions associated with the cultivation and distribution of cannabis (Berkeley Municipal; Code 12.25). A second salient policy consideration related to the needs of low income patients, and thus the requirement that businesses "give back" to the community holding operators accountable to the self-proclaimed belief that if this was all about providing relief to patients, then dispensaries should assist those people who cannot afford this product.

Cannabis Policy at the State Level: California Acts

Running parallel to city of Berkeley activist efforts, various state legislature approved policies such as the Medical Cannabis Regulation and Safety Act (MCRSA) in October 2015, created the framework for state licensing of medical cannabis and, more significantly, in November 2016 the voter approved statewide ballot initiative, Proposition 64, the Adult Use of Marijuana Act (AUMA), legalized adult use and created the framework for state licensing for adult use cannabis In Berkeley, in 2017 the MCRSA and AUMA were combined into MAUCRSA.

In this timeline of public policy, Berkeley was at times ahead of state efforts and at times behind in a figurative game of non-linear policy "leapfrog." The city of Berkeley is now in the position of needing to contemplate the prospects of joint locations or separate locations for medical and recreational dispensaries. Medicinal cannabis, however, has been at the core of the city of Berkeley's efforts from early on, and in some ways, has been a priority and given much attention at all levels.

Whether it be medical or adult use ('recreational"), the city of Berkeley has taken a very deliberate path forward recognizing the broad policy parameters set for by state of California policies and regulations MAUCRSA (MCRSA and AUMA) and the demands of local citizens and activists to provide responsible access to cannabis. Moreover, in so much as to allow for simple access to medical cannabis in July 2014, after much policy discussion amongst the council and commissions, and a stakeholder consensus building process that led to final medical cannabis dispensary regulations, in January 2017 the Berkeley City Council approved commercial *cultivation* regulations, but also set a moratorium on all adult use ("recreational") businesses until final regulations were established.

In July 2017, the Berkeley City Council referred establishment of adult cannabis use regulations to staff to develop. Consistent with the normative policy development process in the city of Berkeley in which there is much back and forth on key policy questions between various commissions, including of course the Cannabis Commission, but also the Community Health Commission and the Planning Commission, as well as ordinary citizens, businesses, non-profits and local school leaders, in 3–4 months, by October

2017, the Berkeley City Council voted to create *temporary* adult cannabis use licenses for existing dispensaries. This action, along with Berkeley City Council actions in February 2018 to reduce the adult use tax from 10 percent to 5 percent, and to pronounce Berkeley as a cannabis sanctuary city, was taken up by the Berkeley City Council separate from the work on the ordinance.

Guiding this process, strongly supported by city staff, the Berkeley City Council has in the recent past, and given the temporary nature of current medical and adult use cannabis licenses, will continue to emphasize specific state driven and local driven considerations, including but not limited to:

- Consistency with state regulations: of tantamount importance to maintain consistency at all levels of government, especially regarding enforcement in light of the city of Berkeley's current feud with the Trump Administration on policies surrounding sanctuary cities and providing protections for "Dreamers."
- Protection of Minors: a top priority amongst Berkeley residents, especially parents of school age children potentially in close proximity to medical and adult use cannabis dispensaries.
- Promoting equity; another hallmark city of Berkeley issue, equity focuses on persons from communities disproportionately affected by the "War on Drugs." These people were adversely impacted (criminal records, loss of income, etc.) by participating in cannabis growing, sales, etc. and now that cannabis is a legal market, are shut out of the market due to lack of capital, criminal background, etc.
- Collection of tax revenues: no public policy of any significance and value should be considered without a careful analysis of the revenues required to implement and sustain over time the effective regulation and enforcement of cannabis operating rules and product quality assurance requirements. Berkeley will need to extract a sales tax rate and business tax rate that covers all costs associated with the responsible regulation of medical and adult use cannabis operations.
- Promoting Public Safety: the city of Berkeley public policy process around both medical and adult use cannabis continuously addressed and continues to address issues around public safety. Highest among the concerns are that dispensaries may become "attractive nuisances" much in the same way that inner city liquor stores have become problematic. Also of concern, the prospects that dispensaries could become victims of crime via "business invasions," or after-hours burglaries.
- Clear Enforcement Guidelines: the Berkeley City Council heard loud and clear from both members of the public concerned about dispensaries in their neighborhoods and dispensary operators that they wanted enforcement of both cannabis specific municipal codes, and codes governing morals, fire and building safety clearly articulated and strictly enforced, with a well-defined schedule of penalties for code violations.
- Potential Impacts on the Community: Berkeley is a gentrifying city. It has one of the highest livability indexes of any city in the country. Home prices are extremely high and taxes relative to other cities are extremely high as well. Consequently, Berkeley tax payers expect a commensurately high degree of

attention paid to community quality of life. The City's Environmental Health Division is specifically charged to inspect dispensaries and manufacturing sites. The ordinance proposes that all cannabis businesses will need an operating permit, but at this writing it has not been determined which city department would be responsible for this.

- Staff capacity to implement regulations: The Berkeley City Council can oftentimes pass resolutions that are simply statements of a specific type of political support, or are relatively minor changes to ordinances that have minimal impact on the use of staff resources. In the case of medical and adult use cannabis, however, the stakes are large in terms of the above considerations, and the City Council will be loath to pass a set of new ordinances and regulations that cannot be responsibly implemented and administered due to the lack of staff resources to do so. That is, on-going staffing costs will need to be assigned to Berkeley's cannabis legislation.

Current Situation

Given Berkeley's vanguard role in California, perhaps a harbinger of sorts for other California cities, other California cities and counties should heed the Berkeley experience and be especially attentive to:

- Licensure: Cities have an inherent role in regulating business and non-business operations that provide a tangible community benefit and at the same time can potentially detract from the quality of life from that very same community. Licensure is far and away the most effective means for accomplishing this.
- Application review: The dispensary selection process was a political process, and the only selection process thus far. The next selection process is still being developed, and could include review by the Berkeley City Council. The role of professional staff is to advise and make recommendations to the Berkeley City Council but the ultimate approval process resides with the City Council.
- Land Use approvals: Ever since the historic Ambler Realty case in 1926, zoning and land use controls have consistently demonstrated to be the most effective and legally defensible means to allow businesses to flourish and yet simultaneously prevent untoward effects of such businesses. The case with Cannabis in Berkeley is no different, and other cities should rightly consider the role of zoning and land use controls as they grapple with the challenges and opportunities associated with medical and adult use cannabis dispensaries.
- Conducting Inspections and Enforcing Local Codes: So far, inspections have come under the purview of the city's Environmental Health Division. Illegal or rogue operators would, as in the recent past, come under the purview of the Code Enforcement Unit in the Neighborhood Service Division in the City Manager's Office, a place rightly so by virtue of high visibility and accountability in the hierarchy of the City.
- Customer Service: the city of Berkeley places a strong emphasis on customer service and has a dedicated centralized 311 telephone number and divisional office within the City's Department of Information Technology to receive

citizen complaints and concerns. The immediate challenge, as of this writing, is that the Customer Service staff be trained by the Environmental Health, Code Enforcement and Legal staff in the nuances of medical and adult use cannabis regulations so as to better understand and respond to community complaints and concerns.

Conclusion, Future Concerns and Challenges

While 3 new dispensaries were selected in 2016, none have opened yet. Currently, Berkeley has three "Retailers" (new term consistent with State language), and two others intend to open in 2018. The sixth Retailer needs to find a suitable location, and it is unclear when that will happen. The city of Berkeley is still in the midst of refining and continuously evaluating its selection process for medical cannabis dispensaries, but more importantly is a leader amongst cities in ensuring that Berkeley is at the vanguard for "clean" cannabis. Since 2015, the city of Berkeley's dispensaries have had to comply with the strictest cannabis contamination regulation in the state, which stipulates allowable limits for pesticides, solvents, molds and mildew. In a city already obsessed with organic food, farm to table, etc., it appears that the same logic will prevail over cannabis.

Presently, as of Spring 2018, the Berkeley City Council will consider a draft ordinance developed by city staff to combine the regulatory and enforcement provisions of both medical and adult use cannabis so as to allow to allow dispensaries to function as both. This is a work in progress.

As the Berkeley City Council moves ahead with this, as in the past, the salient questions of the moment are:

1. License type—Should all license types be permitted? Medical, Adult Use or both? Together or separate?
2. Location—Where should both types of businesses be allowed to locate?
3. Additional limitations—How should the city of Berkeley place local restrictions? Zoning buffers, severe limitations on business operations, etc.?
4. Selection Process—What type of discretionary review should be provided (Administrative Use Permits, Use Permits etc.)?
5. On site Consumption—Should smoking lounges, like hookah bars, be permitted?
6. Outreach—Is more outreach and public process needed? How will this be determined?

These questions and others will dominate the public policy discussion now and in the future. It could make sense for others cities to pay attention to the Berkeley experience and it will behoove Berkeley to look at best and emerging practices elsewhere as well since it seems all local governments are in this together and need to learn from each other on this critical public health and public policy issue.

Elizabeth Greene, Senior Planner, Secretary to the
Cannabis Commission, Planning and Development Department,
City of Berkeley, contributed to this essay.

51. Cloud of Uncertainty Over Legalized Pot as Feds End Obama-Era Accommodation[*]

ANNA GORMAN *and* PHIL GALEWITZ

Three days after California businesses began selling marijuana for recreational use, a policy change by the federal government has sparked uncertainty about the future of legalized cannabis and provoked sharp reactions from officials in the state and around the nation.

U.S. Attorney General Jeff Sessions Thursday rescinded an Obama-era policy that discouraged federal prosecutors from cracking down on the sale and consumption of pot. Sessions issued a memo directing prosecutors to enforce federal marijuana laws to "disrupt criminal organizations, tackle the growing drug crisis and thwart violent crime across our country."

The Obama administration's hands-off approach had paved the way for a growing number of states to legalize cannabis use and boosted the multibillion-dollar marijuana industry.

U.S. House Minority Leader Nancy Pelosi (D–Calif.) said in a tweet that Sessions' decision was "shameful" and an insult to the democratic process.

California Lt. Gov. Gavin Newsom tweeted that Sessions had "destructively doubled down on the failed, costly, and racially discriminatory war on drugs, ignoring facts and logic, and trampling on the will of CA voters." Newsom pledged to "pursue all options to protect our reforms and rights."

The attorney general's announcement did not clarify whether prosecutors would pursue federal charges against marijuana businesses or seek to disrupt the rapidly expanding market. Despite the new policy, California planned to continue issuing licenses to businesses that want to sell pot for recreation. The chief of the state's new Bureau of Cannabis Control, Lori Ajax, said she plans to defend California's law and continue efforts to implement regulations both for medicinal and recreational marijuana.

*Originally published as Anna Gorman and Phil Galewitz, "Cloud of Uncertainty Over Legalized Pot as Feds End Obama-Era Accommodation," *Kaiser Health News*, January 5, 2018. Reprinted with permission of the publisher.

"We expect the federal government to respect the rights of states and the votes of millions of people across America, and if they won't, Congress should act," Ajax said.

Any effort to enforce federal law could undercut California's carefully elaborated marijuana regulations and give rise to an illicit market, warned Josh Drayton, spokesman for the California Cannabis Industry Association, which represents 400 pot-related businesses. "We have worked very hard for the past few years to regulate this industry," he said. "Allowing the federal government to come in ... is going to affect the public safety and public health for the constituents of California."

The health effects of the drug and its legalization are widely debated. Advocates say that cannabis can relieve pain, ease chemotherapy-related nausea for cancer patients and stimulate the appetites of AIDS patients—arguments that have helped propel states to allow marijuana for medicinal purposes.

But critics cite a rise in emergency room visits and impaired driving in states where marijuana is legal for recreational use. In addition, marijuana can affect cognitive functioning, and people who use it long term can suffer from an obscure illness that causes extreme abdominal pain and vomiting.

Drayton said businesses "are trying not to get into a panic" about the policy shift announced by Sessions. MedMen, which operates marijuana stores in New York and California, saw a steep increase in business in California this week with the start of recreational sales, according to company spokesman Daniel Yi. He said the "reality on the ground" has not changed with Thursday's federal announcement. "It has created more uncertainty, but it hasn't created certainty that there will be a crackdown."

State and federal laws have conflicted on marijuana for many years. It remains illegal under the federal Controlled Substances Act, despite the fact that many states have substantially decriminalized its use. Eight states and Washington, D.C., have legalized marijuana for recreational purposes, although the District of Columbia continues to ban sales. A total of 29 states have legalized marijuana for medical use.

The federal government's shift to a more marijuana-adverse stance is unlikely to have a big impact on states that have legalized marijuana, said Robert Mikos, a law professor at Vanderbilt University and an expert on drug law and federalism. That's because Sessions left it up to the country's individual U.S. attorneys, who must decide whether to go after the marijuana industry. Mikos said many U.S. attorneys will be reluctant to crack down on popular marijuana reforms, especially if they have plans to run for higher office.

They also may hesitate to redirect funds from other key priorities, including the opioid crisis, he said.

Mark A.R. Kleiman, a professor at New York University, agreed that not much would change despite Thursday's policy change. The federal government simply lacks the resources to suppress cannabis production and consumption, said Kleiman, co-author of the book "Marijuana Legalization: What Everyone Needs To Know."

The decision by Sessions did not come as a surprise to legislators and others, since he has been openly critical of marijuana legalization. However, President Donald Trump has said in the past that legalization of marijuana was up to the states. On Thursday, his press secretary, Sarah Huckabee Sanders, said that the Justice Department's move "simply gives prosecutors the tools to take on large-scale distributors and enforce federal law."

Opponents of legalized marijuana said that the federal U-turn could stem the growth of the marijuana industry and curb mass marketing.

"It is a good day for public health," said Kevin Sabet, an assistant professor of psychiatry at the University of Florida. Sabet said the Sessions policy is not aimed at individual users but rather the marijuana industry as a whole.

Governors in several states where marijuana is legal issued statements saying that Sessions' new policy subverted the will of voters and committing themselves to uphold their state laws.

Washington Gov. Jay Inslee, a Democrat, said the state has a well-regulated system that keeps "criminal elements" out. "We will vigorously defend our state's laws against undue infringement," he said.

Oregon Gov. Kate Brown, also a Democrat, said the voters in her state were clear when they decided to legalize marijuana, and the federal government shouldn't stand in their way.

"My staff and state agencies are working to evaluate reports of the Attorney General's decision and will fight to continue Oregon's commitment to a safe and prosperous recreational marijuana market," Brown said.

In Alaska, Gov. Bill Walker, an independent, said in a statement that he was disappointed by Thursday's memo and remained committed to "maintaining our state's sovereign rights to manage our own affairs while protecting federal interests."

"I will continue to work with the U.S. Department of Justice and our congressional delegation to prevent federal overreach into Alaska," he said.

Colorado Gov. John Hickenlooper, a Democrat, said his state has created a comprehensive regulatory and enforcement system that prioritizes public health and safety. "We are expanding efforts to eliminate the black market and keep marijuana out of the hands of minors and criminals," he said. "Today's decision does not alter the strength of our resolve in those areas, nor does it change my constitutional responsibilities."

Marijuana is the most commonly used illicit substance in the United States, and the trend of states bucking its prohibition in favor of taxing and regulating it reflects a broad cultural shift toward greater acceptance. That could make it even harder for the federal government to enforce its laws, Kleiman said.

"Cannabis prohibition is over," he said. "We are where we were with alcohol in 1930."

A Gallup poll from late last year found that 64 percent of Americans believed cannabis should be legal. A February survey by Quinnipiac University found that 71 percent of U.S. voters want the federal government to respect state marijuana laws. In that survey, majorities of Republicans, Democrats, independents and every age group agreed the feds should not enforce prohibition on states that have legalized marijuana.

Kaiser Health News is a nonprofit news service covering health issues. It is an editorially independent program of Kaiser Family Foundation that is not affiliated with Kaiser Permanente. KHN's coverage in California is supported in part by Blue Shield of California Foundation.

52. Law, Legalization and the Failed War on Drugs*

DAVID SCHULTZ

What is the best way for the government to control or deter undesirable behavior? Often the solution is to criminalize it, making the behavior illegal and using coercive tools such as the law to punish those who violate proscribed norms. Yet the criminal law solution does not always work, often times producing externalities that make the original problem even worse. This may be the case with drugs.

America has fought a losing war and it is time to end it. No, this is not a reference to Afghanistan or the war on terrorism. It is to the four-decade long war on drugs that has failed miserably. It is time to shift away from a drug policy that criminalizes its use to one that treats it as a public health problem. This is not simply a call for medical marijuana, but for a serious debate on whether to decriminalize drugs in general and to ask if using the law as an instrument of control to address drug usage makes sense.

Richard Nixon launched the "war on drugs" with his presidency in 1968 and coined the phrase in a 1971 speech. Since Nixon, the war on drugs has been a mainstay of Republicans if not bipartisan politics. The 1974 New York Rockefeller Drug laws penalized individuals with sentences of 15, 25 years or even life in prison for possession of small amounts of marijuana. Increased mandatory minimum sentences for crimes were ratcheted up for drugs and the move toward "three strikes and you are out laws" in the 1990s were adopted because of the drive to prosecute drug crimes. In the last decade, the federal government has spent $20-$25 billion annually on drug enforcement with states kicking in at least an additional $10-$15 billion. What has this money purchased?

There is little evidence that drug usage is down. Nearly 40 percent of high school students have reported using illegal drugs, up from 30 percent a decade ago. Some studies suggest 30 million or more Americans use illegal drugs in any given year. Every year, several hundred thousand individuals are arrested for mere use or possession of marijuana. Hard core use is not down. In fact, in some cases it has stabilized or increased. Programs such as DARE show little sign of success and the "just say no" campaign that begin with Nancy Reagan does not seem to have had much impact on drug usage.

If the war on drugs has done little to decrease demand for drugs, it has had powerful

---

*Originally published David Schultz, "Law, Legalization and the Failed War on Drugs," *PA Times*, April 8, 2014. Reprinted with permission of the publisher.

unintended consequences. Interdiction and enforcement has created a significant and profitable market for illegal drugs both in the United States and across the world. Estimates conclude that marijuana is one of the most profitable cash crops in California and the drug violence in Mexico, resulting in approximately 55,000 deaths in the last six years, is tied to American demand for drugs. The price of cocaine is now at record lows, courts are jammed with drug dockets and prison populations are filled with individuals whose only crimes were minor drug possessions.

States are now saddled with overcrowded, bloated and aging prison populations. Lives have been lost due to drug incarceration. Tax dollars that could have been spent on education, roads or simply saved have been wasted on drug enforcement. American politicians never seemed to lose points by ranting against drugs or demanding tougher enforcement. Clearly, they were addicted to our drug policies.

Drug criminalization has failed. This is not to say that drug use is not a problem. In some cases it is. But put into perspective, use of alcohol, tobacco or the consumption of fatty foods and sugary drinks that exacerbate obesity and heart disease are far greater problems in this country. In many cases, recreational use of drugs is harmless, in others, such as with medical marijuana, its uses may be beneficial. For others, personal and occasional use of drugs is a matter of privacy. Yes, one can concede that use of illegal drugs—including abuse of prescription drugs which is perhaps the biggest problem—is a public health issue. Lives can be lost to addiction and families broken up through abuse or neglect. Many of us know of friends or family members who lives read like a drug version of Billy Wilder's 1945 classic The Lost Weekend. These individuals need medical help, not a prison term. Drug policy needs to be decriminalized and shifted to a public health approach. But many oppose decriminalization. Why?

The basis for opposing the use of drugs generally rests on one of two grounds. First, there is the moral claim that drug use is inherently immoral or bad because it alters the mind, debases human nature or reduces the capacity for autonomy. The second claim is social; arguing that the use of drugs and drug related activity produces certain social costs in terms of deaths, black marketing and crime. Another variant of this claim is that drug use diminishes social productivity by sustaining bad work habits or by generating other social cost, including increased health care costs.

One might concede that use of illegal drugs is bad or that it constitutes a public health problem that needs to be addressed. By having acknowledged this, the question is whether the current practice of drug criminalization and using police resources is the most effective policy to addressing this problem. One argument against the decriminalization approach is the sending signals argument. Specifically one major objection to the strategy proposed here is the argument that it would lead to an increase in drug usage and experimentation. Legalizing drugs would send a signal to individuals that drug usage is permissible and therefore more people would use them.

It is just not clear what impact making drugs legal or illegal has on their usage. Conceivably making them illegal creates a "forbidden fruit" aura that encourages their usage and would be abated by legalizing them. The same might be said for tobacco products and teenagers or perhaps for any other products or practices socially shunned. Regardless of the reasons why individuals choose to use drugs, there is little evidence that legalization has resulted in increased usage. In the Netherlands, decriminalization of some drugs has not lead to an increase in usage or in users trading up from soft to harder drugs. Five years after Portugal decriminalized many drugs in 2001, there too was little evidence that it led to increased drug use. Portugal's drug usage rates remain among the lowest in Europe after legalization, while rates of IV-drug user infection rates and other public health problems dropped. In legalization of medical marijuana in California, the decriminalization might have changed attitudes towards the drug but there was no evidence of change in its use. So far, the same is true in Colorado with outright legalized marijuana. There simply is no real evidence that legalization sends a signal that drugs are permissible and therefore more people use them.

The point here is that the war on drugs has failed. It was a political narrative used by politicians for four decades to promote their electoral interests at the expense of public good and taxpayers. The criminal justice-prison industrial complex has gotten addicted to the war on drugs, making billions of dollars off the criminalization of drugs, especially marijuana. If we truly wish to win the war against drugs, whatever that means, jailing people is not the way to do it. It is time to end that narrative and establish a different approach that sees drug usage as a public health issue. The war on drugs may be a terrific example about the limits of the law and its ability to regulate human behavior.

53. As Towns Ban Pot, States Withhold Legalization's Profits[*]

Liz Farmer

Whenever a state legalizes recreational marijuana, there's always a local backlash. Have your drugs, towns and cities say, but keep them away from us. If a municipality bans pot, though, should they reap the financial benefits of it being legal?

Some states just say no.

Oregon has already started keeping marijuana tax revenue from localities that effectively ban the substance. California plans to withhold pot-funded law enforcement and health grants from places with a commercial marijuana ban. And now, an effort is underway in Massachusetts to reduce the amount of money that cities and towns with bans and other restrictions on operations get from the state's 17 percent tax on marijuana sales.

Massachusetts was one of four states that legalized recreational marijuana by popular vote last year. The 2016 election season doubled the number of states with legal weed to eight plus the District of Columbia. The drug is now legal in Alaska, California, Colorado, Maine, Massachusetts, Nevada, Oregon and Washington State.

No hard count exists, but it's not unusual to see about one-third of localities imposing some kind of ban on pot production and sales in any of those states.

By withholding revenue, states are hoping cities will abandon their bans. But it's unclear whether the approach will work.

Initial figures from Oregon's tax revenue distributions suggest the financial hit these cities and towns will take is very small. For starters, the withholding wouldn't affect education aid because 40 percent of marijuana tax revenue in Oregon goes directly to the schools. And, after all the other disbursements of the $84 million in revenue so far, the total left to divvy up between 241 cities was just $8 million—or $2.85 per person, according to the Oregon League of Cities.

Now that the state has imposed its restrictions on that revenue, pro-marijuana places will see a bigger check. But localities with bans likely won't lose enough to incentivize

---

*Originally published as Liz Farmer, "As Towns Ban Pot, States Withhold Legalization's Profits," *Governing*, October 13, 2017. Reprinted with permission of the publisher.

any policy changes, says the league's lobbyist, Wendy Johnson. She thinks allowing for a higher local tax rate, however, could spur changes.

In Massachusetts, observers aren't even sure the approach could be implemented. Geoff Beckwith, executive director of the Massachusetts Municipal Association, says it would unfairly punish jurisdictions for exercising their local control. But either way, figuring out just how much to cut from those localities would be "extremely difficult," he says. "The idea that funding for public schools would be negatively impacted by a community's decision not to allow pot shops," says Beckwith, "is in itself, a laughable solution."

That's because, unlike most other states, Massachusetts' ballot measure didn't earmark large swaths of the potential pot revenue. Whatever marijuana sales tax revenue isn't spent on the cost of regulation and administration is likely to be sent to the state where it will be mixed with general sales tax revenue. It would then be redistributed to localities for spending on things like education and roads.

But there's still time to change that.

Oregon, for one, made major legislative changes to its marijuana tax structure after voters approved legalization in 2014. Cities and counties each were supposed to get 10 percent of the total revenue collected. But the state altered the distribution formula so that localities that limit or ban marijuana sales or production don't receive their portion of that 10 percent slice after July 1 of this year.

Massachusetts could do something similar, says Kamani Jefferson, president of the Massachusetts Recreational Consumer Council, which is pushing the effort to withhold pot tax revenue. He believes the current incentive for localities—the ability to levy their own tax of up to 3 percent on marijuana sales—isn't enough.

"That 3 percent is just not enticing enough for them when they can already get [money] from the state," he says. "If they get no money or a very limited amount of money, then they'd be much more open to saying yes."

54. Cities in Santa Clara County Scramble to Ban Marijuana Sales*

KHALIDA SARWARI

Twenty years after California voters legalized marijuana for medicinal use, they took the next big step at the ballot box last November by deciding it's OK to toke for fun too.

But while 57 percent of the state's voters embraced the recreational use of pot by approving Proposition 64, South Bay cities are sitting back and waiting for the smoke to clear before amending their local laws to let the once forbidden weed openly flourish. Some are even hinting that day may never come.

As a result, anyone who expected to be able to enter a local store starting Jan. 1 and plunk down some green cash for green bud will be out of luck.

Under Prop. 64, recreational marijuana can be sold only at licensed businesses in cities that don't ban them. By the first of the new year, almost all of those businesses will be medical marijuana dispensaries.

The ballot measure also made it legal for anyone 21 years or older to possess, transport, obtain or give away up to an ounce of marijuana or 8 grams of concentrated cannabis and to cultivate up to six plants indoors per household.

Instead of seizing the opportunity to reap a windfall of tax revenue from retail sales of marijuana, South Bay cities are treading gingerly, and many have called for moratoriums or outright bans of marijuana handling within their boundaries.

There are a lot of questions about how this is all going to work, and every city and county is not the same, said Alex Traverso, a spokesman for the states Bureau of Cannabis Control, which has been tasked with developing regulations for the nascent industry. It's really not a one-size-fits-all approach.

I can understand why they want to take a little time, because we've got one shot to put forth a thoughtful ordinance and one that's going to work, and this is not something we want to battle every year.

In Santa Clara County, most cities have passed ordinances banning dispensaries from selling marijuana, either for medicinal or recreational purposes, with the majority opting to outlaw both uses.

---

*Originally published as Khalida Sarwari, "Cities in Santa Clara County Scramble to Ban Marijuana Sales Ahead of Jan. 1," *The Mercury News*, October 5, 2017. Reprinted with permission of the publisher and author.

Campbell residents shouldn't hold their breath for a dispensary in their city anytime soon of the medicinal or recreational kind. City officials there say they need more time to weigh the pros and cons of each.

Interested in more coverage of the California marijuana industry? Head to TheCan nifornian.com or subscribe to The Cannifornian newsletter to get cannabis-related news, features and more.

Three measures went before Campbell voters in a special election this spring. Two were approved, while a third the most divisive was rejected. Voters rejected a measure asking them to let the city license up to three medical marijuana dispensaries and allow patients and caregivers to cultivate cannabis without a license.

Kale Schulte, a consultant who has moved away but lived in Campbell at the time, placed the citizen's initiative that was ultimately rejected on the ballot.

Schulte said he and members of a group called Campbell Green tried negotiating with the city council by presenting options to alleviate its concerns, but he claims their efforts were met with opposition and hostility from city and police officials.

All in all, I was really asking for there to be access for these patients to get their medicine, Schulte said. It just seemed there was no appetite to discuss; there was just an appetite to ban, and I didn't like that because there was no problem.

The election resulted in voters approving the city's competing measure to impose a two-year moratorium on dispensaries to allow more time to study all aspects of the issue, from safety to best practices of neighboring cities, said Campbell city manager Brian Loventhal. When and if they are allowed, Loventhal said, the pot dispensaries will be subject to the same restrictions involving residences, day care centers, schools and parks that tobacco retailers face.

Despite the city's hesitancy to allow dispensaries now, voters approved a measure to levy a 7–15 percent business license tax on marijuana retailers.

According to Loventhal, the operation of three dispensaries could hypothetically generate anywhere from $130,000 to $260,000 in annual revenue money that would go toward city services such as police, fire and code enforcement. But that isn't enough to cover the estimated $958,000 in annual expenses that regulation of those three dispensaries would incur, he added.

We're kind of in the monitor and evaluate stage for our community, he said.

We're trying to be meaningful with our evaluation and do it right the first time, so to speak, and that's difficult because the environment for state laws is changing so rapidly. So we've decided to let the dust settle, so to speak, and then figure out the best path forward.

Until then, Campbell residents with a doctor-approved medical marijuana card can have cannabis delivered to their home from a registered dispensary, an action the council approved in January. For Schulte, that's a silver lining in an otherwise restrictive landscape.

I'm pleased that there is at least delivery, that there is some mechanism, some vehicle that a patient in Campbell can get their medicine without leaving their home, he said.

In Saratoga, the city council early this summer adopted an ordinance permanently prohibiting all marijuana sales and outdoor cultivation the latter which previously had been legal for those with a medical marijuana card citing safety, health and environmental concerns.

The ordinance can help reduce risks of criminal activities and environmental hazards, Mayor Emily Lo said. Our ordinance acts in the interest of protecting public safety in our community.

The new ordinance follows on the heels of an urgency ordinance the city passed, banning all outdoor cultivation immediately after the passage of Prop. 64.

According to Lauren Pettipiece, a spokeswoman for the city, the decision was based on council members belief that outdoor grow sites are potential targets for theft, burglary, trespassing and robbery and that the chemicals and pesticides used on those sites can be harmful to people and the environment. The ban also aligns with the city's tightening smoking laws, said Pettipiece. Deliveries from licensed dispensaries outside Saratoga are legal, however.

While future councils have the discretion to revise the ordinance, this council decided to prioritize public safety and health over potential revenue from marijuana sales, Pettipiece said.

The council's action didn't go over well with all residents. Janet Redman, a longtime Saratoga resident and psychologist who runs a clinic on Fourth Street, said she doesn't understand why the city is going after medical marijuana patients, among them her adult son who has a chronic pain disorder from passing kidney stones frequently and prefers cannabis to opioid drugs.

Prior to the ban, Redman said she grew marijuana for him in her back yard without any issues. She's attended several city council meetings to speak on his behalf, but gotten nowhere. The city's restrictions create a significant hardship for patients, she said, because indoor cultivation can be costly as well as a fire hazard.

It is cheaper to grow marijuana outside than inside the home, where costs can reach $20,000 to set up the right conditions, or to buy it from a dispensary, which can run up to $600 monthly, Redman said.

Personal cultivation also gives patients more control over the safety and cleanliness of the product, she said.

My personal feeling is that the cities are afraid of what Jan. 1 is going to bring, she said. When people are fearful, their natural response is to try and over-control; they want to control everything they can and my feeling is this is what the cities are doing.

The Redman's neighbor, Jonas Persson, spoke before the city council in September in support of lifting the restrictions for chronically ill patients. He said he found the councils position on the issue disappointing and wished that his own father, who died years ago from prostate cancer, had used marijuana for his pain.

It's unclear what triggered (the city council) to make this change, he said. You would think people in this day and age or in Silicon Valley would use data to justify their decision. You have to think about the people who are sick first and who are being helped by this. Of course, there will be someone who'll misuse it, but that's not the end of the world.

The council has offered a number of reasons for the outdoor cultivation ban. In a city staff report from last November, Santa Clara County Sheriff's Capt. Rich Urena said violent confrontations between homeowners and people attempting to take their outdoor marijuana plants have been documented. Urena also told the city that neighbors frequently raise concerns about strong odors, chemical use and pesticides associated with outdoor marijuana cultivation, particularly around children.

The city says outdoor cultivation can result in various code violations and increase the risk of fire in a city already vulnerable to it.

Like Saratoga, Cupertino also chose to extend its urgency ordinance in September to continue banning non-medical marijuana dispensaries, cultivation and cultivation facilities, commercial cannabis activities and transport and deliveries. The moratorium gives city officials another year to come up with a plan for dealing with commercialized marijuana.

Sunnyvale voted on Sept. 26 to ban outdoor personal and commercial marijuana cultivation and non-medical commercial marijuana activity, but like many other cities, it plans to revisit the issue in the future. Councilwoman Nancy Smith said the city is being cautious to retain local control.

The city has prohibited medical marijuana dispensaries since 2010. Last year, it voted to also ban medical marijuana cultivation, delivery and other commercial activities in the city. The recent vote will now include non-medical marijuana in that ban.

Los Gatos has banned the sale, cultivation, transportation and delivery of marijuana for both medical and recreational purposes because of health and safety concerns associated with the drug, according to town manager Laurel Prevetti.

The town's ordinance cites the smell and visibility of marijuana as an attractive nuisance that entices others to the cultivation, and increases the risk of crimes potentially resulting in serious injury or death.

San Jose also does not allow outdoor marijuana cultivation, according to Wendy Sollazzi, a division manager in the police departments medical marijuana control division. While the city does allow medical marijuana facilities to operate it has 16 licensed dispensaries officials are now talking about whether to allow medical marijuana distributors, manufacturers and testing labs to operate in the city, and if so, how many and where, Sollazzi said. It's expected to make some decisions later this year after the state releases its own regulations.

Staff continues to monitor the progress of state regulations, engage with the state agencies, and is working closely with the registered collectives so that San Jose operations will be compliant with state regulatory requirements by Jan. 1, Sollazzi said.

For now, only licensed dispensaries are permitted to deliver medical marijuana in San Jose, with violators subject to closure or fines of up to $50,000 a day per offense. All marijuana businesses are required to pay a 10 percent business tax. Last year, the city reaped roughly $10.5 million from that tax and is projecting $9.35 million for this year, according to Sollazzi.

Matt Lucero, founder and director of Buddy's Cannabis in San Jose, said he's optimistic that San Jose will loosen its restrictions sooner rather than later. With that outlook, he plans to apply for a license to sell marijuana for recreational use at his medical marijuana dispensary as soon as possible.

My thought is to apply for as many licenses as I can and see what the city says, Lucero said.

To me, this is going to give access to more consumers who are wanting this, he added. Obviously, it's going to be good for dispensaries; it's going to end more black market sales. Plus, more sales will mean more revenue for the government.

In anticipation of the changes, he is expanding his 21,000-square-foot indoor grow site and 1,500-square-foot dispensary, hiring more workers, adding more cash registers and offering a delivery service. What he doesn't anticipate changing, he said, are his prices. Because his dispensary cultivates cannabis on site, hes able to keep prices low compared to other dispensaries despite the new taxes.

Alex Nemkov, director at the newly opened Coachella Valley Church in San Jose, says passage of Prop. 64 signals a significant change in attitudes towards marijuana use.

For so long the focus has been on the negative, he said. (This) opens up so many positive things in terms of research on the plant. People already know about the medical uses; now it can actually help save lives, and then the recreational part is great, too. I think what we've shown here is that it can bring people together in a peaceful, positive way.

Nemkov runs Coachella as a nonprofit and hesitates to call it a dispensary, although it does sell marijuana (untaxed) and related products to members who are at least 18 years old. Coachella is also a Rastafarian church that uses marijuana instead of wine for the sacrament. Next to cannabis flowers, smoke pipes and edibles, it sells holy water and crosses.

It's more about the togetherness and love that were promoting more so than the marijuana itself, Nemkov said.

Meanwhile, the state is busy crafting regulations for commercial marijuana retailers with the goal of finalizing them by mid–November and taking online applications in early December, Traverso said. It should be ready to issue permits by Jan. 1.

Retailers will be subject to strict testing of their plants for pesticides and other contaminants. We're going to require that each plant, each edible, go through a pretty rigorous testing process, Traverso said. We've seen stories about cannabis that's out there that wouldn't pass our testing requirements. That's the reason you create a regulatory model so when you have patients coming in purchasing, they know they're getting safe cannabis, clean cannabis.

When cities and counties do come around to allowing dispensaries to sell marijuana for recreational use, they can expect to benefit from a boom in tax revenues.

According to Venus Stromberg, a spokeswoman for the California Department of Tax and Fee Administration, Prop. 64 sets up two new taxes, an excise tax and a cultivation tax. Revenue from both are supposed to reimburse regulatory costs and be disbursed to various agencies.

Some initiatives that stand to benefit from the taxes are a university-led study on the implementation and effects of adult legalization; a study on the protocols for determining impairment to assist law enforcement agencies; programs that support job placement, mental health treatment and substance use disorder treatment; youth education, prevention, early intervention and treatment; environmental restoration and protection; and local and state law enforcement.

55. The Connection Between Power and Pot*

ALAN R. ROPER

The legalization of marijuana will mean large increases in consumer demand. For the savvy business investor, or cannabis producer, the law of supply and demand indicates that there will be a need for increased production. At least this has been the case in states that have voted for legalized recreational marijuana use. And in turn, increased production requires an increase in use of resources. One of the resources marijuana cultivation is hungriest for is electrical power.

Marijuana production currently makes up 1 percent of all U.S. electricity use. Before the passing of Proposition 64 legalizing recreational marijuana use in California, marijuana production accounted for 3 percent of total electric consumption in the state according to Evan Mills, a senior scientist for California's Lawrence Berkeley National Laboratory, who examined the energy use associated with indoor cannabis production (Mills, 2012). This percentage can rise significantly with the opening of recreational outlets in the state beginning in 2018.

Most Californians are familiar with random power blackouts in summer months when air conditioning use is at its highest. Concern for the state's ability to meet increased demand of legalized marijuana cultivation was recently expressed by California Public Utilities Commission president Michael Picker who warned "the grid doesn't have the capacity to generate 1 to 2 percent more electricity to power pot farms, which was the growth in demand Colorado saw when it legalized marijuana for recreational use" (CPUC, 2017).

Looking at California's track record when medical marijuana became legal illustrates how the energy demand can increase. After California legalized medical cannabis cultivation in 1996, Humboldt County experienced a 50 percent rise in per-capita residential electricity use compared to other parts of the state (Lehman and Johnstone, 2010).

Indoor marijuana growing operations in 2012 required $6 billion in energy costs, with warehouse type growing operations consuming as much as $1 million in power a month (Oldham, 2015). In recent years, marijuana has become big business, a rapidly growing 3.5 billion-dollar industry. For agricultural investors, it's a no-brainer. The cash crop value of marijuana production far outpaces others like corn, vegetables, and soybeans.

---

*Published with permission of the author.

Big investors being attracted to this potentially high-profit industry will look to further industrialize marijuana production.

This essay will look at the energy demands of legalized marijuana production, and the anticipated growth trends. This essay will also provide an overview of actions being taken by public utilities and energy producers—and advocacy and cannabis producing associations to cope with current demands, and to plan for the future.

Why Does Marijuana Production Require So Much Energy?

In order to successfully cultivate marijuana, the grower must control environmental conditions. This is an energy intensive process. The most profitable environment for growing cannabis is in a highly controllable indoor environment like a warehouse space. "From the perspective of a producer, the national-average annual energy costs are approximately $5500 per module or $2500 per kilogram of finished product" (Mills, 2012). An example of the retail cost of a kilogram in Colorado is between $5,500 and $7000,–meaning that the cost of energy is around half of the retail value.

Marijuana can be grown outdoors with energy use equivalent to that of producing other crops. However, the demand and profitability may cause the business-wise grower to take the operation indoors. "Growing outdoors yields about two harvests a year. Indoor operations can yield five or even six harvests a year. Indoor production also allows growers to closely control light intensity and spectrum, temperature, nutrients, humidity, and carbon dioxide levels" (Maloney, 2018).

Additionally, the indoor grower has more ability to control consistency. Marijuana grows better in a consistent climate. Weather factors like wind, humidity, and direct sunlight impact growth and can yield lower quality marijuana. The profit-minded grower may choose indoor production as more of a sure path to financial reward. As regulations for products like edibles continue to evolve, standardization and consistency are going to be good for the marijuana production business.

Let's say you want to start producing a cash-crop of marijuana in a state that has legalized recreational or medical use. You'd probably want to set up a growing and cultivation process that produces the greatest profit, and that means setting up an indoor growing operation would be your best path to financial success. Here are some of the components of your operation that will be hungry for large amounts of energy:

For the lighting system, High Pressure Sodium (HPS) or Light Emitting Diodes (LED) grow lights will be used, running on a 12 to 24 hour per day schedule. A typical high-performance indoor growing operation will require 40–50W of artificial light per square foot of garden space. To put this into perspective, a reasonable sized industrial warehouse-type marijuana production facility of 17,000-square-feet set up for maximum yield of marijuana will use a minimum of 680,000 watts of light, or 680 1,000-watt lighting systems.

Cannabis plants require a lot of light, and that can cause a tremendous amount of heat. You will need to install a HVAC system similar to a greenhouse to help program accurate climate control and to ensure the operation maintains ideal growth conditions Without proper ventilation and air exchange, you may ruin your cash crop, or limit your yield due to excess humidity, heat, or oxygen.

In summary, artificial lighting, dehumidification, ventilation, air conditioning, and irrigation control systems all require immense amounts of electricity. From the perspective of a business investor looking for a high-paying cash crop, these expenses can be recovered by the high demand and market price.

However, the companies that generate, transmit, and distribute power may struggle to meet unprecedented spikes in demand.

How Much Energy Will Legalized Marijuana Use?

Okay, we know it takes a lot of power to grow marijuana, and that indoor production using artificial light is the best way to reap high profits. But how can the energy demand be calculated? The Northeast Power Coordinating Council, Inc. (NPCC, 2016) estimates it takes about 5,000 kilowatt hours (kWh) of electricity to grow 1 kilogram of pot.

In Evan Mills' research (2012) done for Lawrence Berkeley National Laboratory, marijuana production in the U.S. accounts for one percent of the entire nation's electrical output—the equivalent of the electricity used by 1.7 million homes at a cost of 6 billion dollars every year. According to industry experts, the average 2,400-square-foot home uses 903 kilowatt hours of power monthly. A marijuana production facility consumes about 360 kWh a month per 25 square feet. During the first year of legalized marijuana production in Colorado, Xcel Energy reported that marijuana facilities in Colorado consumed 200 million kilowatt-hours in 2014.

Portland, Oregon's, Northwest Power and Conservation Council recently completed major planning activities required under the Northwest Power Act. 20-year projections on electrical use in both Washington and Colorado throughout the indoor cannabis production industry suggest an average annual usage of 185–300 megawatts. That's equivalent to the annual electrical use of more than 200,000 homes in the United States (Harrison, 2015).

Denver has a growing number of marijuana growing warehouse operations, which increased with the legalization of recreational marijuana in 2014. "River Rock, which has medical marijuana dispensaries and a major warehouse in Colorado, spends about $21,500 a month on electricity. Another company spends about $100,000 a month, according to River Rock's owner. River Rock expects its sales to 'conservatively' increase by 400%" (Howland, 2014). In Colorado, more than 1,234 licensed grow facilities make up almost half of new demand for power.

Predictions on the growth in demand for power based on the estimated demand for cultivated marijuana vary. According to Jeremy Burke (2017) in the *Business Insider*, the market is expected to hit $3.7 billion in 2018 alone, and that number will increase to over $5 billion in 2019. That number is expected to hit $24.5 billion in sales by 2021. The impact in California will be greater due to its size and population. If the trend seen in Colorado is an indication (with a conservative estimate of 400 percent increase in demand), the current infrastructure for power generation may be sadly unprepared.

How Do Public Utilities Cope with Increased Demand?

Despite the anticipated increase in demand for power due to legalized marijuana, you may ask—why can't we just let utility companies and government regulating agencies take care of it for us?

The producers of marijuana receive their electrical power in the same way everyone else does, from private companies that are regulated at the state level by public service commissions. For example, the State of California regulates the utility companies through the California Public Utilities Commission (CPUC). The CPUC regulates investor-owned electric and natural gas utilities operating in California. This does not necessarily mean that agencies like the CPUC can help ensure infrastructure for increases in energy demands.

Using California as an example, about half of California's total in-state net electricity generation comes from natural gas-fired power plants. Another two-fifths of the state's net electricity generation was from renewable resources, including hydropower (U.S. EIA, 2017). Hydroelectric power's share of the state's net power generation varies with annual precipitation. California is also the top producer of electricity from geothermal energy (generated by heat from the Earth) in the nation with more than 2,700 megawatts of installed capacity and 43 operating geothermal power plants. It's clean and sustainable energy, but is it enough?

California's investor-owned electric utilities may be underprepared for the spike in demand that is predicted from the business side of legalized marijuana. The public regulatory agencies are not responsible for increasing production capacity to meet California's booming legal marijuana market which is expected to soar to $5.1 billion by 2019.

Texas A&M University's Energy Law & Policy Center professor Gina S. Warren examined the problem of energy consumption for the marijuana industry in a recent report published in the Columbia Environmental Law Journal (Warren, 2016). She explains: "Indoor marijuana cultivation is highly energy-intensive. Overall, energy costs account for about one-third of the cost of production. With $6 billion in energy costs annually, marijuana cultivation is one of the most energy-intensive of the major industries in the United States. It consumes six-times as much energy as the pharmaceuticals industry and requires eight-times as much energy per square foot as the average U.S. commercial building."

CPUC President Michael Picker explained that the electrical grid doesn't have the capacity to generate 1 to 2 percent more electricity to deliver electricity to power-hungry marijuana producers (CPUC, 2017). This estimate is based on the growth in demand in Colorado when the state legalized marijuana for recreational use in 2014. Picker (2017) explained "[w]e currently are expecting flat or declining growth in California, so if it starts to go in the other direction, then we're going to have to make sure that the electricity is there for both these uses and everybody else" (CPUC, 2017). Despite these assurances, California has not installed electrical power generating infrastructure that will meet a demand of 1 to 2 percent growth.

Solutions to Powering the Growing Marijuana Industry

There are also opposing opinions that predict the legalization of marijuana for recreational use in California will not impact or even reduce the demand for power. California has a history of marijuana cultivation and warehouse type indoor production, both licensed and unlicensed. Hezekiah Allen, lifelong Humboldt County pot grower turned executive director of the California Growers Association, thinks the legal marijuana industry will consume less power than the black market one did (CPUC, 2017).

Allen suggests that the legalized marijuana market in California will cause operations to move outside, and to go green through solar and wind power.

Grass-roots organizations like the California Growers Association, California Cannabis Industry Association, The National Cannabis Industry Association, and Mendocino County Growers Association are actively engaged in local, State and Federal advocacy. Their constituency represents a base of supporters—farmers, business owners, and cannabis consumers that work together to raise the profile of high priority issues and explore potential solutions.

Allen stated "[o]ur policy framework is agricultural focused. The Department of Food and Agriculture regulates farms, not factories. And I think we're going to see a lot more cannabis on farms than warehouses in a few years" (CPUC, 2017).

There are innovative solutions being tested at the local level. Boulder County (the largest marijuana producing county in Colorado), plans to start charging marijuana producers extra fees for their electricity use. Boulder County cannabis growers will soon have to pay 2.16 cents per kWh as an additional fee which is intended to address the climate impact of production.

The California Public Utilities Commission's Policy and Planning Division convened a workshop in 2017. Some of the questions explored were:

- Should the Commission institute a distinct set of higher energy rates for cannabis cultivation?
- How can the Commission ensure the most effective use of energy efficiency in the cannabis industry, and avoid over-procurement?
- How can the Commission help cities and counties where cannabis is grown meet their sustainability and clean energy goals?

Additionally, they have identified programs in other states like Washington and Oregon which are aimed at identifying effective practices for energy and water use in cannabis facilities (Mulqueen, Lee, & Zafar, 2017).

Conclusion

Legalized marijuana in states like California will impact energy production and demand. The extent of that impact may still be unknown. Work toward sustainable solutions can be shared among public regulatory agencies like the California Public Utilities Commission, and investor-owned electric utilities like Pacific Gas and Electric Company (PG&E) or Xcel Energy Inc. (Holding company for the Public Service Company of Colorado). The planning and cooperation between organizations like Southern California Edison and wind energy producers Alta Wind Energy Center will help meet new demands brought about by legalized marijuana. Grass-roots associations such as the California Growers Association, California Cannabis Industry Association, The National Cannabis Industry Association can help in being thought leaders on emerging cultivation practices, and energy conservation efforts.

The perspective of marijuana production going green predicted by Hezekiah Allen may disagree with the projected 1 to 2 percent growth in demand for electrical power described by CPUC President Michael Picker. From the business investor standpoint, indoor production may yield the greatest profit potential, but will have much more energy demands. The ability to build additional infrastructure to generate more electrical power using conventional methods may not be realistic in the immediate future. Solutions involving conservation, a return to outdoor farming, and sustainable power generation are more achievable.

REFERENCES

Burke, J. (2017), California's cannabis market is expected to soar to $5.1 billion—and it's going to be bigger than beer. Business Insider. Retrieved from http://www.businessinsider.com/california-legalizing-weed-on-january-1-market-size-revenue-2017-12.

CPUC. (2017). CPUC Concerned about marijuana legalization's impact on power grid. CBS Broadcasting, March 1, 2017, Retrieved from http://sanfrancisco.cbslocal.com/2017/03/01/marijuana-legalization-power-grid-cpuc/.

Harrison, J. (2015). Survey: Washington cannabis growers would like help with energy efficiency. NWCounical.org. Retrieved from https://www.nwcouncil.org/news/blog/cannabis-energy-use-update-august-2015/.

Howland, E. (2014). This is the grid. This is the grid on legalized marijuana. Any questions? Marijuana production makes up 1% of U.S. electricity use. Utility Dive. Retrieved from https://www.utilitydive.com/news/this-is-the-grid-this-is-the-grid-on-legalized-marijuana-any-questions/233103/.

Hughes, T. (2014). Power to the pot: Marijuana growers face electric fee. USA Today. Retrieved from https://www.usatoday.com/story/news/nation/2014/11/10/marijuana-power-consumption/18670007/.

Mills, E. (2012). The carbon footprint of indoor Cannabis production. Energy Policy 46 (2012) 58–67. Retrieved from http://evanmills.lbl.gov/pubs/pdf/cannabis-carbon-footprint.pdf.

Mulqueen, A., Lee, R., & Zafar, M. (2017). Energy impacts of cannabis cultivation workshop report and staff recommendations. California Public Utilities Commission, Policy and Planning Division, Workshop Final.

NPCC. (2016). Northeast Power Coordinating Council Inc. Retrieved from https://www.npcc.org/default.aspx.

Oldham, J. (2015). Attention, pot smokers: Weed is not green. *Bloomberg Businessweek* (4457), 42–43.

U.S. EIA, Electric Power Monthly (February 2017). Tables 1.3.B, 1.7.B, 1.10.B, 1.11.B.

Warren, G. (2016). Regulating pot to save the polar bear: Energy and climate impacts of the marijuana industry. Columbia Journal of Environmental Law.

56. How to Keep Marijuana Green*

Alan R. Roper

Marijuana's Environmental Footprint

Just like any other agricultural industry, marijuana cultivation has an effect on the environment. Throughout history, over use of land for farming has resulted in deforestation, the loss of habitat for millions of species, and climate change. As a result, many farming operations are now sustainably managed, protecting watersheds and improving both soil health and water quality. Why is marijuana production so different? There are three main factors that set cannabis cultivation apart from traditional farming. These factors are: (1) unprecedented and rapid expansion of the industry; (2) desirability of indoor production; and (3) incredible potential for profit.

These three factors also contribute to the potential for environmental harm brought about by marijuana production, both indoors and outdoors. The energy demands can result in extreme amounts of carbon dioxide and other carbon compounds emitted into the atmosphere due to use of fossil fuels. Soil and water can be contaminated by use of pesticides, or over farming.

This essay will examine the ways in which the marijuana industry's rapid growth impacts greenhouse gas emissions, and how that can affect air quality. Efforts to protect the environment by state regulatory agencies will also be discussed. This essay will also identify innovative solutions being developed to produce marijuana in a sustainable way.

How Fast Is the Marijuana Industry Growing?

It is widely accepted that marijuana is a fast-growing industry, but just how fast is it growing? How big can it possibly get? On January 1, recreational marijuana became legal in California, and residents of the state lined up at dispensaries ready to buy legal recreational marijuana. One dispensary named 420 Central had already sold $30,000 worth of product by 1:30 in the afternoon on New Year's Day (Schroyer, 2018).

Marijuana is America's number 1 growth sector. According to ArcView Market Research (2012–2017), legal marijuana is the fastest-growing industry in the United States

---

*Published with permission of the author.

223

and if the trend toward legalization spreads to all 50 states, marijuana could outpace the organic food industry. They estimate the total economic output from legal cannabis will grow 150 percent from $16 billion in 2017 to $40 billion by 2021.

The ArcView Market Research Group, a cannabis industry investment and research firm based in Oakland, California, conducted a business study of the marijuana industry. Their findings report that the U.S. market for legal cannabis grew 74 percent in 2014 to $2.7 billion, up from $1.5 billion in the preceding year. They predict U.S. consumer spending on legal cannabis in 2021 will grow $20.8 billion and will generate $39.6 billion in overall economic impact. This will also represent 414,000 jobs, and more than $4 billion in tax receipts.

Other predictions include 35 states expected to legalize marijuana use (medical or recreational) by 2021. In California alone, it is predicted that 99,000 new marijuana industry jobs will be created by 2021. Colorado, one of the first states to legalize recreational marijuana use now has one of the lowest unemployment rates in the nation. Considering the potential surge in tax revenue, economy and employment, it is reasonable to assume many more states will be voting for legal marijuana use in the next few years.

How Does the Growth of the Marijuana Industry Impact Climate and Air Quality?

Rapid growth in an agricultural industry and huge profit potential can be a recipe for trouble for the environment. Marijuana's need for large amounts of electrical energy will burden the dependency on fossil fuel power plants. Rapid growth and profitability can mean that industry expansion can move faster than environmental regulation can keep up with.

Japanese energy economist Yoichi Kaya developed a formula for future emissions calculations known as the *Kaya Identity*. This is considered the industry standard mathematical model that relates human economic activity to carbon dioxide emissions, calculating that the total emission level of the greenhouse gas carbon dioxide can be expressed as the product of four factors: human population, GDP per capita, energy intensity (per unit of GDP), and carbon intensity (emissions per unit of energy consumed) (Kaya, 1997). Using this calculation, it is easy to see that the anticipated growth of the legal marijuana industry is a major threat.

Let's look at this another way. Climate change documentation uses the unit of million metric tons of carbon dioxide equivalents (MMT CO_2) to describe the magnitude of greenhouse gas (GHG) emissions or reductions. To put this in perspective, one MMT CO_2 is equal to about 216,000 passenger cars driven for one year. According to the California Air Resources Board, California's GHG emissions for 2015 were 440.4 MMT CO_2 (CARB, 2017). At the estimated rate of growth in the legalized marijuana industry, the impact on greenhouse gas (GHG) emissions will have a significant impact on air quality.

Considering that about two-thirds of the electricity that marijuana uses will be generated by fossil fuels, we can make the following comparisons: One pound of indoor produced marijuana creates about 1.95 metric tons of carbon dioxide. This is equivalent to 3 cross country trips in a 44-mpg hybrid car, or burning 2,095 lbs. of coal (see *Hard facts* below).

Even before the legalization of recreational marijuana, California has produced more than any other state. In 2010 California produced 8.6 million pounds of marijuana valued at $13.8 billion. With expectations of 150 percent industry growth, and large multinational agricultural interests setting their sights on the lucrative marijuana market, the climate impact could be irreversible.

Hard Facts about Marijuana Production and Greenhouse Gas Emissions

- U.S. marijuana production & distribution energy costs $6 billion, and results in the emissions of 15 million metric tons per year of greenhouse gas emissions (CO_2), equal to the emissions of 3 million average cars.
- U.S. electricity use for cannabis production is equivalent to that of 1.7 Million average U.S. homes or 7 average U.S. power plants.
- California marijuana production and distribution energy costs $ 3 billion, and results in the emissions of 4 million metric tons per year of greenhouse gas emissions (CO_2), equal to the emissions of 1 million average cars.
- A typical 4X4X8-ft production module, accommodating four plants at a time, consumes as much electricity as 1 average U.S. home, or 2 average California homes or 29 average new refrigerators.
- Every 1 kilogram of marijuana produced using national-average grid power results in the emissions of 4.3 metric tons of CO_2, equivalent to 7 cross-country trips in a 44 mpg hybrid car.
- Transportation (wholesale and retail) consumes 226 Liters of gasoline per kg (or $ 1 billion dollars annually), and 546 kilograms of CO_2 per kilogram of final product.

(Mills, 2012)

How Can Regulators Help Keep Marijuana Production Green?

California has a history of innovation and leadership in reducing greenhouse gas emissions and ensuring environmental protection. In 2006, they signed into law Assembly Bill 32 (also known as the Global Warming Solutions Act), which proposes to reduce GHG emissions to 1990 levels by 2020–a reduction of approximately 30 percent, and then an 80 percent reduction below 1990 levels by 2050. The new wave of marijuana producers in California will be operating within these energy-producing boundaries.

The California Department of Food and Agriculture (CDFA) is the state agency responsible for licensing commercial cannabis cultivation. To accomplish this, CDFA proposed the CalCannabis Cultivation Licensing program. In November 2017, the CFDA prepared a Program Environmental Impact Report (PEIR) to provide a transparent, and comprehensive evaluation of the anticipated regulations and the activities that would occur in compliance with the regulations (Horizon, 2018).

Program objectives include:

- Establish minimum requirements for indoor, outdoor, and mixed-light commercial cannabis cultivation operations, as well as nurseries and processors that must be achieved by cultivators in order to obtain a cultivation license from CDFA;
- Establish a license limit for the medium size cultivation categories;
- Require that individual and cumulative effects of water diversion and discharge associated with cultivation do not affect the instream flows needed for fish spawning, migration, and rearing, and the flows needed to maintain natural flow variability;
- Require that cultivation will not negatively impact springs, riparian wetlands, and aquatic habitats;
- Require that cannabis cultivation by licensees is conducted in accordance with applicable federal, state, and local laws related to land conversion, grading, electricity usage, water usage, water quality, woodland and riparian habitat protection, species protection, agricultural discharges, pesticide use, and similar matters

Producing the report and creating these guidelines will work toward sustainable marijuana production and distribution. California already boasts some of the most effective regulation for environmental protection and air quality.

One of the best ways to move toward more ecologically friendly marijuana production is already happening. That is to make it legal. Nikki Gloudeman, a senior fellow at *Mother Jones* magazine, reports that the current system of growing pot is toxic to the environment in many ways. Outlaw growers illegally use remote forest lands for the purpose of marijuana cultivation, often in national parks. These operations use large amounts of pesticides, and set up environmentally hazardous waste and irrigation systems. Legalizing pot would clean things up substantially, as the growing would both eliminate the strain on public lands and meet higher standards for the use and disposal of toxic substances (Scheer & Moss, 2015).

Legalization reduces the environmental impacts of illegal marijuana smuggling across the U.S./Mexico border. This clandestine activity often uses low-efficiency gas generators, diesel storage tanks, and even pesticides and poisons to keep animals away from cannabis storage areas.

Potential policy solutions include promoting outdoor cultivation with tax incentives, and making energy-efficient production a condition of licensing. Innovative policy ideas are emerging that may place responsibility on the producers and consumers of marijuana. Some of these ideas include adjusting the excise tax on indoor-cultivated marijuana to reflect about 9c per gram worth of global warming effect.

Grass-Roots Efforts to Keep Marijuana Green

The intention of increasing the cost of marijuana's use of electrical power through taxation or regulation is to help stimulate new environmentally conscious cultivation technologies. One of these innovations is energy saving LED lighting development (an alternative to energy hungry high-pressure sodium lights).

Other emerging cultivation technologies focused on making indoor growing more efficient include aeroponic growing systems (which use no growing medium), cubic farming using conveyor rotation methods, automated nutrient delivery systems with sensors, lights and a mesh growing, and even all-in-one hydroponics grow boxes. For example, new aeroponic growing systems use less energy and water than hydroponic growing, and can eliminate possible impurities and disease developed from soil" (Hansen, 2016).

Some cannabis retailers are using labels to identify low-GHG marijuana, which will allow the consumer to make environmentally friendly decisions (O'Hare, Sanchez & Alstone, 2013). In the same way that organic food production has become popular, organic and environmentally friendly marijuana production may find a welcome consumer base. An example is the San Francisco Patient Resource Center (Sparc). Last fall, it debuted a new line of cannabis grown outdoors using organic nutrients and no pesticides. Sparc markets this product as *naturally grown*.

The marijuana industry is not eligible for a certified organic label. This requires certification by the U.S. Department of Agriculture, a federal agency. However, in California, the industry has what's called *Clean Green Certify*, which models itself on the USDA's organic program, requiring yearly inspections and pesticide testing (Truong, 2015). The labeling program and identification of naturally grown marijuana may encourage growers to meet the need of the environmentally conscious consumer.

Conclusion

The rapid expansion of marijuana production based on demand and profitability has the potential for dramatic effects on air quality, soil, and water. The environmental footprint of marijuana is already significant. Now that this market is America's number 1 growth sector, the environmental effects can escalate to hazardous conditions rapidly.

Legislative and regulatory actions taken by states like California can help ensure that marijuana is cultivated in a sustainable way. New innovations in growing technology provide an opportunity to reduce the demand for fossil fuel generated energy. Retailers have started using labeling on marijuana products, allowing the consumer to choose organically produced or low GHG produced products.

These solutions can help reduce the impact that the expansion of the marijuana industry will have on the environment. Through a combination of innovative approaches to regulation, marketing, and cultivation technology marijuana can meet growing consumer demands while maintaining environmentally conscious production standards.

REFERENCES

ArcView Group. (2017).U.S. Legal Cannabis: Driving $40 Billion Economic Output. Retrieved from https://arcviewgroup.com/research/.
CARB. (2017). California Greenhouse Gas Emission Inventory–2017 Edition. California Environmental Protection Agency, CA.Gov. Retrieved from https://www.arb.ca.gov/cc/inventory/data/data.htm.
Horizon Water and Environment, LLC. (2018), CalCannabis Cultivation Licensing, Final Program Environmental Impact Report, California Department of Food and Agriculture, Final PEIR, 2018.
Mills, E. (2012). The Carbon Footprint of Indoor Cannabis Production. Energy Policy 46 (2012) 58–67. Retrieved from http://evanmills.lbl.gov/pubs/pdf/cannabis-carbon-footprint.pdf.
O'Hare, M., Sanchez, D., & Alstone, P. (2013). Environmental Risks and Opportunities in Cannabis Cultivation, BOTEC Analysis Corp. Retrieved from https://lcb.wa.gov/publications/Marijuana/SEPA/BOTEC_Whitepaper_Final.pdf.
Salarizadeh, C. (2018). 2018 California Cannabis Forecast, Green Market Report January 2018. Retrieved from https://www.greenmarketreport.com/wp-content/uploads/2018/01/2018-California-Cannabis-Forecast.pdf.

Schroyer, J. (2018). $4B Brave New World: Updates on the Launch of California's Recreational Marijuana Market. MB Daily. Retrieved from https://mjbizdaily.com/4b-brave-new-world-updates-launch-californias-rec-market/.

Scheer, R., & Moss, D. (2015). Is Legalizing Pot Really Beneficial to the Environment? Getting Rid of Dirty Illegal Grow Sites Would Be Just the Beginning. E the Environmental Magazine. Retrieved from https://emagazine.com/legalizing-pot/

Truong, A. (2015). The Bay q Area's Latest Movement: Organic Marijuana. Quartz Media. Retrieved from https://qz.com/334826/the-bay-areas-latest-movement-organic-marijuana/.

57. A "Deal with the Devil"?

*Native American Tribes Push for Marijuana Legalization**

Zoe Sullivan

With 23 U.S. states having legalized marijuana in some form—Oregon became the latest to permit the sale of marijuana for recreational on Thursday—some Native American nations are now also considering the possibility of legalizing the plant, in some cases because it could represent a revenue stream.

Within the past few weeks, two Wisconsin nations, the Menominee and the Ho-Chunk, have registered popular support for such a move, one through a referendum and the other when tribal members voted to adopt a resolution supporting legalization.

Marijuana is not legal in Wisconsin for any use. The relationship of Native American tribes to state and federal governments in the U.S. is complex. Some tribes, such as the Ho-Chunk, are bound by state, federal and tribal law. Others, such as the Menominee, are bound only by federal and tribal law.

A 2014 memorandum from the U.S. Justice Department suggested that U.S. attorneys—the chief federal law enforcement officers for each jurisdiction—have the discretion to decide whether to enforce federal drug laws in Indian country.

That document, however, leaves a great deal of room for interpretation, challenging Native governments to tread carefully as they move forward with any legalization processes.

In order to create functional marijuana projects, tribal governments would have to negotiate agreements with state and local authorities, since marijuana is still illegal under federal law.

"Tribes have to make some kind of deal with the devil," said Gabe Galanda, a Seattle-based attorney focusing on Native American issues.

"Tribal sovereignty means that state and local government have no say in the regulation of on-reservation affairs. Tribes that seek local and, in turn, federal support must either in letter or in spirit cede sovereignty to state and local government," Galanda said.

While the Wisconsin tribes are still in the early stages of determining whether to

---

*Originally published as Zoe Sullivan, "A 'Deal with the Devil'? Native American Tribes Push for Marijuana Legalization," *The Guardian*, October 2, 2015. Reprinted with permission of the publisher.

legalize marijuana, other nations, such as the Flandreau Santee Sioux of South Dakota, have already passed the legislation.

The South Dakota nation approved legalization in June although marijuana is not legal for any purpose in South Dakota.

Seth Pearman, the Santee Sioux's attorney, said that the tribe plans to open a distribution facility by the end of the year that will be open to tribal members and non-tribal members. "The tribe will get direct and immediate economic benefits from the sale of marijuana."

While Pearman declined to comment on the potential magnitude of these benefits, an article in the Cannabist quoted the tribe's president estimating the income at $2m a month. The story describes the facility as a "marijuana resort" that will have a nightclub, bar and food service, and arcade games.

Pearman said that the Santee Sioux didn't consult with local authorities about their initiative, although they did communicate with the U.S. attorney for the district of South Dakota. Asked about enforcement actions, Pearman said he did not expect any.

The tribe is not governed by public law 280, which means that its territory is subject only to tribal law and federal law, not state jurisdiction.

Public law 280 grants states the ability to play a greater criminal justice role on Native American lands. It initially covered six states (Alaska, California, Minnesota, Nebraska, Oregon, and Wisconsin) but other states were allowed to opt in. As a result, while tribal nations may be considered separate legal entities from the state in which their lands are located, public law 280 blurs these lines.

Tribes such as the Menominee, which are not governed by this law, in theory relate directly to the federal government without the state as an interlocutor. In Wisconsin, the Menominee are the only tribe not subject to public law 280. The Ho-Chunk are, and as a result must consider their concurrent jurisdiction with state authorities in matters such as legalizing marijuana.

Asked about the possible reaction the Ho-Chunk nation might expect from Wisconsin authorities in the event that it did decide to move forward with legalization, the tribe's attorney general, Amanda White Eagle, was circumspect. "I don't want to speculate and prejudge anybody's reaction to this."

Wisconsin's attorney general, Brad Schimel, was equally cautious in his email response to inquiries from the Guardian on the issue of legalizing marijuana in Indian country.

"We continue to monitor the situation and we will continue our ongoing discussions with the tribes," he said.

In an August interview with the *Milwaukee Journal-Sentinel*, Schimel was more blunt." We would work to shut it down," he said of marijuana activity on tribal lands, like the Ho-Chunk's, subject to Wisconsin law. "We're not going to sit back and let it happen."

Yet even with the ambiguous memorandum suggesting that federal authorities need not investigate or prosecute marijuana-related activity on Native lands as long as it does not contribute to larger criminal issues, the Menominee are cautious.

Gary Besaw, tribal chairman of the Menominee nation, spoke with the *Guardian* in a phone interview shortly after a referendum on legalization.

The tribe voted in August on two questions related to legalizing marijuana for medicinal purposes and recreational use for individuals over the age of 21. Both passed, with the former winning 76.5 percent of the yes votes, and the latter 57.8 percent.

"I think the idea with any draft legislation, the proof is in the pudding," Besaw said. "How we develop, control and monitor what goes forward really determines how the tribal membership views this and what happens with this. So we have to make sure that as we move forward that we examine all angles and really do our due diligence."

Casinos and Cannabis

At the start of the year, Governor Scott Walker denied permission to the Menominee to open a casino, which would have served the nation as an economic engine.

Walker cited the high cost of the project to taxpayers as his motivation for nixing the project, but other tribes with existing casinos, including the Ho-Chunk, also opposed the deal.

Both the Potawatomi and the Ho-Chunk are the beneficiaries of a pre–Walker era agreement that pledges to reimburse them if a competing casino results in a loss of revenue. The Menominee project, operated by another Native-owned business, Hard Rock International, would have been located on the former site of the Dairyland greyhound park.

According to a Milwaukee Journal-Sentinel report, following Walker's decision, one of the opposing tribes, the Potawatomi, paid the state government $25m in owed casino fees, which they had been withholding since mid–2014 as a result of their objections to the Menominee project.

The move prompted tribal members to march to Madison during the cold month of February in an ultimately unsuccessful effort to convince the governor to change his mind.

Asked whether this decision had prompted the tribe to consider legalizing marijuana, tribal chairman Besaw said: "You know, some people tried to build a case that there is some type of nexus there that is implicating Walker somehow, but the reality is that the governor denied the Kenosha Hard Rock casino, which would have brought much-needed revenue to the reservation and, quite frankly, to the whole north-east Wisconsin region.

"So the fact that he denied that and those revenues are not there, well, that doesn't mean that we roll over and play dead. We still need revenue."

Will Marijuana "Poison" Reservations?

Legalizing marijuana may offer tribes a way of diversifying their income streams, but given the historic challenges Native American communities have faced with alcohol, not everyone is convinced that legalizing marijuana is the best option.

Jerome Brooks Big John lives in northern Wisconsin on the Lac de Flambeau land of the Chippewa nation. He declined to express an opinion about the possibility that nearby nations might legalize cannabis, but he described the "war on drugs" that his community has declared as drug-related deaths have risen into the double digits in recent years.

"Right now we've banished over 80 people from our reservation," he said. "They're not coming back here. They were poisoning our reservation with drugs and preying on our youth and our young adults. They're not welcome back here. We've had enough of it."

For the Santee Sioux, on the other hand, Pearman said the income expected from marijuana sales would help fund treatment programs. "Some of the proceeds from the actual venture itself the tribe wants to use to fund and establish a tribally owned treatment center for some of the epidemics that we see in our area like alcoholism, addiction to prescription drugs, methamphetamines, and some of those current issues we're dealing with."

California's Alturas and Pit River tribes, which were reportedly growing marijuana for medicinal purposes, were raided by authorities in July, but tribal members didn't return calls from the Guardian on the matter.

For Galanda such raids represent one of the very real risks facing tribes that move forward with legalization. "Keep in mind some local law enforcement will not pause to ask whether they have any authority on tribal lands," he said.

This, he said, could have far-reaching consequences. "That raises significant Indian sovereignty implications, potential civil rights violations for those individuals who will find themselves in the cross-hairs of non-tribal cops, and other profound legal consequences."

58. High Praise

Pot Churches Proliferate as States Ease Access to Marijuana*

Barbara Feder Ostrov

Services at the Coachella Valley Church in San Jose, Calif., begin and end with the Lord's Prayer.

In between, there is the sacrament.

"Breathe deep and blow harder," intoned Pastor Grant Atwell after distributing small marijuana joints to 20 worshipers on a recent Sunday afternoon. "Nail the insight down, whether you get it from marijuana or prayer. Consider what in your own life you are thankful for."

A middle-aged man wearing a "Jesus Loves You" baseball cap piped up. "Thank you, God, for the weed," he called out. "I'm thankful for the spirit of cannabis," a woman echoed from the back. "I am grateful to be alive," said another young woman, adding that she had recently overdosed—on what, she did not say—for the third time.

The small room, painted black and gold and decorated with crosses and Rastafarian symbols, filled with pungent smoke after an hour-long service of Christian prayers, self-help slogans and inspirational quotes led by Atwell, a Campbell, Calif., massage therapist and photographer.

Despite its mainstream Christian trappings, the Coachella Valley Church describes itself as a Rastafarian church, something that's tough to define. Rastafari is a political and religious movement that originated in Jamaica. Combining elements of Christianity, pan-Africanism and mysticism, the movement has no central authority. Adherents use marijuana in their rituals.

The church's leaders say they believe that religious freedom laws give them the right to offer marijuana to visitors without a doctor's recommendation—and without having to abide by any other regulations. Some courts and local authorities beg to differ.

As more states ease access to marijuana, churches that offer pot as a sacrament are proliferating, competing with medical marijuana dispensaries and even pot shops in the

---

*Originally published as Barbara Feder Ostrov, "High Praise: Pot Churches Proliferate as States Ease Access to Marijuana," *Kaiser Health News*, January 4, 2018. Reprinted with permission of the publisher.

few states that have legalized recreational weed. While some of them claim Rastafari affiliation, others link themselves to Native American religious traditions.

The churches are vexing local officials, who say that they're simply dispensaries in disguise, skirting the rules that govern other marijuana providers, such as requirements to pay taxes.

In California, which legalized medical marijuana in 1996 and, as of New Year's Day, now allows sales of recreational marijuana, churches tied to marijuana use have recently popped up in Oakland, Roseville, Modesto, San Diego County, Orange County, Los Angeles County and the Southern California desert city of Coachella (no connection to the San Jose church). A few have been shut down by law enforcement.

"I'm not going to say they're not churches, but to the extent that they're distributing marijuana, they're an illegal dispensary, in my view," said San Jose City Attorney Rick Doyle. Doyle has requested a permanent legal injunction to stop the Coachella Valley Church from providing marijuana, and a court hearing is scheduled for Jan. 22. He recently got a court order to shut down operations of a similar church, the Oklevueha Native American Church of South Bay, he said.

Nationally, such churches have opened in Indiana, where marijuana remains illegal, and Michigan, where medical marijuana is allowed. Even in Colorado, which legalized pot in 2012, the "International Church of Cannabis" is testing the limits of state and city rules on consuming marijuana in public.

Marijuana churches typically require people to purchase a membership, then give or sell them marijuana and related products. They may ask for ID such as a driver's license but don't require a doctor's recommendation or medical marijuana identification card.

They're relying on court rulings that made it possible for some groups, including Native Americans, to use federally banned drugs like peyote in their religious ceremonies. (A coalition of Native American churches has disavowed Oklevueha churches that claim marijuana as their sacrament.)

Despite these rulings, courts have thus far rejected religious groups' right to use marijuana, which is still illegal at the federal level, according to Douglas Laycock, a University of Virginia Law School professor specializing in religious liberty issues.

"Marijuana churches have brought religious liberty claims for years, and they have always lost," Laycock said. "Marijuana is a huge recreational drug, and a religious exception … would make enforcement nearly impossible. So the courts have always found a compelling government interest in marijuana enforcement."

Yet, Laycock said, as more states legalize marijuana, courts may regard marijuana churches' rights more favorably.

"Legalization changes everything," he said. "Religious use may not violate state law in some of these states. And if it does, legalizing recreational use but not religious use clearly discriminates against religion."

In California, however, the Coachella Valley Church may not be able to offer its potent sacrament for much longer.

The church operates in a 1925 San Jose mansion that formerly housed the Amsterdam's Garden medical marijuana dispensary, which was shut down last year by San Jose city officials in a citywide crackdown on dispensaries.

City officials have determined that some of the people who ran Amsterdam's Garden now operate the Coachella Valley Church, Doyle said.

Church leaders at first agreed to be interviewed but then did not respond to subsequent emails from California Healthline. A man who was videotaping the recent Sunday service said the church opened in May. The man, who gave his name as Dryden Brite, also goes by Xak Puckett, and has been described in media reports as a former director of Amsterdam's Garden.

"The message is really strong and powerful," Puckett said of the church. "People are craving something new."

He described the back room where marijuana products were sold to members as the church's "gift shop," then declined to answer further questions.

About half of the churchgoers left the black-and-gold worship room immediately after receiving their sacrament, with some heading straight to the gift shop to stock up.

Others remained to finish their joints and chitchat. The man sporting the "Jesus Loves You" cap lingered. He had brought along his dog, Spartan, and a shofar, a ram's horn used in some Jewish ceremonies, which he blew loudly at the end of the service.

"Anytime the word of God is being preached, it's a good thing," said 57-year-old Mark, who declined to give his last name.

Marco, a 29-year-old veterinary technician from San Jose who also declined to give his last name, attended with his husband. He has a medical marijuana card and said marijuana helps him with bipolar disorder, depression and anxiety. He grew up Catholic and felt that the Roman Catholic Church disapproved of his sexual orientation and marijuana use.

"Honestly, this has been the most life-affirming church I've ever been to," Marco said. "Here there are true believers in cannabis—if not the faith."

Kaiser Health News *is a nonprofit news service covering health issues. It is an editorially independent program of Kaiser Family Foundation that is not affiliated with Kaiser Permanente.*

59. Your Grandma's Guide to Grass*

ANA B. IBARRA

Every day, Anna Denny encounters people who know their way around a joint.

Denny owns Elevated 916, a smoke shop in north Sacramento, Calif., that sells tobacco products and smoking accessories. But many of her customers don't limit their smoking to tobacco.

Because they've been there, done that, Denny just can't imagine them using a new state website that offers resources—and plenty of warnings—about the use of marijuana now that lighting up recreationally is legal in California.

"Some of this, I can see it being useful for a grandma who might be interested [in marijuana] and is getting her information from her grandson," Denny said. "In that case, this website is probably a better source."

Grandmas and all other Californians can now visit the "Let's Talk Cannabis" website launched last month by the state Department of Public Health. The site is the first step in the department's public education campaign to inform state residents about the drug as it becomes more widely used and available.

Last November, voters approved Proposition 64, the Adult Use of Marijuana Act, making California one of eight states—plus the District of Columbia—to legalize the drug for recreational use. California's recreational measure immediately made it legal for adults 21 and over to possess up to 1 ounce or 28.5 grams of cannabis, although the state delayed sales by licensed retailers until the beginning of next year. Colorado and Washington were the first to approve recreational use, passing referendums in 2012.

California's website is not a user guide. Instead, it is geared to youth, parents and drivers, mostly focusing on weed's potential risks and harms. Research on its effects has been mixed, but marijuana has been linked to potential cognitive impairments and driving accidents; it may be hazardous for developing fetuses. Today's dope is also two to seven times stronger than it was in the 1970s, according to researchers at the University of Washington.

For novices, the state also helpfully lists the many synonyms for pot, including

---

*Originally published as Ana B. Ibarra, "Your Grandma's Guide to Grass," *Kaiser Health News*, October 9, 2017. Reprinted with permission of the publisher.

"weed, grass, ganga, dope, herb, chronic, bud, trees, broccoli, nuggets, skunk, kief, sticky icky, Mary Jane."

But in general, California is no stranger to Mary Jane.

The state was the first to outlaw it in 1913. In the 1930s and 1940s, anti-weed cultural references were far-reaching and even graced movie posters that warned against the "smoke of hell," linking reefer to crime and "weird orgies."

Since then, illegal use has been widespread. Dope experienced a renaissance in the 1960s when gleeful hippies "turned on" by smoking grass. Now, California's pot industry, legal and illegal, is worth billions of dollars.

Back in 1996, with the passage of Proposition 215, the Golden State became the first of 29 states, plus the District of Columbia, to allow use of marijuana for medical purposes, with authorization from a doctor.

In 2004, the state began issuing medical marijuana ID cards, which allow patients to purchase pot from dispensaries. About 95,000 have been issued so far.

"Getting a card is not that hard," said Denny, whose clients have received medical marijuana cards for ailments including menstrual cramps, difficulty sleeping and depression.

Devonte Legaspi, 20, a student at Sacramento City College, agrees. "There are even apps that let you FaceTime a doctor for your consultation," he said.

Many of his friends have used websites and phone apps to get theirs. "It's so easy," he said.

Legaspi hasn't gotten around to getting his own card. But he turns 21 in February, he said, about a month after licensed retailers will be allowed to sell to the public.

"Right on time," he said.

California's medical marijuana ballot measure didn't require a public education campaign, but this broader law does.

"We are committed to providing Californians with science-based information to ensure safe and informed choices," said Karen Smith, director of the Department of Public Health, in a prepared statement.

The new website provides details about what's legal to buy, sell and give to others.

It's not overtly anti-drug like the infamous "This is your brain on drugs" ads from the 1980s that warned youth that their brains would get fried like eggs if they got high.

The site, however, advises pregnant women that if they get stoned, their babies may be born underweight—putting them at risk for all sorts of medical problems. Pet owners are cautioned that Fido might freak—and in rare cases, suffer potentially deadly poisoning—if he accidentally gobbles a pot brownie.

And parents who find out their teen is getting baked—which remains illegal—are urged to "stay calm. Overreacting may lead youth to rebel, feel resentment or take greater risks," the state advises.

The website has a resource page specifically for youth, but Legaspi doesn't think it will be the first stop for curious teens and young adults.

"You ask your friends first, then Google," he said. "I think we've been exposed to it for a while. ... We know almost everything there is to know about it."

Still, there are things that some young adults want to see on the website. Aatiqah Murdoc, 22, is Legaspi's friend. She wants information about possible ingredients in marijuana products, such as brownies and candies.

The site doesn't offer that. But it does warn that "edibles may have higher concentrations of tetrahydrocannabinol (THC). If you eat too much, too fast you are at higher risk for poisoning."

THC is the chemical responsible for providing marijuana's high.

Tamara Cross, who works at Broham Smoke Shop in Sacramento, said she might share the website link with customers who walk in with questions, mostly around legality.

"I have a lot of questions myself, so it's good to know this exists," Cross, 24, said. Some customers already ask her when they'll be able to buy marijuana for recreational use, or whether their access to medical pot will change with the new law.

Sharon Duplechan, 65, who helps care for four of her grandchildren, voted against legalization last year, she said.

As she watched her grandchildren play at a Sacramento park, she said she wishes that the precautions offered on the state website had been more widely available when Californians were deciding how to vote. Now she worries that her grandchildren are growing up in an era when pot is more available and accepted.

"The warnings are a little late," she said. "You don't put the cart before the horse."

Kaiser Health News *is a nonprofit news service covering health issues. It is an editorially independent program of Kaiser Family Foundation that is not affiliated with Kaiser Permanente. This story was produced by* Kaiser Health News, *which publishes California Healthline, an editorially independent service of the California Health Care Foundation.*

60. Officials Argue for Medical Marijuana*

DAVE BOUCHER

Advocates and some doctors agree marijuana can alleviate symptoms of some medical conditions.

But the federal government doesn't, and that gives some West Virginia lawmakers pause when contemplating state legislation to legalize medical marijuana.

Explaining how states negotiate the situation played a central role in two presentations given Wednesday during a joint state Senate and House health committee meeting.

Karmen Hanson, a health policy expert with the National Conference of State Legislatures, and Matt Simon, a lobbyist and analyst with the Marijuana Policy Project, presented ways other states have handled legalizing marijuana for medical purposes.

At the moment, the federal government classifies marijuana as a Schedule I drug. That classification is reserved for substances that offer no medicinal benefits and have a high propensity for abuse, Simon said.

Twenty states and Washington, D.C., have legalized marijuana for medical use, and President Barack Obama's administration has said it will not try to criminally prosecute people who follow the laws in that state. Still, the federal classification makes West Virginia lawmakers uneasy.

"I would like to see the feds get on board with us," said Delegate Joe Ellington, R–Mercer.

"If the FDA were to say, 'Hey, there are some medical reasons to use this' and back us up, then I think (state legalization is) not an unreasonable thing."

Ellington, a physician, is the vice chairman of the House Health Committee.

Delegate Don Perdue, D–Wayne, chairs the committee and sponsored a resolution calling for the study of medical marijuana legalization. After the hearing Wednesday he also said the federal stance, while frustrating, is a concern for some lawmakers.

That's why it's so important to learn what other states are doing and see if something similar could work for West Virginia, Perdue said.

Republican delegates Daryl Cowles of Morgan County and Kelli Sobonya of Cabell

*Originally published as Dave Boucher, "Officials Argue for Medical Marijuana," *Charleston Daily Mail* (West Virginia), September 26, 2013. Reprinted with permission of the publisher.

County asked about the classification. Taking it a step further, Sobonya postulated that states ignoring federal drug classifications could also open a door for states to ignore rules from the Environmental Protection Agency or aspects of the Affordable Care Act.

Federal drug experts have tried to change the classification in the past: Simon pointed to a 1988 ruling from a Drug Enforcement Agency official who favored reclassifying marijuana. The ruling was overturned, leading states to find their own solutions, Simon said.

Regulations in each of those states vary greatly, but Hanson said there are similar aspects in most states.

—Typically, states have registries for patients, growers or caregivers—the entities that produce the marijuana—and dispensaries that sell it. Growers and dispensaries are licensed by the state, and typically fall under the jurisdiction of that state's department of health, Hanson said.

—Most states require patients to have some sort of relationship with prescribers, in order to avoid fraudulent prescriptions, Simon said.

—Some states also allow patients to grow their own marijuana, but set a limit on the number of plants they can have or grow at any given time.

Each state sits on a regulation spectrum, Simon said. California is considered to have the fewest regulations. New Jersey, where patients are still not readily able to receive marijuana several years after it was legalized, might have too many regulations, Simon said.

An advocate and registered lobbyist, Simon believes West Virginia can find a happy medium.

Although some states use legalization as a way to make tax revenue, Simon said the focus should be on finding a way to help patients who can't find a suitable form of treatment. There are states that earn money from legalization, but the law is revenue neutral in many states, Simon said.

Ellington said he thought the two presentations were beneficial. He said he learned about strains of marijuana that had more of the drug's active medicinal ingredient and less of "THC," the active intoxicant in marijuana.

Although he said he decided not to support a legalization bill during the last legislative session, Ellington thinks some patients could benefit from using marijuana.

"Personally, I am a physician. I believe there may be some medical use," Ellington said.

"If it's done properly, we may be able to implement something. I don't want to see it deteriorate and see a lot of people getting high on pot and going to other drugs and things like that."

The concept of marijuana as a gateway drug bothered other lawmakers as well. Sen. Ron Stollings, a Boone County Democrat and a physician, questioned whether there was a conclusive study that linked marijuana usage to using other drugs.

Hanson said she did not know of a study, but Perdue said he and others believe it can be a gateway drug.

Perdue, a retired pharmacist, said many drugs have the capacity for abuse. Weighing potential benefits needs to be part of that conversation, he argued.

During the committee meeting Sobonya also asked about if legalizing medical marijuana led to increased arrests for impaired driving, and if there was any particular form of consumption included in any laws.

Hanson said she had not seen any conclusive data that showed legalization of medical marijuana directly caused increased impaired driving citations. In states that have legalized marijuana, it's consumed in a variety of different ways, from smoking to inhaling vapor to eating products that include marijuana, Hanson said.

It's going to take lawmakers asking questions and receiving information for a medical marijuana legalization bill to pass the Legislature, said Delegate Mike Manypenny, D–Taylor.

For the last three years Manypenny has introduced a legalization bill. Although there was practically no formal support for those measures, Manypenny said recently he's noticed a change in attitudes among lawmakers.

After introducing the measure and still winning re-election, Manypenny thinks other lawmakers see it's not political suicide to support medical marijuana. In fact, he's confident the measure has a real chance of passage in the near future.

"I think this year we'll at least get it through a committee, if not two committees," Manypenny said.

"I'd like to see it go to the floor for a vote. I anticipate if it doesn't, it'll be one more year, and I'm sure we can have it passed by 2015."

Ellington thought lawmakers still had plenty of questions, but the measure is potentially moving forward. Perdue said he still needed to speak with other lawmakers to see where they stood. He could support a legalization measure, but only if it had the support of others.

"If the citizens of the state of West Virginia seem to be headed in that direction and the Legislature is going along with them, then yes, I could be comfortable in taking up legislation like that," Perdue said. "But if it is just an exercise in futility, no, I can't justify that."

Perdue didn't say how many other lawmakers it would take to convince him to move forward with the bill. With legislators facing an election next fall, whipping up support could be difficult during the 2014 session, Perdue has said.

Appendix A. Glossary
of Legalized Marijuana Terms*

ALAN R. ROPER *and* JOAQUIN JAY GONZALEZ III

ADAM: Arrestee Drug and Alcohol Monitoring

Administer: to apply a controlled substance, whether by ingestion, inhalation, injection, or other means, directly to a patient's body.

Advertising: the indirect or direct act of providing promotional materials for publication, dissemination, solicitation, or circulation to induce a person to patronize a marijuana business or to purchase a particular marijuana product.

Agent: a person or business authorized to act on behalf of or at the command of a manufacturer, distributor or dispenser.

AMA: American Medical Association

Angel Investor: an investor who provides personal capital for small startups or entrepreneurs.

Applicant: a person whose application for licensure has been accepted for review, but has not been approved or denied by the state's licensing authority.

Associated Key License: an occupational license for an individual who is owns a medical marijuana business.

Batch Number: a distinct group of numbers, letters, or symbols, combined by a retail marijuana facility or manufacturer to designate a specific harvest or production batch of marijuana.

BHO: Butane hash oil and is a potent concentrate of cannabinoids made by dissolving marijuana in its plant form in a solvent (usually butane).

CADCA: Community Anti-Drug Coalitions of America

Cannabidiol (CBD): a compound in cannabis that has medicinal effects with reduced psychoactivity. It does not make users feel high, but it is effective treatment for debilitating medical conditions.

Cannabinoids: essential chemical compounds that are the active principles in medical marijuana.

Cannabis indica: a species of cannabis that often produces a relaxed and social high for users.

Cannabis Product: a product that contains cannabis or cannabis extracts. In Washington,

---

*Published with permission of the authors.

this designation indicates a product has a THC concentration more than three-tenths of 1 percent.

Cannabis ruderalis: a species of cannabis that has a lower amount of THC, but a higher amount of cannabidiol. Its characteristics make it a good candidate for medical marijuana.

Cannabis sativa: a species of cannabis that often produces an inspirational and lively high for users.

CB1: Cannabinoid Receptor 1: one of two receptors in the brain's endocannabinoid (EC) system associated with the intake of food and tobacco dependency.

CBD: The abbreviation for cannabidiol, (See *Cannabidiol* above), one of the at least 85 cannabinoids found in cannabis and the second only to THC when it comes to average volume. Recently, CBD has gained support for its use as a medical treatment as research has shown it effectively treats pain, inflammation, and anxiety without the psychoactive effects (the "high" or "stoned" feeling) associated with THC.

CBN Cannabinol. A degraded version of THC. Causes sedation.

Child-resistant: opaque, sealable and labeled packaging that is challenging for a child under five to open, yet not difficult for the average adult to open.

CMCR: Center for Medicinal Cannabis Research

Collective Gardens: Gardens shared by qualified patients that produce and process cannabis for medicinal use.

Container: the sealed and labeled package in which marijuana or marijuana products are sold.

Controlled Substance: a drug or substance included in Schedules I through V of the U.S. Controlled Substance Act (CSA) as classified by federal and state governments.

Controlled Substance Analog: a substance whose chemical structure is noticeably similar to the chemical structure of a controlled substance included in Schedule I or II of the U.S. Controlled Substance Act (CSA) as classified by federal and state governments.

CO2 oil: A cannabis concentrate, made from the Supercritical CO2 extraction process. Supercritical CO2 is a fluid state of carbon dioxide held at or above the critical point of temperature and pressure, which can be used as a solvent in the cannabis extraction process.

DASIS: Drug and Alcohol Services Information System

DEA: Drug Enforcement Administration

Denied Applicant: a person whose application for licensure was accepted for review, but later denied by the state's licensing authority.

Designated Provider: in Washington, a person eighteen years of age or older; has been designated in a signed and dated written document by a qualifying patient to serve as a designated provider in compliance with RCW 69.51A.040. (look up).

Dispense: to select, measure, compound, package, label, deliver or retail cannabis as a licensed dispenser to a qualifying patient or legal recreational user.

Distribute: to deliver a controlled substance, excluding administering or dispensing.

Distributor: an entity that distributes a controlled substance.

Division Approved Sampler: In Colorado, a person who has satisfied all approval requirements related to training, examination and continuing education in accordance with the Marijuana Enforcement Division.

Drug Enforcement Administration: an agency within the U.S. Department of Justice that enforces federal laws and regulations regarding controlled substances, investigates potential violators, prosecutes the accused and supervises the seizure and forfeiture assets related to illegal drug trafficking.

Edible Medical Marijuana-Infused Product: a product infused with medical marijuana that is meant for oral consumption by way of food, drink or pill.

Edible Retail Marijuana Product: any retail marijuana product that is meant for oral consumption by way of food, drink or pill.

Exit Package: a sealed package or container supplied at the retail point of sale in which the individually packaged marijuana product is placed.

FDA: Food and Drug Administration

Flowering: reproductive state of cannabis when it is beneficial for the plant to be in a light cycle so the production of flowers, trichromes and cannabinoids are stimulated.

Food and Drug Administration: an agency within the U.S. Department of Health and Human Services that governs the oversight of medical products, tobacco, foods, veterinary medicine, global regulatory operations and policy.

Food-Based Medical Marijuana Concentrate: produced by extracting cannabinoids from medical marijuana through the use of propylene glycol, glycerin, butter, olive oil or other cooking fats.

Food-Based Retail Marijuana Concentrate: produced by extracting cannabinoids from retail marijuana through the use of propylene glycol, glycerin, butter, olive oil or other cooking fats.

Harvest Batch: an explicitly classified quantity of processed marijuana that has strain, pesticide and agricultural uniformity as well as being produced in a concurrent harvest.

Hashish (hash): product of compressing the collected trichromes, stalked resin glands, from the flowers of the cannabis plant. It has a higher concentration of THC and comes in a solid or paste-like form depending upon how it was prepared. Color ranges from light to dark brown, but can also appear yellowish tan, black or red.

Hedge Fund: an aggressively managed and largely unregulated speculative fund for high-risk investments attempting to generate large capital gains.

HIV: Human Immunodeficiency Virus

Hydro: hydroponic cannabis grown in water enriched with nutrients instead of soil enriched with nutrients. The plant's roots are suspended in water, or inside a soilless medium, a sterile medium not containing soil, (e.g., clay pebbles, coir, perlite).

Identity Statement: the name of a business as it is commonly known and used in marketing materials.

Immature Plant: a nonflowering marijuana plant that is neither taller than eight inches nor wider than eight inches; produced from a cutting, clipping or seedling planted in a cultivation container.

INCB: International Narcotics Control Board

Industrial Hemp: all parts and varieties of the cannabis plant that contain less than .3 percent of tetrahydrocannabinol (THC). Hemp production is controlled and regulated by the U.S. Drug Enforcement Administration; it is illegal to grow hemp without a permit from the DEA.

IOM: Institute of Medicine

IOP: Intraocular Pressure

Key License: an occupational license for an individual who performs duties that are key to the operation of a marijuana business and has the highest level of responsibility.

Licensed Premise: the premise identified in a licensure application in which the licensee is authorized to cultivate, manufacture, distribute, sell, or test marijuana products in the state.

Licensee: a person licensed to cultivate, manufacture, distribute, sell, or test marijuana.

Limited Access Area: the restricted and secure area under control by the licensee on the licensed premise where marijuana is grown, cultivated, stored, weighted, packaged, sold, possessed for sale, displayed for sale or processed for sale.

Local Licensing Authority: a local jurisdiction that has adopted local licensing requirements in addition to state licensing requirements.

Lot: a definite quantity of marijuana, useable marijuana or marijuana-infused product identified by a lot number for labeling purposes.

Lot Number: a number used to identify the licensee's marijuana establishment for labeling purposes.

LSD: Lysergic Acid Diethylamide

Manufacture: the production, preparation, propagation, compounding, conversion or processing of a controlled substance.

Marijuana: all parts of the cannabis plant, whether growing or not, with a THC concentration greater than .3 percent on a dry weight basis, which also includes its seeds, resins, compounds and derivatives.

Marijuana Enforcement Division (MED): responsible for providing the operational rules for the legal marijuana industry in Colorado.

Marijuana-Infused Products: products containing marijuana or marijuana extracts intended for human use.

Marijuana Retailer: a person or entity licensed by the state to sell useable marijuana and marijuana-infused products in a retail outlet.

Material Change: a change that would require a fundamental change to a marijuana business' modus operandi.

Medical Marijuana: marijuana that is grown and sold according to a state's medical code.

Medical Marijuana Business: a licensed medical marijuana center, a medical marijuana-infused products manufacturer or an optional premises cultivation operation.

Medical Marijuana Center: a business licensed to sell medical marijuana to registered patients or primary caregivers in compliance with a state's medical code.

Medical Marijuana Concentrate: a specific subcategory produced by extracting cannabinoids from medical marijuana. Types include food-based, solvent-based and water-based medical marijuana concentrates.

Medical Marijuana-Infused Products: products infused with medical marijuana (e.g., edibles, ointments, and tinctures).

Medical Marijuana-Infused Products Manufacturer: a business licensed to operate a manufactory that infuses products with medical marijuana.

MITS: Marijuana Inventory Tracking Solution

MJ: commonly accepted abbreviation for marijuana

MMJ: commonly accepted abbreviation for medical marijuana

Mobile Distribution Center: a vehicle other than a common passenger vehicle with a short wheel base used to carry more than one ounce of marijuana.

Monitoring: the continuous and uninterrupted electronic security surveillance of licensed marijuana establishments.

Monitoring Company: a provider of electronic monitoring services for licensed marijuana establishments.

MS: Multiple Sclerosis

NIDA: National Institute on Drug Abuse

NMSS: National Multiple Sclerosis Society

NORML: National Organization for the Reform of Marijuana Laws

Notice of Denial: a written statement explaining the reasons why an applicant has been denied.

NSDUH: National Survey of Drug Use and Health

Occupational License: a license granted to an individual for an associated key license, a key license or a support license.

ONDCP: Office of National Drug Control Policy

Operating Fees: fees that may be charged by a local jurisdiction for costs associated with inspection, administration and enforcement of marijuana regulations.

Optional Premises Cultivation Operation: an establishment licensed for optional premises to cultivate marijuana.

Over-the-Counter Bulletin Board (OTCBB): the National Association of Securities Dealers' (NASD) regulated electronic trading service whose companies do not have to meet any listing standards so they are not required to have a minimum market value or an independent board of directors.

Owner: the person or establishment whose beneficial interest in the license is such that they bear risk of loss other than as an insurer, and have an opportunity to gain profit from the operation or sale of the marijuana establishment.

Practitioner: a physician licensed, registered, or otherwise permitted within licensing laws, to distribute, dispense, research or administer controlled substances in a professional capacity.

Prescription: an order for a controlled substance issued by a practitioner authorized by law to prescribe controlled substances within his or her professional practice for a legitimate medical purpose.

Production Batch: any amount of marijuana concentrate of identical category, extraction method, modus operandi and harvest batch; or any amount of marijuana product of identical type, ingredient, modus operandi and production batch of marijuana concentrate.

Proficiency Testing Samples: samples tested, analyzed and compared to ensure uniformity.

Propagation: reproduction of marijuana plants by seeds, cuttings or grafting.

Proposition 64 The Adult Use of Marijuana Act of 2016, which legalized pot over the counter for adults 21 and older in California.

Proposition 215 The Compassionate Use Act of 1996, which created medical defenses against prosecution for pot patients in California.

Public Stocks: stocks that are traded in the public markets and have daily liquidity

Restricted Access Area: a designated and secure area under control by the licensee on the licensed premise where marijuana and marijuana-infused products are grown, cultivated, stored, weighted, packaged, sold, possessed for sale, displayed for sale or processed for sale.

Retail Marijuana: marijuana cultivated, manufactured, distributed or sold by a licensed retail marijuana establishment.

Retail Marijuana Concentrate: an explicit subcategory of retail marijuana produced by extracting cannabinoids from the plant. Types include food-based, solvent-based and water-based retail marijuana concentrates.

Retail Marijuana Cultivation Facility: an entity licensed to cultivate, prepare and package retail marijuana for sale to retail marijuana establishments, but not directly to consumers.

Retail Marijuana Establishment: a retail marijuana store, cultivation facility, products manufacturer or testing facility.

Retail Marijuana Products: products infused with medical marijuana (e.g., edibles, ointments, and tinctures).

Retail Marijuana Products Manufacturing Facility: an entity licensed to operate a manufactory that purchases, manufactures, prepares and packages retail marijuana products; and sells retail marijuana and retail marijuana products to other licensed manufacturing facilities and stores, but not directly to consumers.

Retail Marijuana Store: an entity licensed to purchase retail marijuana and products from retail marijuana cultivation and manufacturing facilities and licensed to sell retail marijuana and products directly to consumers.

Retail Marijuana Testing Facility: a public or private laboratory licensed and certified, or approved by the state, to conduct research and analyze retail marijuana, products and concentrates for contaminants and potency.

Sample: In Colorado, anything collected from a medical or retail marijuana business by Marijuana Enforcement Division personnel or division approved samplers.

Shipping Container: a container or wrapping specifically used to transport marijuana or marijuana-infused products in bulk.

Solvent-Based Medical Marijuana Concentrate: a concentrate that is produced by extracting cannabinoids from medical marijuana through the use of a solvent.

Solvent-Based Retail Marijuana Concentrate: a concentrate that is produced by extracting cannabinoids from retail marijuana through the use of a solvent.

Standardized Graphic Symbol: a graphic image or small design adopted by a licensee to identify business.

State Licensing Authority: the agency formed for the purpose of regulating and controlling the licensing of the cultivation, manufacture, distribution, sale and testing of retail marijuana within the state.

Street Marijuana Names (or a.k.a.): 420, Acapulco gold, BC bud, Buddha, Cheeba, Chronic, Damo, Dope, Ganja, Green Goddess, Herb, Homegrown, Hydro, Indo, KGB (killer green bud), Kindbud, Locoweed, Mary Jane, Shake, Sinsemilla, Skunk, Wacky tabacky

Support License: a license for an individual who performs duties that support the operations of a marijuana business. A support license indicates the licensee must conduct himself or herself professionally, he or she has restricted authority and reports to a supervisor with an associated key license.

TEDS: Treatment Episode Data Set

THC: Tetrahydrocannabinol, the main psychoactive substance found in the marijuana plant

THCA: tetrahydrocannabinolic acid

Test Batch: a group of samples concurrently submitted to a marijuana testing facility.

Tincture: A liquid cannabis extract usually made with alcohol or glycerol that is often dosed with a dropper. Tinctures can be flavored and are usually placed under the tongue, where they are absorbed quickly. Effects can be felt within minutes.

USSC: United States Sentencing Commission

Vaporizer An electrical device that gently heats cannabis to release its active ingredients without burning the plant.

Vegetative: the state of the cannabis plant during which the plant does not produce resin or flowers, and is bulking up to an ideal production size for flowering.

Water-Based Medical Marijuana Concentrate: produced by extracting cannabinoids from medical marijuana through of use of only water, ice or dry ice.

RESOURCES

Chambers, R. (2013). Leafly Glossary of Cannabis Terms. Retrieved from https://www.leafly.com/news/cannabis-101/glossary-of-cannabis-terms.

Downs, D. (2017). A Glossary of Marijuana Terms. *San Francisco Chronicle*, March 16, 2017. Retrieved from https://www.sfchronicle.com/science/article/Feed-Your-Head-A-glossary-of-marijuana-terms-11004259.php.

Glossary of Cannabis Terms. (2016). Marijuana Industry News. Retrieved from http://mjinews.com/glossary-cannabis-terms/.

Appendix B: City of Portland Ordinance No. 186857

Passed October 22, 2014

Establish a tax on the sale, transfer, mixing, handling or serving of recreational marijuana and recreational marijuana-infused products in the City (Ordinance; add Code Chapter 6.07)

The City of Portland Ordains:

Section 1. Council finds:

1. The City has incurred and will continue to incur substantial costs related to the legalization of medical marijuana and likely incur additional ongoing expenses if and when recreational marijuana becomes legalized in Oregon.
2. The City is an Oregon home-rule municipal corporation having the authority under the terms of its Charter to exercise all powers and authority that the constitutions, statutes, and common law of the United States and of the State of Oregon expressly or impliedly grant or allow as fully as though each such power were specifically enumerated therein.
3. The City desires to tax the sale, transfer, mixing, handling or serving of recreational marijuana and marijuana-infused products within the City. The tax is imposed to raise general revenues and to offset increased costs to the City of police enforcement and other City services.
4. The City's estimated costs to administer this new tax will be significantly less than the tax proceeds expected from this new tax. The Revenue Division of the Bureau of Revenue and Financial Services estimates that this new tax will raise $1.7 million to $4 million in annual general fund revenues. The Revenue Division also estimates that to collect the tax, ongoing costs will be $280,000 and one-time costs will be $150,000.</LIST>

NOW, THEREFORE, the Council directs:

a. A new chapter, 6.07 Marijuana and Marijuana-Infused Products Tax, establishing a tax on the sale, transfer, mixing, handling or serving of recreational marijuana and recreational marijuana-infused products is hereby added to Title 6 "Special Taxes" of the Portland City Code as follows:

6.07.010 Purpose

For the purposes of PCC 6.07, every person who sells, transfers, mixes, handles or serves recreational marijuana, or recreational marijuana-infused products in the City is exercising a taxable privilege. The purpose of PCC 6.07 is to impose a tax upon the sale, transfer, mixing, handling or serving of recreational marijuana and recreational marijuana-infused products.

6.07.020 Definitions

When not clearly otherwise indicated by the context, the following words and phrases as used in PCC 6.07 have the following meanings:

A. "Director" means the director of the Revenue Division of the Bureau of Revenue and Financial Services or his/her designee.

B. "Gross Taxable Sales" means the total amount received in money, credits, property or other consideration from sale, transfer, mixing, handling or serving of recreational marijuana and recreational marijuana-infused products that is subject to the tax imposed by PCC 6.07.

C. "Marijuana" means all parts of the plant of the Cannabis family Moraceae, whether growing or not; the resin extracted from any part of the plant; and every compound, manufacture, salt, derivative, mixture, or preparation of the plant or its resin, as may be defined by Oregon Revised Statutes as they currently exist or may from time to time be amended. It does not include the mature stalks of the plant, fiber produced from the stalks, oil or cake made from the seeds of the plant, any other compound, manufacture, salt, derivative, mixture, or preparation of the mature stalks (except the resin extracted there from), fiber, oil, or cake, or the sterilized seed of the plant which is incapable of germination.

D. "Oregon Medical Marijuana Program" means the office within the Oregon Health Authority that administers the provisions of ORS 475.300 through 475.346, the Oregon Medical Marijuana Act, and all policies and procedures pertaining thereto.

E. "Person" means a natural person, joint venture, joint stock company, partnership, association, club, company, corporation, business, trust, organization, or any group or combination acting as a unit, including the United States of America, the state and any political subdivision thereof, or the manager, lessee, agent, servant, officer or employee of any of them.

F. "Purchase or Sale" means the retail acquisition or furnishing for consideration by any person of marijuana within the City and does not include the acquisition or furnishing of marijuana by a grower or processor to a Seller.

G. "Retail Sale" means the transfer of goods or services in exchange for any valuable consideration and does not include the transfer or exchange of goods or services between a grower or processor and a Seller.

H. "Seller" means any person who is required to be licensed or has been licensed by the state to provide, mix, handle, or serve marijuana or marijuana-infused products to purchasers for money, credit, property or other consideration.

I. "Tax" means either the tax payable by the Seller or the aggregate amount of taxes due from a Seller during the period for which the Seller is required to report collections under PCC 6.07.

J. "Taxpayer" means any person obligated to account to the Director for taxes collected or to be collected, or from whom a tax is due, under the terms of PCC 6.07.

6.01.030 levy of tax

A. Every Seller exercising the taxable privilege of selling, mixing, handling or serving recreational marijuana and recreational marijuana-infused products as defined in PCC 6.07 is subject to and must pay a tax for exercising that privilege.

B. The amount of tax levied is as follows: Ten percent (10%) of the gross sale amount paid to the Seller of recreational marijuana and recreational marijuana-infused products by persons who are purchasing recreational marijuana and recreational marijuana-infused products. This tax would not apply to sales made under the provisions of the Oregon Medical Marijuana Program.

6.07.040 Deductions

The following deductions are allowed against sales received by the Seller providing marijuana:

A. Refunds of sales actually returned to any purchaser;

B. Any adjustments in sales that amount to a refund to a purchaser, providing such adjustment pertains to the actual sale of marijuana or marijuana-infused products and does not include any adjustments for other services furnished by a Seller.

6.07.050 Seller responsible for payment of tax

A. Every Seller must, on or before the last day of the month following the end of each calendar quarter (in the months of April, July, October and January) make a return to the Director, on forms provided by the Revenue Division, specifying the total sales subject to PCC 6.07 and the amount of tax collected under PCC 6.07. The Seller may request, or the Director may establish, shorter reporting periods for any Seller if the Seller or Director deems it necessary in order to ensure collection of the tax. The Director may require further information in the return relevant to the payment of the tax. A return is not considered filed until it is actually received by the director.

B. At the time the return is filed, the Seller must remit to the Director the full amount of the tax collected. Payments received by the Director for application against existing liabilities will be credited toward the period designated by the Taxpayer under conditions that are not prejudicial to the interest of the City. A condition considered prejudicial is the imminent expiration of the statute of limitations for a period or periods.

C. The City will apply non-designated payments in the order of the oldest liability first, with the payment credited first toward any accrued penalty, then to interest, then to the underlying tax until the payment is exhausted. Crediting of a payment toward a specific reporting period will be first applied against any accrued penalty, then to interest, then to the underlying tax.

D. If the Director, in his or her sole discretion, determines that an alternative order of payment application would be in the best interest of the City in a particular tax or factual situation, the Director may order such a change. The Director also may require additional information in the return relevant to payment of the liability. When a shorter return period is required, penalties and interest will be computed according to the shorter return period. Returns and payments are due immediately upon cessation of business for any reason. Sellers must hold in trust all taxes collected pursuant to PCC 6.07 on the City's behalf until the Seller makes payment to the Director. A separate trust bank account is not required in order to comply with this provision, unless the Director determines one necessary to ensure collection of the tax.

E. Every Seller must keep and preserve in an accounting format established by the Director records of all sales made by the Seller and such other books or accounts as the Director may require. Every Seller must keep and preserve for a period of three years after the tax was due or paid, whichever is later, all such books, invoices and other records. The Director has the right to inspect all such records at all reasonable times.

6.07.060 Penalties and interest

A. Any Seller who fails to remit any portion of any tax imposed by PCC 6.07 within the time required must pay a penalty of 15 percent of the entire amount of the tax, in addition to the amount of the tax.

B. If any Seller fails to remit any delinquent remittance on or before a period of 30 days following the date on which the remittance first became delinquent, the Seller must pay a second delinquency penalty of 15 percent of the entire amount of the tax in addition to the amount of the tax and the penalty first imposed.

C. If the Director determines that the nonpayment of any remittance due under PCC 6.07 is due to fraud, a penalty of 25 percent of the entire amount of the tax will be added thereto in addition to the penalties stated in PCC 6.07.060A and PCC 6.07.060B.

D. In addition to the penalties imposed, any Seller who fails to remit any tax imposed by PCC 6.07 must pay compound interest at the rate of one percent per month or fraction thereof on the amount of the tax, inclusive of penalties, from the date on which the remittance first became delinquent until paid.

E. Every penalty imposed, and any interest that accrues under the provisions of PCC 6.07.060, becomes a part of the tax required to be paid.

F. All sums collected, including penalty and interest, will be distributed to the City's general fund.

G. Penalties for certain late tax payments may be waived or reduced pursuant to policies and processes adopted by the Director. However, the Director is not required to create a penalty waiver or reduction policy. If the Director does not create a policy for waivers or reductions, no waivers or reductions are allowed.

6.07.070 Failure to report and remit tax—determination of tax by director

A. If any Seller fails to make any report of the tax required by PCC 6.07 within the time provided in PCC 6.07, the Director will proceed to obtain facts and information on which to base the estimate of tax due. As soon as the Director procures such facts and information upon which to base the assessment of any tax imposed by PCC 6.07 and payable by any Seller, the Director will determine and assess against such Seller the tax, interest and penalties provided for by PCC 6.07.

B. If the Director makes a determination as outlined in PCC 6.07.070A, the Director must give notice to the Seller of the amount assessed. The notice must be personally served on the Seller or deposited in the United States mail, postage prepaid, addressed to the Seller at the last known place of address.

C. The Seller may appeal the determination as provided in PCC 6.07.080. If no appeal is timely filed, the Director's determination is final and the amount assessed is immediately due and payable.

6.07.080 Appeal

A. Any Seller aggrieved by any decision of the Director with respect to the amount of the tax owed along with interest and penalties, if any, may appeal the decision to the Business License Appeals Board as created under PCC 7.02.295.

B. The Seller must file the appeal within 30 days of the City's serving or mailing of the determination of tax due. The Seller must file using forms provided by the City.

C. Upon receipt of the appeal form, the City will schedule a hearing to occur within 90 calendar days. The City will give the Seller notice of the time and date for the hearing no less than seven days before the hearing date. At the hearing the Business License Appeals Board will hear and consider any records and evidence presented bearing upon the Director's determination of amount due and make findings affirming, reversing or modifying the determination. The Director and the appellant may both provide written and oral testimony during the hearing. The findings of the Business License Appeal Board are final and conclusive. The City will serve the findings upon the appellant in the manner prescribed above for service of notice of hearing. Any amount found to be due is immediately due and payable upon the service of notice.

6.07.090 Credits/Refunds

A. The City may credit to the Seller any tax, interest or penalty amount under any of the following circumstances:
   1. The Seller has overpaid the correct amount of tax, interest or penalty; or
   2. The Seller has paid more than once for the correct amount owed; or
   3. The City has erroneously collected or received any tax, interest or penalties.

B. The City may not issue a credit under PCC 6.07.090 unless the Seller provides to the director a written claim under penalty of perjury stating the specific grounds upon which the claim is founded and on forms furnished by the director. The Seller must file the claim within one year from the date of the alleged incorrect payment to be eligible for a credit.

C. The Director has 30 calendar days from the date of the claim's receipt to review the claim and make a written determination as to its validity. After making the determination, the Director will notify the claimant in writing of the determination by mailing notice to the claimant at the address provided on the claim form.

D. If the Director determines the claim is valid, the claimant may take as credit against taxes collected and remitted the amount that was overpaid, paid more than once, or erroneously received or collected by the city.

E. In cases where a there is no future filing to claim the credit or other circumstances where a credit amount should be refunded, the claimant may petition the director to have the credit amount refunded to the claimant.

F. The City will not pay a refund unless the claimant establishes by written records the right to a refund and the Director acknowledges the claim's validity.

G. The Director may, upon request of the claimant or the Revenue Division, extend the deadlines to file a refund/credit claim or review a refund/credit claim by up to 60 additional days for good cause.

6.07.100 Actions to collect

Any tax required to be paid by any Seller under the provisions of PCC 6.07 is a debt owed by the Seller to the city. Any tax collected by a Seller that has not been paid to the City is a debt owed by the Seller to the City. Any person owing money to the City under the provisions of PCC 6.07 is liable to an action brought in the name of the City of Portland for the recovery of the amount owing. In lieu of filing an action for the recovery, the City, when taxes due are more than 30 days delinquent, may submit any outstanding tax to a collection agency. So long as the City has complied with the provisions set forth in ORS 697 .105, if the City turns over a delinquent tax account to a collection agency, it may add to the amount owing an amount equal to the collection agency fees.

6.07.110 Violation infractions

A. All violations of PCC 6.07 are also subject to civil penalties of up to $2,000 per occurrence. It is a violation of PCC 6.07 for any Seller or other person to:
1) Fail or refuse to comply as required herein;
2) Fail or refuse to furnish any return required to be made;
3) Fail or refuse to permit inspection of records;
4) Fail or refuse to furnish a supplemental return or other data required by the director;
5) Render a false or fraudulent return or claim; or
6) Fail, refuse or neglect to remit the tax to the City by the due date.

B. The remedies provided by PCC 6.07 are not exclusive and do not prevent the City from exercising any other remedy available under the law.

C. The remedies provided by this section do not prohibit or restrict the City or other appropriate prosecutor from pursuing criminal charges under state law or city ordinance.

6.07.120 Confidentiality

Except as otherwise required by law, it is unlawful for the City, any officer, employee or agent to divulge, release or make known in any manner any financial information submitted or disclosed to the City under the terms of PCC 6.07. Nothing in PCC 6.07.120 prohibits any of the following:

A. The disclosure of the names and addresses of any person who is operating a licensed establishment from which marijuana is sold or provided; or
8. The disclosure of general statistics in a form which would not reveal an individual Seller's financial information; or
C. Presentation of evidence to the court, or other tribunal having jurisdiction in

the prosecution of any criminal or civil claim by the Director or an appeal from the Director for amounts due the city under PCC 6.07; or

D. The disclosure of information to a collection agency in order to collect any delinquent tax amount; or

E. The disclosure of records related to a business' failure to report and remit the tax when the report or tax is in arrears for over six months or when the tax exceeds $5,000. The Council expressly finds that the public interest in disclosure of such records clearly outweighs the interest in confidentiality under ORS 192.501 (5).

F. The Revenue Division may also disclose and give access to information described in PCC 6.07.120 to:

1. The City Attorney, his or her assistants and employees, or other legal representatives of the City, to the extent the Revenue Division deems disclosure or access necessary for the performance of the duties of advising or representing the Revenue Division, including but not limited to instituting legal actions on unpaid accounts.

2. Other employees, agents and officials of the City, to the extent the Revenue Division deems disclosure or access necessary for such employees, agents or officials to:

   a. Aid in any legal collection effort on unpaid accounts,
   b. Perform their duties under contracts or agreements between the Revenue Division and any other department, bureau, agency or subdivision of the City relating to the administration of PCC 6.07, or
   c. Aid in determining whether a Revenue Division account is in compliance with all city, state and federal laws or policies.

6.07.130 Audit of books, records or persons

The City may examine or may cause to be examined by an agent or representative designated by the City for that purpose, any books, papers, records, or memoranda, including copies of Seller's state and federal income tax return, bearing upon the matter of the Seller's tax return for the purpose of determining the correctness of any tax return, or for the purpose of an estimate of taxes due. All books, invoices, accounts and other records must be made available within the city limits and be open at any time during regular business hours for examination by the director or an authorized agent of the director. If any Taxpayer refuses to voluntarily furnish any of the foregoing information when requested, the Director may immediately seek a subpoena from the court to require that the Taxpayer or a representative of the Taxpayer attend a hearing or produce any such books, accounts and records for examination.

6.07.140 Forms and regulations

A. The Director is authorized to prescribe forms and promulgate rules, policies and regulations to aid in the making of returns, the ascertainment, assessment and collection of the marijuana tax and to provide for:

1. A form of report on sales and purchases to be supplied to all Sellers;
2. The records that Sellers providing, mixing, serving, or handling marijuana and marijuana-infused products must keep concerning the tax imposed by PCC 6.07.

6.07.150 Invalidity

If any section, clause, phrase, sentence or part of this Chapter shall for any reason be adjudged unconstitutional, invalid or unenforceable, it shall only void that part, clause, phrase or section so declared and the remainder shall remain in full force and effect.

Appendix C: U.S. Drug Enforcement Agency Drug Fact Sheet

Overview: Marijuana is a mind-altering (psychoactive) drug, produced by the Cannabis sativa plant. Marijuana contains over 400 chemicals. THC (delta-9-tetrahydrocannabinol) is believed to be the main chemical ingredient that produces the psychoactive effect.

Street names: Aunt Mary, BC Bud, Blunts, Boom, Chronic, Dope, Gangster, Ganja, Grass, Hash, Herb, Hydro, Indo, Joint, Kif, Mary Jane, Mota, Pot, Reefer, Sinsemilla, Skunk, Smoke, Weed, Yerba

Looks like: Marijuana is a dry, shredded green/brown mix of flowers, stems, seeds, and leaves from the Cannabis sativa plant. The mixture typically is green, brown, or gray in color and may resemble tobacco.

Methods of abuse: Marijuana is usually smoked as a cigarette (called a joint) or in a pipe or bong. It is also smoked in blunts, which are cigars that have been emptied of tobacco and refilled with marijuana, sometimes in combination with another drug. Marijuana is also mixed with foods or brewed as a tea.

Affect on mind: When marijuana is smoked, the THC passes from the lungs and into the bloodstream, which carries the chemical to the organs throughout the body, including the brain. In the brain, the THC connects to specific sites called cannabinoid receptors on nerve cells and influences the activity of those cells. Many of these receptors are found in the parts of the brain that influence pleasure, memory, thought, concentration, sensory and time perception, and coordinated movement. The short-term effects of marijuana include problems with memory and learning, distorted perception, difficulty in thinking and problem-solving, and loss of coordination. The effect of marijuana on perception and coordination are responsible for serious impairments in driving abilities. Long-term chronic marijuana use is associated with Amotivational Syndrome, characterized by apathy, impairment of judgment, memory and concentration, and loss of motivation, ambition and interest in the pursuit of personal goals. High doses of marijuana can result in mental confusion, panic reactions and hallucinations. Researchers have also found an association between marijuana use and an increased risk of depression; an increased risk and earlier onset of schizophrenia and other psychotic disorders, especially for teens that have a genetic predisposition.

Affect on body: Short-term physical effects from marijuana use may include sedation, blood shot eyes, increased heart rate, coughing from lung irritation, increased appetite, and decreased blood pressure. Like tobacco smokers, marijuana smokers experience serious health problems such as bronchitis, emphysema, and bronchial asthma. Extended use may cause suppression of the immune system. Because marijuana contains toxins and carcinogens, marijuana smokers increase their risk of cancer of the head, neck, lungs and respiratory track. Withdrawal from chronic use of high doses of marijuana causes physical signs including headache, shakiness, sweating, stomach pains and nausea, as well as behavioral signs including restlessness, irritability, sleep difficulties and decreased appetite.

Drugs causing similar effects: Hashish and hashish oil are drugs made from the cannabis plant that are like marijuana, only stronger. Hashish (hash) consists of the THC–rich resinous material of the cannabis plant, which is collected, dried, and then compressed into a variety of forms, such as balls, cakes, or cookie like sheets. Pieces are then broken off, placed in pipes or mixed with tobacco and placed in pipes or cigarettes, or smoked. The main sources of hashish are the Middle East, North Africa, Pakistan and Afghanistan. Hashish Oil (hash oil, liquid hash, cannabis oil) is produced by extracting the cannabinoids from the plant material with a solvent. The color and odor of the extract will vary, depending on the solvent used. A drop or two of this liquid on a cigarette is equal to a single marijuana joint. Like marijuana, hashish and hashish oil are both Schedule I drugs.

Overdose effects: No death from overdose of marijuana has been reported.

Legal status in the United States: Marijuana is a Schedule I substance under the Controlled Substances Act. Schedule I drugs are classified as having a high potential for abuse, no currently accepted medical use in treatment in the United States, and a lack of accepted safety for use of the drug or other substance under medical supervision. Marinol, a synthetic version of THC, the active ingredient found in the marijuana plant, can be prescribed for the control of nausea and vomiting caused by chemotherapeutic agents used in the treatment of cancer and to stimulate appetite in AIDS patients. Marinol is a Schedule III substance under the Controlled Substances Act. Schedule III drugs are classified as having less potential for abuse than the drugs or substances in Schedules I and II, and have a currently accepted medical use in treatment in the U.S., and abuse of the drug may lead to moderate or low physical dependence or psychological dependence.

Common places of origin: Marijuana is grown in the United States, Canada, Mexico, South America and Asia. It can be cultivated in both outdoor and in indoor settings.

Appendix D: Federal Trafficking Penalties for Marijuana, Hashish and Hashish Oil, Schedule I Substances

Marijuana

1,000 kilograms or more marijuana mixture or 1,000 or more marijuana plants

First Offense: Not less than 10 yrs. or more than life. If death or serious bodily injury, not less than 20 yrs., or more than life. Fine not more than $10 million if an individual, $50 million if other than an individual.

Second Offense: Not less than 20 yrs. or more than life. If death or serious bodily injury, life imprisonment. Fine not more than $20 million if an individual, $75 million if other than an individual.

Marijuana

100 to 999 kilograms marijuana mixture or 100 to 999 marijuana plants

First Offense: Not less than 5 yrs. or more than 40 yrs. If death or serious bodily injury, not less than 20 yrs. or more than life. Fine not more than $5 million if an individual, $25 million if other than an individual.

Second Offense: Not less than 10 yrs. or more than life. If death or serious bodily injury, life imprisonment. Fine not more than $8 million if an individual, $50million if other than an individual.

Marijuana

50 to 99 kilograms marijuana mixture,
50 to 99 marijuana plants

First Offense: Not more than 20 yrs. If death or serious bodily injury, not less than 20 yrs. or more than life. Fine $1 million if an individual, $5 million if other than an individual.

Second Offense: Not more than 30 yrs. If death or serious bodily injury, life imprisonment. Fine $2 million if an individual, $10 million if other than an individual.

Hashish

More than 10 kilograms

Hashish Oil

More than 1 kilogram

Marijuana

less than 50 kilograms marijuana (but does not include 50 or more marijuana plants regardless of weight)
1 to 49 marijuana plants
First Offense: Not more than 5 yrs. Fine not more than $250,000, $1 million if other than an individual.
Second Offense: Not more than 10 yrs. Fine $500,000 if an individual, $2 million if other than individual.

Hashish

10 kilograms or less

Hashish Oil

1 kilogram or less

Appendix E: VA and Medical Marijuana— What Veterans Need to Know

Several states in the U.S. have approved the use of marijuana (cannabis) for medical and/or recreational use. Veterans should know that federal law classifies marijuana—including all derivative products—as a Schedule One controlled substance. This makes it illegal in the eyes of the federal government.

The U.S. Department of Veterans Affairs is required to follow all federal laws including those regarding marijuana. As long as the Food and Drug Administration classifies marijuana as Schedule One VA health care providers may not recommend it or assist Veterans to obtain it.

Veteran participation in State medical marijuana program does not affect eligibility for VA care and services. VA providers can and do discuss marijuana use with Veterans as part of comprehensive care planning, and adjust treatment plans as necessary.

Some things Veteran need to know about medical marijuana and the VA:

- Veterans are encouraged to discuss marijuana use with their VA providers.
- Veterans will not be denied VA health services because of marijuana use.
- VA health care providers will record marijuana use in the Veteran's VA medical record in order to have the information available in treatment planning. As with all clinical information, this is part of the confidential medical record and protected under patient privacy and confidentiality laws and regulations.
- VA clinicians may not recommend medical marijuana.
- VA clinicians may not complete paperwork/forms required for Veteran patients to participate in state-approved marijuana programs.
- VA pharmacies may not fill prescriptions for medical marijuana.
- VA will not pay for medical marijuana prescriptions from any source.
- The use or possession of marijuana is prohibited at all VA medical centers, locations and grounds. When you are on VA grounds it is federal law that is in force, not the laws of the state.
- Veterans who are VA employees are subject to drug testing under the terms of employment.

October 2, 2017, https://www.publichealth.va.gov/marijuana.asp

About the Contributors

Juliet **Akhigbe** is a member of the Ontario Public Health Association's Cannabis Task Group.

Michelle **Andrews** is a *Kaiser Health News* contributing columnist who writes the series *Insuring Your Health*, which explores health care coverage and costs.

Rebecca **Beitsch** writes about energy and environment for *Stateline*.

Marcel O. **Bonn-Miller** is an adjunct assistant professor of psychology in psychiatry at the University of Pennsylvania.

Dave **Boucher** is a capitol reporter with the *Charleston Gazette*, West Virginia.

Sarah **Breitenbach** writes about the business of government for *Stateline*.

Van **Bustic** is an assistant cooperative extension specialist and adjunct professor at the University of California Berkeley's Department of Environmental Science Policy and Management.

John **Carnevale** is the president and CEO of Carnevale Associates and has served three administrations and four "drug czars" within the executive branch of the U.S. government.

Gary A. **Craft** is a retired chief district attorney investigator for the Monterey County District Attorney's Office and has four decades of experience working marijuana related investigations.

Vash **Ebbadi** is a member of the Ontario Public Health Association's Cannabis Task Group.

Liz **Farmer** is *Governing*'s public finance reporter, covering state and local budgets, pensions and other public-sector fiscal issues.

Michele **Frisby** is the director of public information at the International City/County Management Association in Washington, D.C.

Phil **Galewitz**, *Kaiser Health News* senior correspondent, covers the intersection of health policy, health economics, public health and consumer health.

Dereck **Glover**, a Golden Gate University executive master of public administration student, is an Ohio native who joined and retired from the Army with a passion for the pursuit of knowledge and fair, equitable treatment of individuals.

Stephen **Goldsmith** is a professor of practice at the Harvard Kennedy School and director of the Innovations in American Government Program.

Joaquin Jay **Gonzalez** III is the Mayor George Christopher Professor of Public Administration at the Edward S. Ageno School of Business of Golden Gate University.

Paula **Gordon** is an educator, analyst, and online publisher with websites on public administration and on drug abuse and past consultant to the National Institute of Mental Health.

Anna **Gorman** is a senior correspondent with *Kaiser Health News* and writes about all things health: policy, reform and disparities.

Kevin **Harper** is a managing partner of Kevin W. Harper CPA & Associates, Castro Valley, California.

Dylan Woolf **Harris** is a staff writer for the *Elko Daily Free Press* in Elko, Nevada.

Katie **Huynh** is a member of the Ontario Public Health Association's Cannabis Task Group.

Jim **Hynes** is an adjunct professor at Golden Gate University's Public Administration Department and 30-year executive manager with the City of Berkeley.

Ana B. **Ibarra** is a web reporter at *Kaiser Health News*.

Joe **Jarret** is a public sector manager, attorney and mediator who lectures full-time on at the master of public policy and administration program at the University of Tennessee.

Donald F. **Kettl** is a former dean of the School of Public Policy at the University of Maryland and a nonresident senior fellow at the Volcker Alliance and the Brookings Institution.

Beau **Kilmer** is a senior policy researcher at the RAND Corporation, where he codirects the RAND Drug Policy Research Center.

William **Kirchhoff** a long-time local government manager and now management adviser, Coronado, California and the author of *Managing Medical Marijuana in Local Government*.

James **Leckie** is a member of the Ontario Public Health Association's Cannabis Task Group.

Douglas **Levy** is a journalist and editor who was previously web editor and a writer for the *Michigan Lawyers Weekly*.

Shefali **Luthra** is a reporter covering health and health policy for *Kaiser Health News*.

Maria **Major** is a member of the Ontario Public Health Association's Cannabis Task Group.

Ben **Markus** is a business reporter with Colorado Public Radio.

Henry **McCann** is a research associate at the Public Policy Institute of California Water Policy Center, where he manages research projects and provides core research support.

Mickey P. **McGee** is an associate professor of public administration at the Edward S. Ageno School of Business of Golden Gate University.

Andy **Metzger** writes for the State House News Service and contributes to the *Berkshire Eagle*, covering all of Berkshire County in Massachusetts.

Patrick **Murphy** is the research director and senior fellow at the Public Policy Institute of California. He is also an adjunct professor of politics at the University of San Francisco.

National Institute on Drug Abuse is a federal-government research institute whose mission is to lead the U.S. in bringing the power of science to bear on drug abuse and addiction.

Gordon **Oliver** is the business editor for *The Columbian*.

Stephanie **O'Neill** is an award-winning health care journalist and a 2013–2017 NPR/*Kaiser Health News* health policy reporting fellow.

Barbara Feder **Ostrov** is a former *San Jose Mercury News* medical writer free-lancing for *Kaiser Health News*.

Rosalie Liccardo **Pacula** is a senior economist at the RAND Corporation and a professor at the Pardee RAND Graduate School.

Samira J. **Perry** is an active entrepreneur and social justice advocate in the Monterey Peninsula and is an executive master of public administration graduate of Golden Gate University.

Seth **Poe** is a graduate student in the executive master of public administration program at the Edward S. Ageno School of Business of Golden Gate University.

Sophie **Quinton** writes about fiscal and economic policy for *Stateline.*

Diane **Raver** is an assistant editor of *The Herald-Tribune*, in Batesville, Indiana.

Cara **Robinson** is a member of the Ontario Public Health Association's Cannabis Task Group.

Carmen Heredia **Rodriguez** is a reporter for *Kaiser Health News.*

Alan R. **Roper** is a senior adjunct professor at Golden Gate University, and instructional designer/curriculum developer for the University of California, Office of the President.

Glenna S. **Rousseau** is an assistant professor of psychiatry at Dartmouth's Geisel School of Medicine.

Khalida **Sarwari** is a cover writer/arts and entertainment writer for the Bay Area News Group's Silicon Valley Community Newspapers.

David **Schultz** is a professor in the department of political science at Hamline University and is the editor of the *Journal of Public Affairs Education.*

Dylan **Scott** is a staff writer with *Governing,* covering education reform movements in state and local government.

John **Sepulvado** reports for KQED's *The California Report* and has written for *Government Technology.*

William **Smith** contributes to *The Hawk Eye* in Burlington, Iowa.

Michelle **Suarly** is a member of the Ontario Public Health Association's Cannabis Task Group.

Zoe **Sullivan** is a photographer, independent multimedia journalist focusing on gender and social equity issues who has reported for *The Guardian*, NPR, Marketplace, and many other news outlets.

Deborah **Sutton** is a beat reporter for the *Deseret News* writing weekly in-depth pieces on personal finance, financial policy, and money smarts.

U.S. Department of Veterans Affairs is a federal government agency providing health care services and other benefits to eligible veterans and their dependents.

U.S. Drug Enforcement Agency (or DEA) is a federal law enforcement agency under the U.S. Department of Justice, tasked with combating drug smuggling and use.

U.S. Food and Drug Administration is a federal agency of the U.S. Department of Health and Human Services.

Sarah **Varney** is a senior correspondent for *Kaiser Health News.*

Daniel C. **Vock** is *Governing*'s transportation and infrastructure reporter.

Nora D. **Volkow** is the director of the National Institute on Drug Abuse at the National Institutes of Health, supporting research on the health aspects of drug abuse and addiction.

David **Wasserstein** is a member of the Ontario Public Health Association's Cannabis Task Group.

J.B. **Wogan** is a *Governing* staff writer reporting on public programs aimed at addressing poverty.

Ted **Yoakum** is the managing editor with the *Tryon Daily Bulletin* and was previously community editor of the *Dowagiac Daily News.*

Stephen **Zimney** is the president of Zimney Associates in New York.

Index